MICROSCOPY HANDBOOKS 33

Modern PhotoMICROgraphy

Royal Microscopical Society MICROSCOPY HANDBOOKS

Modern PhotoMICROgraphy

Brian Bracegirdle
Cold Aston Lodge, Cold Aston,
Cheltenham, Glos. GL54 3BN, UK

Savile Bradbury
61 Hill Top Road,
Oxford OX4 1PD, UK

βIOS
SCIENTIFIC
PUBLISHERS

In association with the Royal Microscopical Society

A CIP catalogue for this book is available from the British Library.

ISBN 1 85996 09 01

BIOS Scientific Publishers Ltd
9 Newtec Place, Magdalen Road, Oxford, OX4 1RE, UK
Tel. +44 (0) 1865 726286. Fax. +44 (0) 1865 246823

DISTRIBUTORS

Australia and New Zealand
  DA Information Services
  648 Whitehorse Road, Mitcham
  Victoria 3132

Singapore and South East Asia
  Toppan Company (S) PTE Ltd
  38 Liu Fang Road, Jurong
  Singapore 2262

India
  Viva Books Private Limited
  4346/4C Ansari Road
  New Delhi 110002

USA and Canada
  Books International Inc.
  PO Box 605, Herndon, VA 22070

Typeset by AMA Graphics Ltd, Preston, UK.
Printed and bound in Great Britain by Biddles Ltd, Guildford and King's Lynn.

Contents

Abbreviations

ASA	American Standards Association
CAD	computer-assisted design
CAM	computer-assisted manufacture
CCD	charge-coupled device
CCTV	closed-circuit television
CD	compact disc
CI	contrast index
DIC	difference interference contrast
FN	field of view number
ISO	International Organization for Standardization
mired	micro-reciprocal degree
NA	numerical aperture
OTF	off-the-film
SLR	single lens reflex
TTL	through-the-lens
WORM	write once, read many

Preface

This book is a totally rewritten successor to Thomson and Bradbury's *An Introduction to Photomicrography* (RMS Microscopy Handbook 13, 1987). That book had a section on macro-range photography, but this has now been omitted as the subject is covered in detail by Bracegirdle's *Scientific PhotoMACROgraphy* (RMS Microscopy Handbook 31, 1995). The two works have been written to be read in conjunction in order to provide a modern account of photography with the microscope.

The subject remains an essentially practical one, 'hands-on' experience alone providing the fine tuning which allows good results to be achieved as a norm. Our short approach is intended to provide all that is necessary for modern workers to achieve such consistent good results. That there is still need for such a treatment is proven by the routine appearance of substandard photomicrographs in the literature. They cost just as much to print as good ones, while failing in their prime duty of communication.

B. Bracegirdle and S. Bradbury

1 Introduction

Photographs of microscopical images have been made almost from the very beginning of photography, and many books and papers from about 1850 onwards gave advice on the techniques required. The books tended to be preoccupied with difficulties of illumination, and with exposure estimation, and the whole process remained esoteric, perhaps unnecessarily so, until about 1900. By this time, the theory of the instrument was well known, dry plates were well established and much had been experienced. Most of the standard textbooks included a section on making photomicrographs, but plenty of special texts had been published. One of the most satisfactory at the turn of the century was that by Spitta (1899), while Pringle (1890) had written a full account also; both have excellent halftones and line illustrations.

By this time, the two forms of apparatus, vertical and horizontal, were well established, and sold by the leading makers (see *Figures 1.1* and *1.2*). The very authoritative J.E. Barnard FRS (1911) wrote an excellent manual, and joined with Welch to write two further editions, in 1925 and 1936; a comparison of the editions shows that progress in the source of illuminant was the most critical factor during these 25 years, closely followed by improved photographic materials. The eyepiece camera had made its appearance also, courtesy of Leitz.

Shillaber wrote a very practical account in 1944, still useful for any who use older apparatus and, after World War II, Michel produced a very full treatment in 1957, which contrasts with the predominantly practical account of Lawson (1960), which he completely rewrote (without losing the practicality) in 1972. This last book also remains useful for those using older equipment. In 1970, however, the two-volume work by Loveland had appeared, and this was to overshadow all other texts for a long time afterwards. The series of very well-illustrated shorter books published by Kodak (see, for example Delly, 1988) is also a landmark in publishing on photomicrography.

Finally, two general works on microscopy require mention, for their treatment of photomicrography. Needham (1958) remains an excellent text for immediate post-World War II instruments and their associated techniques, while Richardson (1991) is an up-to-date account with very clear treatment.

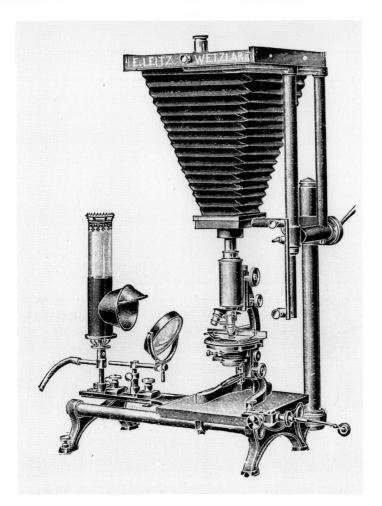

Figure 1.1: Leitz photomicrographic apparatus, in vertical mode (1910).
A gas lamp is used, with adjustable collector lens. A bellows camera is attached to a vertical pillar, above a stand resting on a platform. Reproduced from Barnard (1911), p. 114.

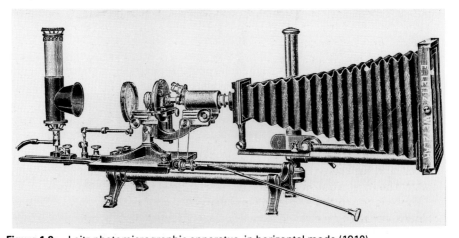

Figure 1.2: Leitz photomicrographic apparatus, in horizontal mode (1910).
The same equipment as in *Figure 1.1* is shown, with the camera swung to the horizontal on its pillar. The remote-acting fine adjustment is now in use, and the collector has been rearranged to act without need of the substage mirror. Reproduced from Barnard (1911) p. 115. The apparatus represented the state of the art at the time.

Most ordinary photographs are taken of people and/or places, where the subject is much further away from the lens than its focal length. All cameras are designed to make such pictures, but some can be used closer to the subject, until it is about life-size on the film (when the camera lens is twice as far from the negative as its own focal length). Beyond this limit of close-up photography special techniques and equipment are needed, to work at photoMACROgraphy (see Bracegirdle, 1995). Such a discipline takes magnifications to about 50× and, beyond this, a compound microscope is needed, using the techniques of photoMICROgraphy. In the past, a text describing the equipment and techniques of this subject would have been quite lengthy, as we have noted above. In this present account the authors have been able to describe the procedures and point out the pitfalls in much shorter compass, by concentrating on the modern apparatus and materials, which have been developed to the point where excellent results can be obtained by all those who are prepared to take minimal trouble.

The process begins with a determination to get the best possible microscopical image before making the exposure. Even with the most costly integrated modern equipment, it is possible to obtain and photograph a poor image, but one almost has to try to do so. The image must be evenly illuminated, with the magnification obtained so as to produce the required definition, free from glare, and of proper contrast. Given a basic understanding and perhaps a little more time, an older stand put together with a suitable lamp and an available camera for occasional use can be made to produce excellent results, and the whole may even be more flexible in application than some modern very expensive integrated equipment (see *Figure 1.3*).

Much of this older equipment used a monocular microscope with a long extension horizontal camera, perhaps of large format. Focusing was checked by inspection of the ground glass screen with a magnifier, and it was often the case that no eyepiece was used. At long extensions, an auxiliary focusing rod worked on the distant fine adjustment knob from the camera back position. Nowadays, if such equipment is to hand *with modern objectives and matching eyepieces*, it can still produce good results, in spite of being cumbersome and slow in use. Long extensions of the bellows are *not* nowadays required (an eyepiece is always used, as some of the corrections to the system might be carried out by its means), and large formats are not needed (4 × 5 in is as large as any now normally used, and that only for special work). A roll-film adapter to allow 120 mm films to be used on a plate back is ideal with such apparatus. Older objectives and eyepieces (pre-1960) are best avoided, as they will probably not be coated and (in spite of being the best of their day) they will certainly not match the image quality of even modest ranges of optics nowadays.

There is much to be said for mounting the microscope below a bellows camera vertically mounted above it (see *Figure 1.4*). This allows a choice of format if the highest quality work is to be produced, but most routine photomicrography has been carried out on 35 mm film since the 1950s.

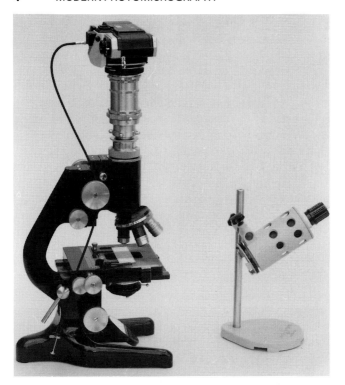

Figure 1.3:   A basic photomicrographic apparatus.
   A Watson 'Bactil' stand of about 1960 has a 1970s Russian lamp (with focusing collector, and iris) as its illuminant. The draw-tube is fitted with a clamp to prevent it sliding downwards under the weight of the 1980s Olympus OM4Ti camera, carried on a simple tube fitting directly to the eyepiece tube. Such an arrangement provides Köhler illumination and (once calibrated) controllable automatic exposure for those needing occasional 35 mm transparencies. The image size on the frame can be varied only by using different powers of eyepiece, or by using longer extension tubes. Note the use of a long cable release.

Simple adapter tubes to fit a 35 mm camera to most stands remain universally and cheaply available, and the simplest way to obtain photomicrographs is still to use a (lensless) single lens reflex (SLR) camera with through-the-lens (TTL) built-in metering, focusing directly on the screen. A step onwards is to mount on the microscope eyetube a beam-splitting cube below a shutter block to carry an ordinary 35 mm camera back, thus allowing viewing and focusing, with metering, even during the exposure (see *Figure 1.5*).

The most usual format is still 35 mm, even for the several attached camera backs which the most modern universal stands now carry. The format is small, but has a relatively high information content capacity, and the medium is ideal for illustrating lectures. Larger formats on roll-film or sheet-film are used when much better quality is required (often for book illustrations in colour), and the largest modern integrated stands include such a port. Much information from the microscope is now stored

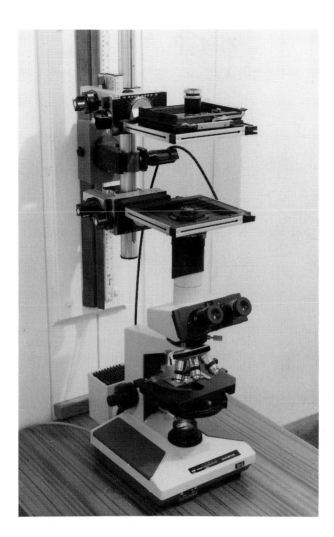

Figure 1.4: A versatile modern apparatus.

An Olympus BHS stand, with built-in Köhler illumination and widely interchangeable optics, is fitted with a trinocular head. It stands on a heavy levelled table 300 mm above floor level, under a 4 × 5 in Sinar P camera carried on a truly vertical optical bench. This arrangement allows the camera to be centred to the stand, moved bodily vertically as required, and the bellows length adjusted to frame the subject precisely. The picture was made with a split exposure, to reveal the relay lens resting behind the shutter inside the bellows. In use, the image is optimized, and focused on the ground glass not by turning the fine adjustment but by moving the relay lens (on the camera front) up and down; the shorter the extension, the longer the excursion required. This accounts for the very long light-trap sleeve (cut away at the bottom to accommodate the tilt of the trinocular head). The merest final touch on the fine adjustment ensures that the image is in focus (checked by the 8× lens on the aerial image provided by the clear centre spot of the ground glass) without destroying the corrections of higher power objectives.

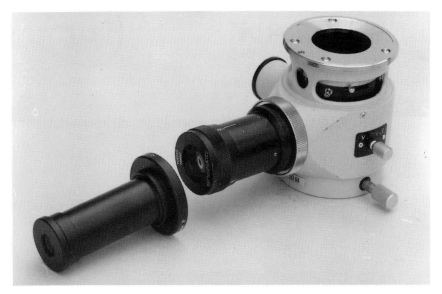

Figure 1.5: Olympus manual beam-splitter.
The Olympus PM-10M manual exposure beam-splitter clamps to an eyepiece adapter which carries a choice of photo eyepiece (2.5×, 3.3×, 5× or 6.7×). It has a prism which can be moved to divert 100% of the light to the focusing telescope, or 100% to the meter port, or 80% to the film and 20% to the telescope. The telescope focuses on a graticule, and has an attachable focusing magnifier to prevent accommodation of the eye interfering with focusing at low powers. The meter port accepts an integrating meter probe. A mechanical shutter is mounted in rubber, and has speeds from 1/250 sec to 1 sec plus B. The rear of the unit may carry a 35 mm camera, a 4 × 5 in back or a Polaroid back.

as digitized images, perhaps for image analysis, and relatively few hard copies may be made in some departments. This trend is likely to increase in future, but the rigour required for the proper setting up of the instrument, the selection of the field to be recorded, the optimization of the image obtained and the proper noting of the picture content will not change, and it is with this that the present book is concerned.

References

Barnard JE. (1911) *Practical Photo-micrography*. Edward Arnold, London.
Barnard JE, Welch FV. (1925) *Practical Photo-micrography*. Edward Arnold, London.
Barnard JE, Welch FV. (1936) *Practical Photo-micrography*. Edward Arnold, London.
Bracegirdle B. (1995) *Scientific PhotoMACROgraphy* (RMS Handbook no. 31). BIOS Scientific Publishers, Oxford.
Delly J. (1988) *Photography through the Microscope*, 9th edn. Publication P-2. Eastman Kodak, Rochester, NY.
Lawson DF. (1960) *The Technique of Photomicrography*. Newnes, London.

Lawson DF. (1972) *Photomicrography*. Academic Press, London.

Loveland RP. (1970) *Photomicrography: a Comprehensive Treatise*. John Wiley & Sons, New York.

Michel K. (1957) *Die Mikrophotographie*. Springer-Verlag, Vienna.

Needham GH. (1958) *The Practical Use of the Microscope Including Photomicrography*. Thomas, Springfield, OH.

Pringle A. (1890) *Practical Photo-micrography: by the Latest Methods*. Scovill & Adams, New York.

Richardson JH. (1991) *Handbook for the Light Microscope*. Noyes Publications, Park Ridge, NJ.

Shillaber CP. (1944) *Photomicrography in Theory and Practice*. John Wiley & Sons, New York.

Spitta EJ. (1899) *Photo-micrography*. Scientific Press, London.

2 Obtaining the Image

2.1 Illumination

Some specimens for the microscope are opaque and must be examined with reflected light (epi-illumination). Many specimens, however, are thin enough so that transmitted light passing through them is used. In both transmitted and epi-illumination the light may be axial or oblique. If the obliquity of the illuminating rays is such that no direct light can enter the microscope objective then the object will be visible only by light which it diffracts. This gives a high-contrast image with the object appearing bright upon a dark background (dark ground illumination).

In epi-illumination with low power objectives (with their large working distances), the focused light may be directed on to the specimen from a lamp or lamps positioned to one side of the microscope stage. Such illumination will necessarily be oblique. For higher power objectives, the light is directed on to the specimen by reflection through a specialized beam-splitter prism block above the objective. The objective then serves as its own condenser, directing the light on to the specimen. This arrangement is now almost universally used, not only in materials science, but also for fluorescence microscopy in which the short-wave exciting radiation is isolated via a suitable filter. The longer wavelength fluorescence emission passes through the beam splitter, above which is a barrier filter to eliminate any of the exciting radiation which has been reflected by the specimen.

Transmitted illumination involves the use of a separate condenser placed between the illuminating source and the specimen stage of the microscope. There has been much theoretical discussion during the last 100 years, especially as to the merits of two main methods of arranging the illumination. The first of these, now obsolescent, is 'source-focused' illumination, which uses a uniform light source imaged into the specimen plane. Often, a mains voltage flashed-opal electric bulb is used, mounted in a housing fitted with a series of stops or an iris diaphragm close to it. These 'field stops' are focused by the substage condenser into the plane of the object to limit the size of the illuminated area and to control glare

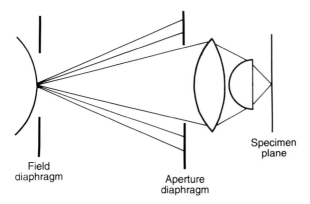

Figure 2.1:   A diagram of source-focused illumination.
   A homogeneous light source (such as the surface of an opal lamp bulb) shown on the left, has a field-limiting diaphragm immediately in front of it. Light is focused into the specimen plane by the microscope condenser, the solid angle of the cone of light accepted being controlled by the aperture diaphragm placed in the front focal plane of the microscope condenser.

(*Figure 2.1*). The principal problem with this simple system is ensuring that the light source is sufficiently large to cover the required illuminated field area when working at low powers. It is possible to use a simple diffusing screen in the plane of the field stop to extend the area of the light source, but this often means losing intensity of illumination. If the diffuser is placed too close to the condenser then unacceptable glare may be introduced. Baker and Bell (1951) showed that excellent illumination will be obtained even if the lamp is not focused into the plane of the object, provided that the field stop is so focused.

   The second method of illumination, proposed by August Köhler (1893) specifically for photomicrography and named after him (see *Figure 2.2*), is intended to provide a bright, evenly illuminated field from a small light source. This latter is imaged by a lamp condenser or collector lens into the front focal plane of the microscope condenser. The collector then serves as a uniform secondary light source and is imaged in turn by the microscope condenser into the plane of the object. A diaphragm immediately in front of the lamp collector acts as a field diaphragm controlling the area of the object which is illuminated. The condenser diaphragm acts as an aperture diaphragm controlling the solid angle of the cone of light entering the objective. Köhler's method has the advantage that a small structured source of light, such as the filament of a low-voltage bulb, may be used since its structure will not appear in the field of view. The lamp collector must be well corrected, since if it has much spherical aberration then it may not be possible to obtain a uniformly lit field at the object. The drawbacks of Köhler illumination are that the optical axis of the lamp plus its collector lens must be aligned with the optical axis of the microscope itself and (when a separate lamp and collector is used) there are

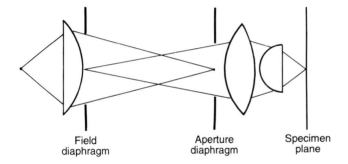

| Field | Aperture | Specimen |
| diaphragm | diaphragm | plane |

Figure 2.2:   A diagram of Köhler illumination.
Light from the source (which usually is not homogeneous) is focused by the lamp collector lens into the front focal plane of the condenser where the aperture diaphragm is placed. An image of the source is thus formed here (see *Figure 2.14*). The lamp collector lens acts as an apparently homogeneous source of light which is imaged by the microscope condenser into the specimen plane. The area of the specimen which is illuminated is controlled by the field diaphragm, whilst the aperture diaphragm controls the solid angle of the illuminating cone of light.

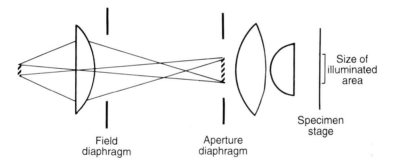

Size of
illuminated
area

Specimen
stage

| Field | Aperture |
| diaphragm | diaphragm |

Figure 2.3:   Köhler illumination at low power.
For low-power microscopy, a large area of the specimen must be illuminated. which needs a large lamp collector lens of low power; the image of the filament (shown cross-hatched) in the front focal plane of the microscope condenser is thus small and so the full working aperture of the system is not available with a standard microscope condenser or lamp collector. The large illuminated area is often achieved by the use of a condenser whose focal length may be altered by removing the upper element from the optical path.

restrictions in the range of magnifications over which the system gives correct illumination.

At low powers, one needs a large field of view evenly lit with a small solid cone of light (i.e. of low numerical aperture); at high powers the converse is true (a high numerical aperture but a relatively small illuminated area). A single lamp collector lens is often not able to satisfy both of these conditions. If it is large enough to give a full field of illumination at low powers then it will have a long focal length and only provide a cone of small numerical aperture (NA) (see *Figure 2.3*) and the image of the

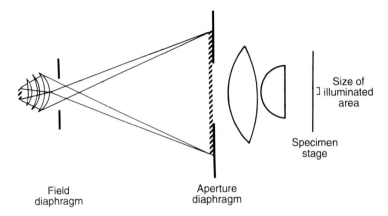

Figure 2.4: Köhler illumination at high power.
With high powers of the microscope, only a small area of the specimen needs to be illuminated but the cone of light must fill the working aperture of the system. In order to achieve this, a large image of the lamp filament (shown here cross-hatched) must be formed in the front focal plane of the microscope condenser. This is done by means of a small, high-power lamp collector lens system.

filament only occupies a small part of the plane of the condenser aperture. If a cone of light of high NA is needed then the lamp collector must provide a large image of the source and will have short focus and a small diameter and so can only light a small area of the specimen (see *Figure 2.4*). Either several condensers of differing focal lengths must be used or the condenser may have its top lens unscrewed. A 'flip top' condenser has a lever which moves the top element out of the optical path to provide this larger area of illumination needed for the low-power objectives. Köhler illumination is now universal on all microscopes in which the illumination is built-in. A useful discussion of the merits of the different systems of obtaining transmitted illumination for the microscope is provided in a paper by Hartley (1974).

2.2 Microscope lamps

2.2.1 Separate lamps

In the past almost all microscopes had a mirror and used a separate lamp (see *Figure 2.5*). This arrangement, still often used where cost or simplicity is a prime consideration, has the merit of great flexibility. Provided that care is taken in the alignment, a separate lamp is perfectly satisfactory. In order to help maintain the alignment, the lamp and microscope may be mounted on a board to hold both in the correct position. An external lamp

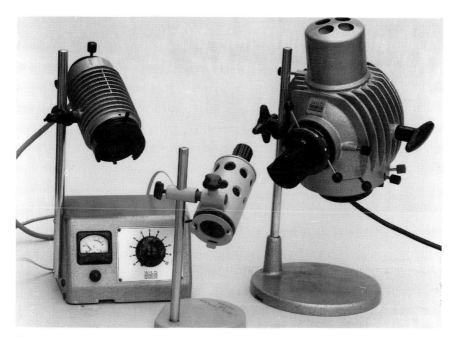

Figure 2.5:   Representative microscope lamps.
  In front, the small Russian lamp (still current) has a corrected collector, focusing (but not centring) lampholder, and lamp iris, with a compact 8 V tungsten filament. It is a very useful and inexpensive small lamp. On the left is shown the Wild compact lamp, with built-in power supply, and 6 V 30 W compact tungsten filament bulb in centring focusing holder with iris. This remains a high-quality source. On the right is the Wild Universal lamp, fitted here with a 12 V 100 W tungsten–halogen lamp, in centring holder with focusing quartz collector lens. A concave mirror behind the lamp is also centrable, and the lamp has built-in swing-in frosted and UV barrier filters, as well as an auxiliary filter holder, and one (tiltable) also for interference filters. Interchangeable with the tungsten–halogen socket is one for the HBO 200 mercury source, and one for the XBO 150 xenon burner. A Metz electronic flash, carrying a tungsten lamp, could also be inserted. These three lamps are representative of others by other makers, and demonstrate increasing sophistication of sources.

mounted in a simple housing without any lens will serve for source-focused illumination. A separate lamp with collector lens is needed for Köhler illumination. Such lamps usually have a low-voltage tungsten filament bulb operating from a transformer, with a rheostat to control the brightness. The lamp house is vented and the bulb holder is fitted with centring screws and a means of height adjustment. The field iris diaphragm is fitted immediately in front of the collector lens, which should be well corrected and capable of focusing an image of the filament.

There are several types of low-voltage bulb which may be fitted to this type of lamp. Some have only a single linear coil filament which when focused into the condenser tends not to fill its aperture. Bulbs which have several parallel rows of tungsten coils are much better. These, when focused, provide a much larger patch of light capable of filling the condenser aperture completely. An example of this was the bulb fitted to the

Vickers 'Intense' lamp (now no longer available) which had five such rows. All conventional tungsten filament bulbs suffer, however, from blackening of the glass envelope as the bulb ages, due to evaporation of tungsten metal from the filament; further, unless they are 'over-run', the colour temperature of their light is below that necessary for the use of colour film and correction by filtration is needed (see Section 6.3).

Nowadays tungsten–halogen (sometimes called quartz–iodine) bulbs are standard. These bulbs are very small, have a compact, flat filament and contain halogen vapour inside the quartz envelope. This reaches a high temperature (over 600°C) during operation so their lamp houses require adequate venting and heat filters to protect the collector lens. Like conventional tungsten lamps, the colour temperature of tungsten–halogen bulbs varies with the applied voltage and, if operated at their nominal voltage, they emit radiation which is rich in the shorter wavelengths. They may, therefore, be used for exciting some of the fluorophores which are in current use.

All lamps fitted with a collector lens require that the filament is centred to the collector and, as these lamps have an optical axis of their own, this axis must also be in line with that of the microscope itself. Bulb alignment may be checked by focusing a filament image with the collector lens on to a white surface a few metres from the lamp housing. The bulb centring screws and height adjustment are then adjusted to make the filament image symmetrical and central in the illuminated area. Setting up Köhler illumination with a separate lamp and a microscope with a mirror is described in Section 2.4.

2.2.2 Built-in lamps

The majority of current microscopes have the lamp built into some part of the stand, either in its body or in the base, and have complex, often highly corrected, collector lens systems to provide the best possible illumination of the specimen.

In specialist instruments for use with fluorescence techniques there is often more than one light source. One lamp may be used for direct transmission microscopy, whilst a second is provided for incident illumination for exciting the fluorescence. This second source may be a tungsten–halogen lamp or, if ultraviolet radiation is needed, it could be a mercury arc. These latter are seldom used for visual observation because they do not emit a continuous spectrum, but a line spectrum. That of the mercury arc is strong in radiations of 546 nm in the green, 577 nm in the yellow and 366 nm and 253 nm in the ultraviolet. To transmit the ultraviolet wavelengths, such lamps have quartz envelopes and must be provided with rather bulky power units, since, although the running voltage is relatively low, a high-voltage pulse is need to start the lamp.

It is possible to combine tungsten light sources for visual observation with a flash tube for photomicrography. Electronic flash has the great advantage of providing a light pulse of extremely short duration, so that if the subject is active (e.g. aquatic organisms) sharp images are still obtained.

2.3 Microscope optics

A transmitted light microscope for photomicrography consists of the light source with its collector lens, a substage condenser, the objective and an eyepiece, in addition to any optics needed to produce a real image in the film plane of the camera. If the instrument is operating solely in incident light then no substage condenser is used, but there is a semi-reflective plate or a beam-splitting prism arrangement above the objective to direct the light down to the specimen through the objective which acts as its own condenser.

In many microscopes, the objective produces a real image in the primary image plane located in the microscope tube. The eyepiece diaphragm is placed in this plane and thus the eyepiece produces a virtual image. The refractive system of the observer's eye provides the final real image on the retina. The basic ray path of such an instrument is shown in *Figure 2.6*.

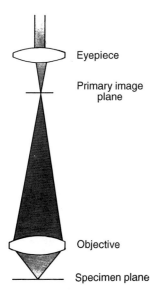

Eyepiece

Primary image
plane

Objective

Specimen plane

Figure 2.6:   Ray paths in a traditional microscope system.
The shaded area represents the rays from a point in the specimen being converged by the objective to produce a real primary image. The rays emerging from the eyepiece are parallel and are converged by the refractive apparatus of the eye to form the final real image on the retina.

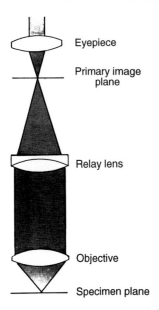

Eyepiece

Primary image
plane

Relay lens

Objective

Specimen plane

Figure 2.7:   Ray paths in an infinity-corrected microscope.
The shaded area represents the rays from a point in the object. Note that they are parallel until converged by a separate relay lens to form the real primary image. The eyepiece acts as in a traditional system.

Some of the most modern microscopes, however, have their optics arranged so that the objective does not produce a real image but a parallel beam path (*Figure 2.7*). An additional relay lens in the system then provides a real primary image for the eyepiece and may serve with the objective to correct some chromatic aberrations (see Section 2.4.2). There are several advantages to this so-called 'infinity-corrected' arrangement. For instance, the dependence on a set mechanical tube length is abolished, giving freedom to introduce other optical elements into the beam path between the objective and the tube lens. Phase plates or Wollaston prisms for differential interference contrast may be placed here.

In any optical system there are planes which are equivalent; an object placed in one of these will appear sharply imaged in any subsequent plane of that series. These are called conjugate planes, and a knowledge of them in the microscope is essential to the photomicrographer so that graticules may be inserted in the correct place or correct adjustment of the illumination obtained. There are two separate sets of conjugate planes called the illuminating series and the image-forming series. Their locations are summarized in *Table 2.1* and illustrated in *Figure 2.8*.

The two series of conjugate planes are separate, so that an image of the lamp filament, although appearing in focus in all subsequent planes of its own series, will never appear in any of the planes of the other series. A measurement graticule, which must appear in focus at the same time as the image of the object, is normally placed for convenience in the primary

Table 2.1:   Conjugate planes

Illuminating series	Image-forming series
Lamp filament	Field diaphragm (lamp iris diaphragm)
Front focal plane of condenser (aperture iris)	Specimen plane
	Primary image plane
Back focal plane of the objective	Retina of the eye
Exit pupil of the eyepiece (Ramsden disc)	

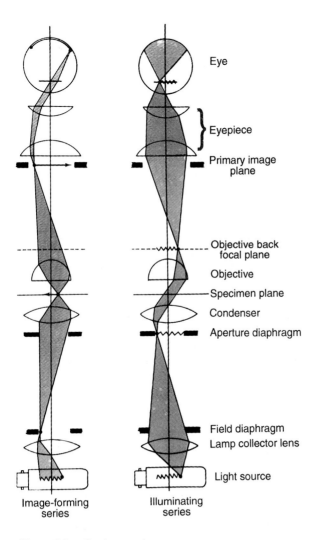

Eye

Eyepiece

Primary image plane

Objective back focal plane

Objective

Specimen plane

Condenser

Aperture diaphragm

Field diaphragm

Lamp collector lens

Light source

Image-forming series   Illuminating series

Figure 2.8:   Conjugate planes.
A diagram to illustrate the two series of conjugate planes in the microscope. On the left is the image-forming series, whilst the illuminating series is shown on the right. See *Table 2.1* for a listing of the individual planes in each series.

image plane. It would also be possible to place it in the plane of the field iris diaphragm, when it would still appear in focus along with the specimen. With conventional microscopes a phase plate is usually placed in the back focal plane of the objective and the correct size of annulus is then fitted in the preceding conjugate plane of its series (the front focal plane of the condenser), so its image is superimposed upon the phase plate. This ensures that all the direct light passes through a predetermined path in the objective back focal plane.

2.3.1 The condenser

All microscopes intended for serious work with transmitted light are fitted with a substage condenser. This not only increases the intensity of the light from the lamp but, more importantly, focuses an image of the field diaphragm into the plane of the specimen. The most important function of the condenser, however, is to provide a cone of light which matches the NA of the objective lens. This is achieved by altering the opening of the aperture iris diaphragm which is located in the front focal plane of the condenser. Use of too small an illuminating cone results in loss of resolution of the objective and the appearance of diffraction rings surrounding objects. The resulting, useless, image (often called a 'rotten' image) is unsuitable for either visual observation or photography (*Figure 2.9*). In some cases, a careful, controlled closure of the aperture iris (checked by observation of the appearance of the image) is permissible, since this will increase contrast in the image. This may be needed when the object is transparent and other contrast techniques cannot be used. The use of too large an illuminating cone of light will also degrade the image as a result of glare. With older objectives, uncoated and less well corrected than current ones, the recommendation is to reduce the aperture of the illuminating cone of light to about 80% of that of the objective (a four-fifths cone, see *Figure 2.10*). With the greatly improved computations and coatings of modern objectives, the angle of the cone of light from the condenser may be set to almost match that accepted by the objective.

To reduce the possibility of glare degrading the contrast of the image, it is important to limit the *area* of the specimen which is illuminated to that which is seen or photographed. This is done by closing the field diaphragm, an image of which is conjugate with that of the specimen plane.

The simplest type of condenser available is the Abbe, consisting basically of two highly curved but uncorrected lenses. It suffers from both spherical and chromatic aberration and normally can only deliver a cone of light of numerical aperture of about 0.7. This type of condenser is usually fitted to microscopes intended for student use, but may appear on more advanced models also. A much improved achromatized version may be fitted with a swing-out top lens and can provide a cone of light of up to 0.9 NA. The top lens is removed from the optical path to increase the focal length of the condenser when it is required to illuminate fully the field of

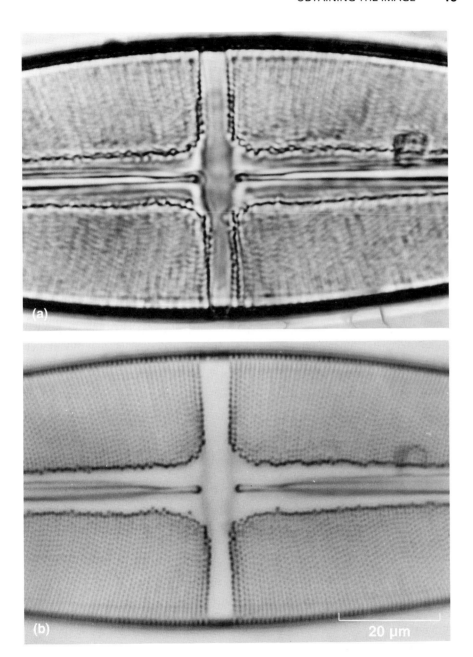

Figure 2.9: Images of the diatom *Navicula lyra.*
(a) An example of an image produced when the numerical aperture of the objective was reduced dramatically. Note the very strong black and white borders to the frustule produced by diffraction effects and the loss of resolution of the fine detail. This is often called a 'rotten image'. (b) The image produced by the same objective operated at its full numerical aperture. The diffraction halos are no longer present and the puncta on the frustule are clearly resolved.

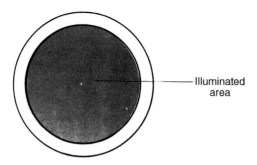

Figure 2.10:   The appearance of the back focal plane of an objective.
 This diagram shows the appearance of the back focal plane of an objective as seen when the eyepiece of the microscope has been removed or with an auxiliary telescope. The hatched area represents a four-fifths cone of light.

view of a low-power objective. There are, however, special condensers available from most microscope makers, computed to work with very low-power objectives of initial magnifications of ×1 or ×2.

For microscopy involving high resolution, makers supply an achromatic/aplanatic condenser. This works well and, if immersed to the under surface of the slide, will illuminate an oil immersion objective of the highest quality and with a NA of up to 1.4. Many of the common techniques available for introducing contrast into a specimen, such as dark ground, phase contrast and differential interference microscopy, require special condensers, although some makers now supply what they term 'universal' condensers into which several different combinations of optical elements are fitted in a rotating turret, to allow rapid changeover between different observation methods.

Dark ground condensers are designed to illuminate the specimen plane with a cone of light rays which falls outside the acceptance angle of the objective. In the absence of a specimen, no light enters the objective and the field of view remains dark. Any object on the stage will diffract light, some of which will be accepted by the objective so that the object is seen in reverse contrast, that is bright upon a dark background. For objectives of up to 0.8 NA this is done by fitting a central opaque stop in the condenser which is used 'dry'. For objectives of higher numerical apertures the dark ground condenser contains two mirror systems, one spherical, the other a cardioid of revolution. This condenser is used in oil immersion contact with the underside of the slide when the NA of the innermost part of the oblique cone of light which it gives is about 1.2. This means that since most oil immersion objectives have an NA *greater* than this, in order for them to give dark ground they must have their NA reduced to this figure. Older objectives used an inserted metal cone for this but modern immersion objectives intended for dark ground have an iris diaphragm built into their back focal plane. Further details are to be found in Bradbury (1989).

All condensers have a tray fitted, usually below, which is intended for the insertion of glass or resin filters. If the image is to be photographed in monochrome, especially with an objective of perhaps average quality, then a green filter which restricts the wavelength of the light to a narrow band centred on 550 nm will often improve the resolution by eliminating any slight residual chromatic aberrations. The use of colour filters to modify the tonal range or to enhance the contrast of a stained specimen is much more important. Without a filter, areas of the specimen of the same brightness may reproduce as similar grey tones, even though to the eye they are of different colour, so giving a print lacking in contrast. This defect is easily remedied. Any feature in the specimen may be given more contrast (i.e. will print darker) by the use of a filter of a complementary colour. A blue object will be darkened by photographing it through a yellow or orange filter, red or magenta filters will darken green, and blue–green or blue filters will darken reds. Conversely, objects will have their tones made lighter if they are photographed through a filter of the same colour (see Bradbury, 1985). Suitable Kodak 'Wratten' filters for use in photo-micrography are listed in the Kodak monograph P-2 (Anon, 1988). The filter tray may also be used for neutral density filters if these are required to moderate the intensity of the illumination.

2.3.2 The objective

The objective is the most important component in the imaging system of the microscope. It alone provides the resolution of fine detail and the initial magnification. All objectives contain lenses made from different types of glass and other material; they are computed so that the image defects of chromatic and spherical aberration, astigmatism, curvature of field and coma are minimized. In recent years, both lens design and the control of their manufacture have been done by computers. This has led to objectives becoming very complex, with as many as 14 lens elements in several groups. Such objectives are necessarily very expensive but do provide excellent performance for those who need it. Objectives with the highest possible standard of corrections are called apochromats. Such lenses have the red, yellow and blue regions of the spectrum brought to almost identical focal planes whilst the other aberrations are so small that, for practical purposes, they may be ignored. Older apochromats suffered from excessive field curvature but modern apochromats possess a truly flat field. Simpler objectives (called achromats) suffice for most routine work, the modern examples having good correction of axial chromatic aberration. The image formed by rays at the extremes of the spectrum are brought to a common focal plane by combining lenses made from glasses with different disper-sions. The image formed by the intermediate wavelengths is at a slightly different plane of focus and appears as a greenish 'residual colour' ap-parent around contrasty objects. Spherical aberration and coma are cor-rected for the intermediate wavelengths, so that if the objective is used

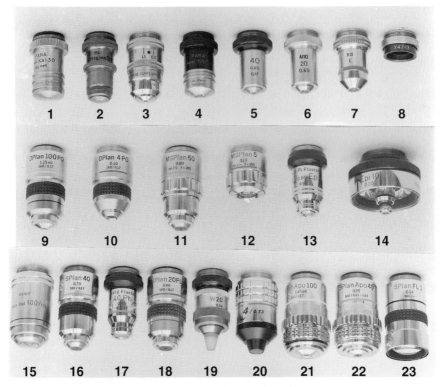

Figure 2.11: Group of objectives to show the barrel markings.
(*Note*: the markings engraved on the barrels are listed in this legend in **bold** type and their meaning is given by comments in square brackets). 1. Watson achromat, of about 1955. **WATSON B 37841 PARA** [achromat (Watson used the term Parachromatic to designate achromats)], **2MM** [focal length], **NA 1.30, OIL IMM.** [homogenous immersion], ×100. 2. Reichert achromat, of about 1940. **C.REICHERT WIEN 18b** [type number], **Homog.imm.,** **1/12"** [focal length], **Apert.1.30** [NA]. 3. Leitz apochromat, of about 1965. **Ernst Leitz Wetzlar Germany A = 0.95** [NA], **45:1** [magnification], **Apochromat 4MM.** [type and focal length]. 4. Watson achromat, of about 1955. **WATSON 43664 PARA** [achromat], **4MM NA 0.70 ×40.** [focal length, NA and magnification]. 5. Zeiss Jena achromat, of about 1955. **CARL ZEISS JENA 179601 40** [magnification], **0,65** [NA], **0,17** [thickness of cover-glass to be used]. 6. Russian apochromat, of 1991. **LOMO 910041 AПO** [apochromat], **20** [magnification], **0.65** [NA]. 7. Leitz achromat, of about 1960. **E.LEITZ WETZLAR 3** [type number], **10**× [magnification]. 8. Watson achromat, of about 1965. **WATSON PARA ×4/.13** [type, magnification and NA].

9. Olympus planachromat for polarizing work, of about 1985. **OLYMPUS JAPAN DPlan 100 PO** [flat-field achromat×100 strain-free] **1.25 oil 160/0.17** [NA 1.25, oil immersion, tube length 160 mm, for cover glasses 0.17 mm thick]. 10. Olympus planachromat for polarizing work, of about 1985. **OLYMPUS JAPAN DPlan 4 PO** [flat-field achromat strain-free], **0.10 160/0.17** [NA 0.10, tube length 160 mm, for cover glasses 0.17 mm thick]. 11. Olympus flat field metallurgical objective, of about 1988. **OLYMPUS JAPAN 105292 MSPlan 50** [highly corrected wide-field objective, magnification 50×], **0.80 ∞/0 f = 180** [NA 0.80, infinity-corrected, no cover glass, focal length of corrector lens]. 12. Olympus flat field metallurgical objective, of about 1988. **OLYMPUS JAPAN 106054 MSPlan 5** [highly corrected wide-field objective, magnification 5×], **0.13 ∞/– f = 180** [NA 0.13, infinity-corrected, no cover glass, focal length of corrector lens]. 13. Wild flat field fluorite epi-objective, of about 1970. **WILD HEERBRUG SWITZERLAND 284394 Wild Pl.Fluotar 40/0.65 Epi d = 0.** [flat field fluorite 40×, NA 0.65, epi-illumination, no cover glass]. 14. Wild epi-objective, of about 1969. **WILD HEERBRUG SWITZERLAND Epi 10 0.25** [epi-objective (in non-RMS mount to permit dark ground illumination) 10×, NA 0.25].

15. Leitz plan-apo oil immersion objective, of about 1963. **Leitz WETZLAR C20994 GERMANY 170/0.17 Pl Apo Oel 100/1.32** [tube length 170 mm, cover thickness 0.17 mm, planapochromat oil immersion, 100×, NA 1.32]. 16. Olympus planachromat, of about 1985. **OLYMPUS JAPAN 116518 SPlan 40 0.70 160/0.17** [planachromat, 40×, NA 0.70, tube length 160 mm, cover thickness 0.17 mm]. 17. Wild phase-fluorite, of about 1965. **WILD HEER-BRUG SWITZERLAND 12008 Wild Fluotar 40 Ph 0.75 d = 0.17** [fluorite phase objective, 40×, NA 0.75, cover thickness 0.17 mm]. 18. Olympus plan phase objective, of about 1986. **OLYMPUS JAPAN 801085 SPlan 20PL 0.46 160/0.17** [planachromat phase objective with positive-low contrast, 20×, NA 0.46, tube length 160 mm, cover thickness 0.17 mm]. 19. Nikon water-immersion objective, of about 1970. **Nikon 67945 LENS MADE IN JAPAN W20 0.33** [water-immersion achromat, 20×, NA 0.33. *Note*: the lens has a dipping cone attached to its front element; this is immersed in the water in use]. 20. Nikon water-immersion objective, of about 1990. **Nikon JAPAN 104062 4/0.13W 160/–** [4×, NA 0.13, water immersion, tube length 260 mm, no cover. This objective also has a dipping cone]. 21. Olympus planapo objective, of about 1983. **OLYMPUS JAPAN 100849 SPlan Apo 100 1.40 oil 160/0.17** [planapochromat, 100×, NA 1.40, oil immersion, tube length 160 mm, cover thickness 0.17 mm. The milled ring on the mount works an internal iris diaphragm]. 22. Olympus planapo objective, of about 1983. **OLYMPUS JAPAN 103067 SPlan Apo 40 0.95 160/0.11– 0.23** [planapochromat, 40×, NA 0.95, tube length 160 mm, cover thickness variable between 0.11 and 0.23 mm. The milled ring on the mount is the correction collar, varying the separation of the components of this high NA dry lens to provide correction for this wide variation in cover thickness]. 23. Olympus plan fluorite objective, of about 1984. **OLYMPUS JAPAN 100472 SPlan FL1 0.04 160/–** [plan fluorite, 1×, NA 0.04, tube length 160 mm, no cover correction. This last means that the focal length/numerical aperture combination is such that the lens is not sensitive to cover thickness, and can be used on covered and uncovered preparations].

under the correct conditions the image in the central area is of high quality. Many achromats now have these simple corrections improved by adding flatness of field. The characteristics of an objective are engraved on the lens barrel (see *Figure 2.11*). Firstly there is usually a series of letters denoting the type of objective. These vary from maker to maker. Typical examples (from the Olympus range) would be:

- UPLANAPO – universal plan apochromats. These have the very best corrections and offer the highest quality of resolution, contrast and field flatness over their entire field, and which are suitable for different types of contrast techniques;
- PLANAPO – plan apochromats with corrections nearing those of the UPLANAPO series and suitable for transmitted light brightfield microscopy;
- UPLANFL – universal plan semi-apochromatic objectives whose corrections, although excellent, are not as good as the apochromatic series;
- PLAN – achromatic objectives corrected for a flat field;
- ACH – achromatic objectives best suited for routine work.

Objectives for phase contrast usually have the letters 'PH' added and, if the lens is intended for use on an uncovered specimen, then this will be indicated also, either by a letter or by replacing the cover thickness specification with a '–'. Oil immersion objectives are often marked 'OEL'. Other makers may use the words 'OIL' or 'HOMOGENEOUS IMMER-SION'. All objectives carry markings to indicate their initial magnification and numerical aperture, followed by the tube length and the thickness of cover for which they are corrected. On an achromatic objective a typical marking might be

×40/0.65 initial magnification of 40 times, NA of 0.65,
∞/0.17 infinity-corrected, for 0.17 mm thick cover.

For photomicrography, an important requirement is flatness of field, so ideally objectives should be of the 'PLAN' type. Older objectives, especially apochromats, suffered from excessive curvature of field and are not really suitable for photographic work. Modern objectives are so good, however, that very satisfactory results are possible from almost any objective provided it is used correctly. Semi-apochromats generally have higher numerical apertures than achromats of corresponding focal length and initial power so that they are particularly useful where image brightness is low, as in fluorescence microscopy.

One problem with older microscope objectives was that lenses of different magnifications and of different types were often mounted in barrels of differing length. Changing from one magnification or type of objective to another required great care on the part of the user; it was only too easy to rotate an objective turret and bring an apochromatic 'dry' objective into contact with the slide itself! Most new objectives are parfocal so that there is little risk of a high-power objective hitting the slide after first focusing with a low-power objective.

Most modern 'dry' objectives of low initial magnifications (up to ×40) are for use with a standard coverslip thickness of 0.17 mm. If the thickness is incorrect, severe spherical aberration may be introduced into the image. Some 'dry' objectives of high NA are provided with a correction collar to allow the user to adjust for variations in cover thickness. In the case of oil immersion objectives, spherical aberration due to the use of a cover glass of the wrong thickness does not arise. However, the coverslip thickness must not be so great as to prevent the lens focusing on the object plane if the immersion objective has a short working distance. A discussion of the importance of NA and the advantages and drawbacks of 'dry' and immersion objectives is given in Bradbury (1989).

No matter how good the objective, the user may completely ruin its image quality if the microscope adjustments are incorrect. In particular, spherical aberration may be introduced which will destroy image contrast and sharpness. As we have seen above, the use of an incorrect thickness of cover slip with a 'dry' objective of high NA may destroy the resolution (see *Figure 2.12*), but use of an immersion medium with the wrong optical characteristics can also easily impair the performance, as can defocusing to place the image on the film. If specimens such as metal surfaces are studied without any coverslip with a 'dry' lens intended for work with covered objects, then so much spherical aberration will be introduced that a sharp image cannot be formed. Special objectives are made for examining uncovered objects; conversely, if these objectives are used on a traditional

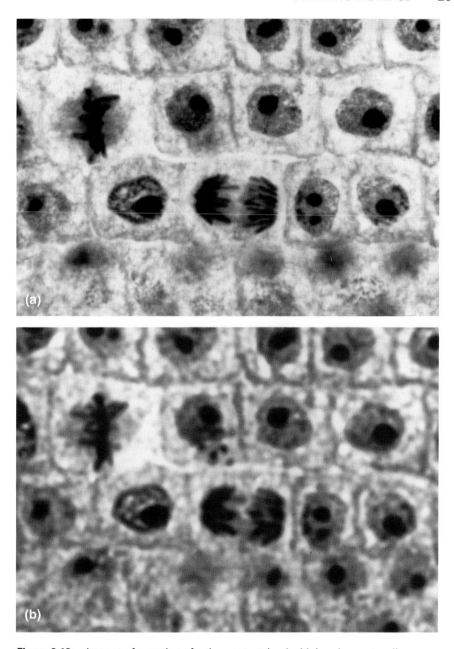

Figure 2.12: Images of a section of onion root, stained with iron haematoxylin.

These micrographs of the same area of the section were taken with an apochromatic objective of 0.95 NA fitted with a correction collar. (a) Micrograph photographed with the collar set at the correct value (0.17) of cover thickness. Note the image of the chromosomes and nuclei is sharp. (b) The same field photographed with the correction collar set to an extreme of its range. The detail in the image has become blurred due to the uncorrected spherical aberration.

slide with a coverslip then sharp images will not be obtainable. One prominent maker has currently over 100 different objectives of various initial magnifications and numerical aperture in his catalogue, grouped into series for the various specialist users.

Even the highest quality conventional objectives still retain some aberrations in their primary image plane, especially lateral chromatic aberration (sometimes called chromatic difference of magnification). When this is present, the images formed by light of different wavelengths are brought to a focus in the same plane but are of different sizes. If this difference can be made equal for all of the objectives of the series then it may be corrected by using eyepieces which have lateral chromatic aberration of the same amount but of the opposite sense deliberately introduced.

With an infinity-corrected system, the removal of the final lateral chromatic aberration is done with a 'corrector' lens introduced between the objective and the relay lens, an innovation introduced in 1971 by Carl Zeiss in their 'Axiomat' series of microscopes. A later development from the same maker produced a new series of objectives, all of which have the same degree of lateral chromatic aberration so that the relay lens itself serves as the corrector lens. Objectives and other optical parts of modern microscopes are no longer interchangeable between makers or even between different series from the same maker.

2.3.3 Relay lenses and eyepieces

The eyepiece not only converts the real primary image into a virtual image for the observer's eye, but is also responsible for adding extra magnification to the image, and for providing a place for the insertion of measuring or framing graticules. In older microscopes, the eyepiece also completes the correction of image aberrations, especially the removal of lateral chromatic difference of magnification and the final flattening of the field of view.

There are two main classes of eyepiece – the Huygenian and Ramsden. The former (see *Figure 2.13a*) has its diaphragm between the eye lens and the field lens, both of which have only a single element. This type of eyepiece provides good corrections for residual chromatic aberrations in the image and for residual coma. It is most often used with older achromatic objectives but has the drawback that the eye point is close to the upper surface of the eye lens, a fault which becomes more apparent as the magnification of the eyepiece is made greater. For this reason, it is rare to find a Huygenian eyepiece with a greater magnification than ×10. The Ramsden eyepiece has its diaphragm below the field lens (*Figure 2.13b*) and generally has a high eye point; older eyepieces with magnifications greater than ×10 were generally of this type. The Ramsden eyepiece corrects the residual aberrations well, a property which is even more pronounced in a Kellner eyepiece in which the eye lens is an achromatic

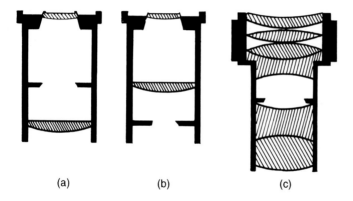

(a)   (b)   (c)

Figure 2.13:   Diagrams of the structure of three types of eyepiece.
(a) Huygenian eyepiece with internal diaphragm. (b) Ramsden eyepiece with the diaphragm located below the field lens. A Kellner eyepiece is similar but has an achromatized
doublet as the eye lens. (c) A 'Periplan' type of eyepiece as used in a modern microscope.
This gives exceptional corrections and a very wide field of view.

doublet. Some eyepieces were made with adjustable separations between
the eye and field lenses to allow the user either to make the final correction
of lateral chromatic aberration or to project an image on to a negative.
Other types of special eyepiece, designed with special high eye points, are
intended for use by spectacle wearers. With the most modern eyepieces,
this type is no longer needed, since the eyepiece is fitted with a flexible
collar which locates the observer's eye at the correct distance from the top
lens; a spectacle wearer has only to fold down this collar and can then use
the microscope without removing his or her glasses.

Whatever type of eyepiece is used, the observer is able to examine only
a finite area of the primary image. This area is represented by the 'field of
view number' [often abbreviated to the 'field number' (FN)]. For a Rams-
den-type eyepiece, this number is simply the diameter in millimetres of
the opening in the eyepiece field diaphragm. For a Huygenian eyepiece,
the FN is obtained by multiplying this diameter by the ratio of the focal
length of the eyepiece as a whole divided by the focal length of the eye lens
alone. A typical value of the FN for a modern eyepiece would be 20–25.
Eyepieces (see *Figure 2.13*c) intended for use with infinity-corrected objectives contain several optical elements to provide the large, flat field now
required, even though they do not complete the correction of residual
chromatic aberration.

Eyepieces have provision for insertion of a graticule (now more usually
termed a 'reticle') in the plane of the primary image, so it is seen in sharp
focus at the same time as the image. The graticule may have a simple
linear scale for measurement of objects or it may show the area of the field
which will be recorded on the photographic film. Other graticules are
available for special purposes, such as particle size comparisons and
stereological estimations.

2.4 Setting up the microscope to get the best image

Before using any type of microscope, it must be set up correctly so that it will provide the best image of which it is capable. This involves both mechanical and optical adjustments for the illumination system, and for the imaging and contrast provision.

With older microscopes used with a separate lamp and Köhler illumination, the following procedure is recommended, after checking the cleanliness of the optical surfaces of lamp collector, microscope condenser, objectives and eyepieces. Such cleaning may be done by wiping gently with lens tissue moistened with isopropyl alcohol.

1. Use a well-stained preparation as the specimen and focus with the ×10 objective.
2. Place the lamp at a suitable height about 250 cm in front of the microscope mirror, tilting the lamp housing so that a focused image of the lamp filament is centred on the mirror and reflected on to the front focal plane of the condenser. Check by closing the condenser iris and adjust the lamp collector focus if necessary. Ideally the filament image should occupy most of the area of the condenser aperture (*Figure 2.14*). This is easier to achieve with the solid-source type of filament rather than with the single coiled tungsten filament of some lamps. The lamp to microscope distance may be increased to enlarge this image if necessary. Open the condenser diaphragm fully.
3. Move the mirror until the light passes through the condenser and appears in the field of view of the microscope.
4. Close the field diaphragm until its image (possibly blurred and off-centre) appears in the field of view. Centre by moving the mirror.
5. Use the condenser focus knob to bring the image of the field iris into sharp focus on the image of the section.
6. Open the field iris to illuminate the field fully and make minor alterations to the mirror and lamp alignment to obtain even illumination. Centre the image of the field diaphragm with the condenser centring screws if necessary .
7. Remove the eyepiece (or insert the Bertrand lens) and close the condenser aperture diaphragm until the back focal plane is almost filled with light. Traditionally 4/5ths of the diameter of the back focal plane should be illuminated, but with current objectives this may be exceeded. With older lenses (or with low contrast specimens) it may need to be reduced. Replace the eyepiece and adjust the brightness of the light to a comfortable level for viewing by means of the lamp rheostat. *Never* close the aperture diaphragm in order to reduce the light, since this will degrade the image as shown in *Figure 2.9*.

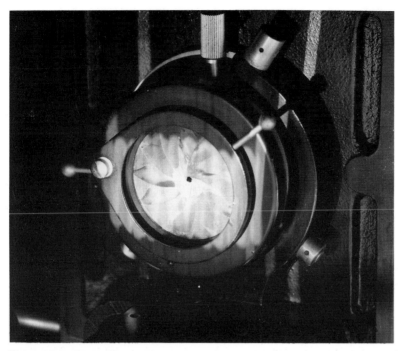

Figure 2.14: Lamp filament imaged on substage iris.
In setting up Köhler illumination, the lamp filament is focused at infinity, and then imaged on the substage iris via the mirror, thus providing a visual check for centration and that the image fills the aperture.

If using a binocular microscope, alter the separation of the eyepiece tubes to suit your interocular distance. Set the dioptre adjustment by closing one eye and focusing with the fine adjustment on some detail in the image with the other eye. Now use the other eye and bring the same detail into focus by altering the dioptre ring. If necessary, the process may be repeated with the other eyepiece. If the microscope has a built-in illuminator, setting up for Köhler will probably involve only focusing the specimen, adjusting the focus of the field diaphragm, checking its centring and setting of the aperture diaphragm to suit the numerical aperture of the objective in use.

The adjustments for use with a microscope using incident light are similar but, since the objective is acting as its own condenser, focusing the image will also ensure the specimen is at the focus of the lamp collector. If a separate lamp is used this is set horizontally, pointed at the side arm of the incident light attachment which contains the field and aperture diaphragms. Note that in many attachments for incident light work the relative positions of the field and aperture diaphragms are reversed; unlike a transmitted light instrument, the aperture diaphragm is generally *nearest* the lamp. Minor adjustments may need to be made to the focus and centration of the diaphragms, but setting the field diaphragm size and the working aperture is done as in steps 6 and 7 for transmitted light.

With several of the newer modular research microscopes the base may contain both field and aperture diaphragms as well as filter holders, separate from the actual stand with the stage and optical elements. As a preliminary to setting up the system, it will be necessary to read the instruction manual and locate the relevant controls which may not necessarily be where a cursory inspection suggests!

2.5 Obtaining a real image in the film plane

The microscope used visually provides parallel rays from the eyepiece which are converged by the eye to produce a real image on the retina (see *Figure 2.15a*). In order to take a photomicrograph these rays must produce a real image at some finite distance from the eyepiece. There are several ways in which this can be done, which are detailed in Evennett (1989). The simplest way is to refocus the microscope so that the real primary image is formed at a lower level in the eyepiece, below its focal plane (*Figure 2.15b*), so that converging rays leave the eyepiece and form a real image. Such refocusing is not ideal, especially with high-power objectives, since the distance between object and the objective is greater and that between the objective and primary image is shorter than that for which the system was computed. Image degradation due to the introduction of spherical aberration is inevitable. Such a method is, however, simple and serves well if the magnification is low (objectives of NA no greater than 0.25) and the eyepiece to film distance is long, so that the refocusing required is minimal. This may be the case if large format film is in use with a bellows camera. This technique is used with the simplest camera adapter tubes which are sold for attachment to a monocular microscope tube. These are fitted with an adapter to carry the body of an SLR camera and the refocusing of the microscope is controlled by observing the image through the camera's own reflex focus mechanism.

Another simple method to obtain a real image which avoids refocusing the objective is to raise the eyepiece in the tube by adding a simple collar (*Figure 2.15c*). Altering the separation between the components of the eyepiece has also been used to produce a real image in the film plane (*Figure 2.15d*). The use of a moveable eye lens was the basis of the so-called 'photographic' or 'projection' eyepieces available from the 1920s to the 1960s.

The most satisfactory method of achieving a real image, however, is to add above the eyepiece an extra relay lens which acts in the same way as

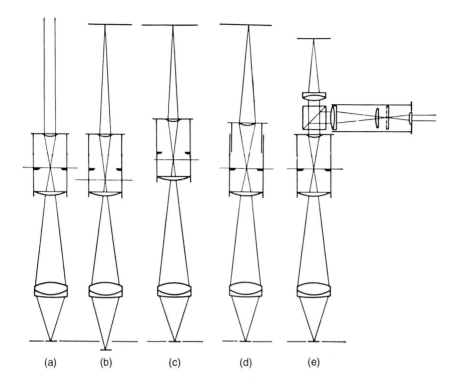

(a)   (b)   (c)   (d)   (e)

Figure 2.15: Methods of obtaining a real image on a photographic film.
(a) The arrangement of the microscope for visual observation. The rays emerging from the eyepiece do not form a real image. (b) Refocusing the microscope so that the primary image is lowered and falls below the focal plane of the eyepiece. Rays from the eyepiece now converge and form a real image but the objective performance will be impaired. (c) Specimen and primary image are in their correct positions but the eyepiece is raised to increase the primary image–eye lens distance, again forming a real image. (d) A projection or photographic eyepiece with variable field/eye lens distance may be used to form a real image. (e) The microscope settings are as for visual work but an extra relay lens in the photomicrographic camera provides the real image in the film plane. Redrawn from Evennett (1989) by permission of Oxford University Press.

the refractive media of the eye. When this is used in the large integrated photomicrographic stands in use today, the optics are so arranged that the image is framed and focused with the aid of a graticule in one of the normal eyepieces. For more occasional use with a standard microscope, the extra relay lens may be incorporated into the simple adapter tube intended to carry an SLR camera. If the extra lens forms part of a dedicated 'add-on' eyepiece camera (as in *Figure 2.15e*), then an additional beam-splitting cube and focusing telescope are usually added in the optical path.

2.6 An overview of photomicrographic equipment

A very wide variety of photomicrographic apparatus is available and, although the frequent user often has the advantage of using modern equipment where the microscope and camera are often fully integrated and all functions are automated, there are often occasions when older equipment has to be used. Given care in the adjustments, and accepting that the user has to determine the exposure and operate the film advance, such equipment is capable of producing micrographs of the highest quality. An overview of the older equipment is given in Chapter 1.

The current major makers all provide facilities for adapting their microscopes to take photomicrographs. With some monocular student microscopes this may be only a simple tube which fits on to the microscope tube and contains the eyepiece. The other end of the adapter has a fitting for the attachment of the body of an SLR camera (see *Figure 1.3*). This

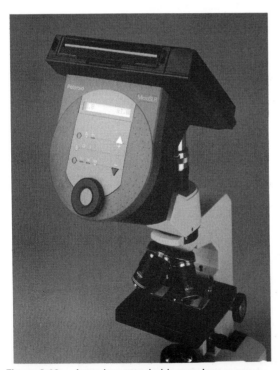

Figure 2.16:   A modern attachable eyepiece camera.
   This is the SLR66 from Polaroid which can be attached to almost any microscope. It carries the film pack in a magazine and provides fully automatic exposure. Photograph provided by courtesy of Polaroid (UK) Ltd.

allows the focusing of the image to be carried out on the screen of the camera itself. This may be done on the camera's standard screen but it is easier if the camera has interchangeable screens. A suitable screen is plain glass with simple lines engraved on it with a plain centre spot to allow the focus plane to be defined. In use, an extra magnifier is used to focus these lines and the microscope image is then focused by adjusting the microscope focus. The point of correct focus is achieved when there is no lateral movement between the image and the focusing lines when the eye is moved from side to side (i.e. when there is no parallax). If the camera has integral

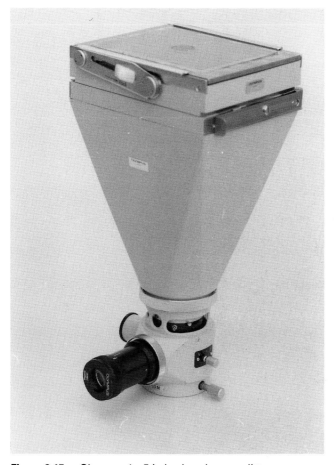

Figure 2.17:   Olympus 4 × 5 in back on beam-splitter.
   The beam splitter-shutter assembly (see also *Figure 1.5*) is shown carrying the 4 × 5 back. A ground-glass screen has been made up, and carries a central cover glass, cemented to the underside of the glass, to allow for viewing the aerial image. A pencilled cross on the ground surface provides a reference focus for the 8× magnifier used to inspect the focus. This set up is good in use, apart only from an inability to vary the extension; change of field size is obtained in discrete steps only by varying the power of the projection eyepieces used.

metering the problem of exposure determination is eliminated. If no such facility is present then the exposure must be determined by some other method (see Section 7.2). With all of these systems, however, the exposure is often made with the camera's own focal plane shutter. This might occasionally cause image unsharpness problems as a result of shutter vibration but, if so, this can be eliminated by making the exposure manually, using a card to interrupt the light path of the microscope whilst the camera shutter is held open on the 'bulb' setting. Some more sophisticated microscopes are fitted with a 'trinocular head'. This allows visual observation through the binocular eyepiece with the camera on a vertical photomicrographic tube which is left permanently in position.

For occasional photomicrographs, where rapid results are required, a completely self-contained attachment camera is now available which fits on to an eyepiece tube. This is the Polaroid MicroSLR (*Figure 2.16*) which

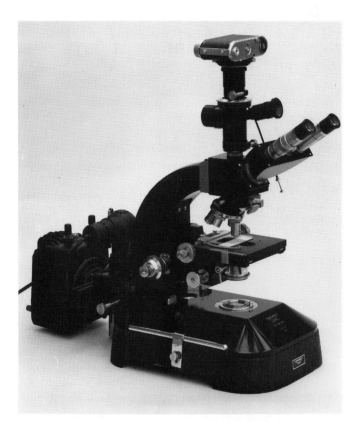

Figure 2.18: Reichert Zetopan stand with attached camera.
A typical advanced stand of the late 1950s, with dual lamp housings, and camera tube carrying a beam-splitting head with viewing and exposure estimating ports, below a rather basic manual-wind 35 mm camera back. At this time, the provision of photomicrographic facilities even on the most advanced stands was still far from comprehensive or integrated.

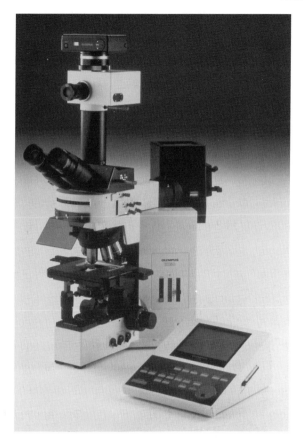

Figure 2.19: The Olympus BX50 research microscope.
This is one of the latest models of research microscope from Olympus and is shown fitted with the PM30 fully automatic photomicrographic camera. The beam-splitter housing carries a single 35 mm body in this illustration, although other format housings may be fitted. The exposure control unit with its LCD display is seen to the right of the microscope.

is fully automatic and simply requires the user to select the film type (colour or black and white), focus and expose. The exposure will be made and the print will eject and develop automatically.

It is possible to obtain attachment cameras from most of the current makers. Examples are the Nikon Microflex series and the Olympus PM10, PM20 or PM30 systems. These, although usually intended primarily for use with 35 mm film, may accept larger format materials with roll-film backs or sheet-film holders (see *Figure 2.17*). The simpler versions are manually operated but many are provided with sophisticated electronic control boxes which provide automatic exposure, measure colour temperature and give automated film wind-on. In some systems the focus is achieved through the normal microscope binocular head which is fitted for

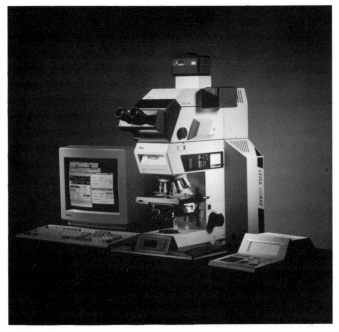

Figure 2.20:   The Leica DM RD research microscope. Photograph provided by courtesy of Leica UK Ltd.

this purpose with a special 'framing eyepiece' replacing one of the normal microscope eyepieces. It is also possible for a separate ocular finder, often with its own special focusing magnifier, to be attached to the main body of the camera. The aim in these systems is to achieve maximum flexibility so that provision is usually made for the attachment of a video camera on a separate port; it may also be possible to attach a cine camera with intervalometer.

In the 1950s, firms began to produce large integrated photomicrographic systems. One of the first of these was the Reichert MeF inverted model, primarily intended for metallographic use. This was soon followed by the Reichert 'Zetopan' (see *Figure 2.18*), a conventional stand which had an attachable illuminating base and a manually operated camera attachment. The large research microscopes now available from all makers all have completely integrated photomicrographic units. For example, the 'Axiophot' series of microscopes from Zeiss, the Leica DM RD photosystem and the Olympus BX series (see *Figure 2.19*) fitted with the PM30 photo system are all capable of the most sophisticated photomicrography. All of these modern instruments have multi-coated optics which provide flat fields and excellent colour corrections, so that if correctly adjusted they will provide high contrast images with the best possible resolution of detail. These integrated photomicroscopes provide the choice of several different methods of exposure estimation, such as integrated field or spot measurement, the ability to use special protocols for difficult situations (such as dark ground microscopy) and the ability to mount up to three separate cameras at any one time (see *Figure 2.20*). Automation has been carried a very long way with these instruments, and the ability to take excellent photomicrographs by several different contrast techniques in rapid succession is a great advantage.

With any of these automated systems there is the provision for setting the exposure manually so that, if desired, the operator can effect some control. The main disadvantage of such integrated systems is their very high cost.

References

Anon. (1988) *Photography Through the Microscope*. Kodak Monograph P-2.

Bell AS, Baker, JR. (1951) Experiments on the illumination of microscopical objects. *J. Quekett Microsc. Club*, *Ser 4* **III**, 261–275.

Bradbury S. (1985) Filters in microscopy. *Proc. R. Microsc. Soc.* **20**, 83–91

Bradbury S. (1989) *An Introduction to the Optical Microscope*. (RMS Handbook no. 1). Oxford University Pres, Oxford.

Evennett PJ. (1989) Image recording. In *Light Microscopy in Biology: a Practical Approach* (ed. AJ Lacey). Oxford University Press, Oxford, pp. 61–102.

Hartley WG. (1974) Microscope illuminating systems for transmitted light. *Proc. R. Microsc. Soc.* **9**, 167–179.

Köhler A. (1893) Ein neues Beleuchtungs fahren für microphotographische Zwecke. *Z. Wiss. Mikrosk.* **10**, 433–440. Translated and reprinted in full in *Proc. R. Microsc. Soc.* (1993) **28**, 181–186. This issue contains other papers on the same subject.

3 Imaging Methods in Current Use

Many methods of recording various kinds of image have been developed, some old and some recent and very specialized. They are then disseminated in a wide variety of ways, for the whole purpose of capturing an image is to show it to others. The methods may be summarized as follows.

3.1 Graphical methods

These include older techniques, and require a skilled and trained artist to capture the original image in some way. Formerly, a skilled engraver was also then required to transfer the picture to a plate for printing. Robert Hooke remains the greatest exponent of such art, the plates in his *Micrographia* of 1665 never having been surpassed. Artists today use many media to capture images, including line (made with pens but perhaps including machine-made sheets of tint and stipple), watercolour and/or oil colours (applied with brushes and perhaps spatulas), air-brush (achieving precise effects of light and shade), scraper-board (giving a positive or negative effect, with or without colour) and some other colour effects obtained with pastels or pencils. Much expertise and 'feel' is required to achieve sometimes stunning results, and the profession of medical artist includes some notable exponents of such work.

All require reproduction, and processes include letterpress (now being superseded), gravure (expensive but exquisite) and lithography (using various media), with a variety of screening techniques to produce apparently continuous tones. Ink-jet systems and dye sublimation systems are also now being developed to a high state of perfection for shorter runs of larger copies of high quality from digitized originals.

3.2 Photographic silver halide imaging

Images may be in monochrome or colour, and chromogenic or not. Traditional methods of black and white photography are still widely used to make prints and slides from negatives, but instant materials also have wide usage. Colour chromogenic systems produce colour output from electronic images, and non-colour chromogenic systems produce instant colour prints and transparencies, while dye bleach materials are noted for their good archival qualities.

3.3 Chemical imaging

This is mainly used to produce end results, rather than capture the immediate image, but is included here for completeness. Photopolymer and resist systems are used mainly for circuit boards and chips, while diazo systems are used in addition for overheads and microfilms. Dye imaging is mainly used for duplicates, and thermal systems for overheads and non-impact printing.

3.4 Electronic imaging

Electronic imaging now plays a great part in capturing the original image in much scientific work, especially with various kinds of microscopes. Medical cathode-ray tube applications, and remote sensing (with infrared and radar wavelengths as well as visible), are also widely used. The result is displayed on the familiar monitor screen, in real time or from tape or diskette or from compact disc (CD)-recorded images. Computer-generated images such as word processors, computer-assisted design/manufacture (CAD/CAM), facsimile and the like, are widespread. The image may be analogue which is then scanned to digitize it, or focused on to a charge-coupled device (CCD) chip, to give a pixel output direct. Once an image is generated or stored in digital form, it is susceptible to manipulation, and more is said of this in Chapter 6. Such images require a further process to produce a hard copy, of course.

3.5 Electrophotographic imaging

Xerographic copying has revolutionized the office, while laser scanning xerography and a variety of electrostatic, dielectric and magnetostatic systems are widely used in non-impact printing.

3.6 Criteria for assessing the behaviour of imaging systems

With new kinds of microscopy and image recording being developed, it is worth considering a variety of assessment criteria before adopting a new system of image recording, or continuing with a previously used system.

(i) Does it image in real time, or is access delayed? If so, by how long? Does this matter for the work in hand?

(ii) What is the sensitivity of the receptor? Does it need a high level of energy input to record detail?

For example, the sensitivity of four systems is summarized here:

System	ISO speed (median)	Exposure required in lux (for lux/sec at 1/60 sec)	Photons/pixel or grain area/cm^2
Photopolymer	0.001	48 000	3×10^{14}
Xerography	1	48	3×10^{11}
Silver halide	100	0.48	3×10^{9}
Electronic	10 000	0.0048	3×10^{7}

(iii) What is its nature? If the equipment is very bulky or very expensive, or requires much cooling or high maintenance, such factors might militate against its adoption in a particular situation.

(iv) What is its wavelength response? Much information can be gained from non-visible parts of the spectrum.

(v) Does the system form a latent image, and if so is it stable?

(vi) How great an amplification does the system yield? Compare with conventional photography, which yields about $\times 10^6$.

(vii) What is the nature of any noise recorded?

(viii) What is the nature of the final image? Is it digitized?

(ix) What is its modulation transfer function? (See Ray, 1994 for a discussion of this measure of optical quality.)

(x) What is the stability of the final image? Does this matter for the purpose in hand?

Answers to many of these criteria are not always easy to obtain. More photographic information is provided by Stroebel *et al.* (1990), and Stroebel and Zakia (1993), while much information on television is offered by Fink and Christiansen (1982). Coote (1993) has a lot to say on the history and technicalities of colour photography, and Hunt (1987) should be consulted for television/photographic reproduction of colour. Camera systems are reviewed by Ray (1983), and optics by the same author (1994). Burden (1973) and Croy (1972) are worth consulting on graphic arts processes.

References

Burden JW. (1973) *Graphic Reproduction Photography*. Focal Press, London.

Coote JH. (1993) *The Illustrated History of Colour Photography*. Fountain Press, London.

Croy P. (1972) *Graphic Design and Reproduction Techniques* (2nd edn). Focal Press, London.

Fink DG, Christiansen D. (eds) (1982) *Electronic Engineers' Handbook* (2nd edn). McGraw-Hill, New York.

Hunt RWG. (1987) *The Reproduction of Colour in Photography, Printing and Television* (4th edn). Fountain Press, Tolworth.

Ray SF. (1983) *Camera Systems*. Focal Press, London.

Ray SF. (1994) *Applied Photographic Optics* (2nd edn). Focal Press, London.

Stroebel L, Compton J, Current I, Zakia R. (1990) *Basic Photographic Materials and Processes*. Focal Press, London.

Stroebel L, Zakia R. (1993) *Focal Encyclopaedia of Photography* (3rd edn). Focal Press, London.

4 Recording the Image Using Graphics Methods

4.1 Introductory remarks

Although drawing a microscopical image was for a long time the only way to record it, only occasionally nowadays will an image be recorded directly using graphics methods. However, such methods still have a considerable part to play in helping to interpret images captured in other ways.

The advantages are considerable, one of the principal ones being that one picture can be synthesized from several images. This may merely allow a greater effective depth of field to be obtained if several image planes are combined, or (given a competent artist) very different pictures are to be combined in one. For example, Paul Peck, a medical artist who specialized in this work, was able to combine a gross view of a vertebra with one derived from a low-power stereo microscope, together with another from an optical section, with electron microscope details added, to form a highly original, harmonious and informative whole. More mundane possibilities include merely omitting confusing details, or emphasizing others, and above all providing a clear carrier for labels. Such drawings are thus vehicles for interpretation as well as for recording.

The main difficulty to be overcome is to obtain accurate outlines in pencil of the whole area to be portrayed. A second stage is to add whatever finer detail is necessary, using higher powers on smaller areas of the whole, in ink. Several methods of obtaining such outlines are available, especially for transmitted-light work. These techniques have much to commend them, as even a beginner who is no artist can produce professional looking results with their aid.

A suitable set of drawing pens is needed, of the Rotring type, capable between them of producing a range of accurate widths of line (see *Figure 4.1*). The pens are held vertically in use, with definite controlled movements (see *Figure 4.2*) – at all costs sketchiness must be avoided in scientific work, for if a drawing becomes a sketch the reader may be deterred from considering the actual content of a picture, due to mere irritation intervening. Lines of definite and consistent width are used to suit and accurately to match definite structures in the original, and to

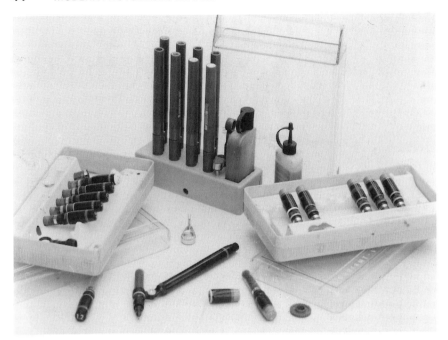

Figure 4.1: A selection of drawing pens.
Two older sets by Rötring are shown, producing between them definite thicknesses of line varying from 0.1 mm to 1.2 mm, and 2 mm to 10 mm. The adapter to keep the pen upright (principally for use with lettering stencils) is included, as is a compass adapter and bottle of ink. A later set by Staedtler is also shown, covering line thicknesses from 0.18 to 1.4 mm.

provide consistent emphasis. All drawings are made larger than the size finally required, by a definite factor to be agreed with the publisher beforehand. This makes a big difference to the final quality as printed (see *Figure 4.3*).

It is highly desirable to make the photomicrograph first, and to have it to hand during the drawing. Not only is this a guide to the amount of detail required, but it does ensure that photomicrograph and drawing have the same orientation! Always leave wide margins round the actual area covered by the drawing itself, to allow for putting in lead lines and labels (which are usually printed and stuck on), as well as an additional width for handling – so that when the drawing is dropped at the printers the bending of its edge will not affect it. General remarks on drawing for publication are offered by Hill (1915), Lamb (1962) and Staniland (1952).

4.2 Inking over a photographic print

A very easy way to obtain accurate outlines of the whole subject is to make a matching *faint* and non-contrasty but still detailed bromide print of the

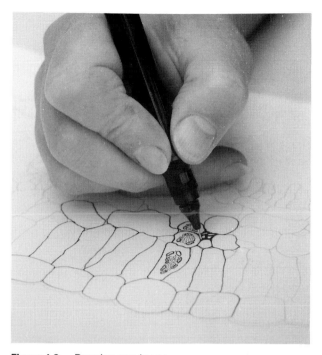

Figure 4.2:   Drawing pen in use.
A drawing outlined in pencil using the drawing tube at lower power is being completed at higher power using a Rötring pen. This is being held less upright than is desirable, just within the limit at which the line thickness would otherwise vary. Photograph made with the kind co-operation of Mrs P.H. Bracegirdle.

final size required, and then ink over the lines in the manner described above using *genuine waterproof indian ink*. The print is allowed to dry for at least 1 h, and then the photographic image is bleached out with one of the standard formulae (Jacobson *et al.*, 1988). Either a negative is used to make the print or, if a large specimen is being recorded, the slide itself is used.

Details can be added or omitted (the title must make this clear), and as much shading, stippling or dotting added as is needed to convey the desired information clearly. For large areas of shading, mechanical tints are available in sheets, to be cut and applied to particular areas; this not only saves much time but looks good in the final publication.

4.3 Using a projection mirror or drawing tube

Pre-World War II, the camera lucida was used to allow the eye at the eyepiece to see also the point of the pencil, to trace accurate outlines; such devices came in several patterns, and that by Abbe was still being sold in

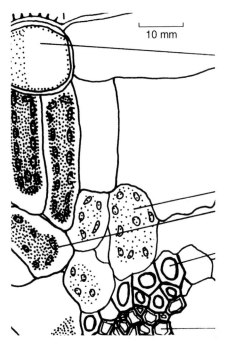

Figure 4.3:   Close view of an original line drawing.
This section of an original drawing made for reproduction by the methods described, shows varying thickness of line, the varying methods of emphasizing detail and the precise termination of lead lines (here shown without their original labels). This photograph is of drawing 102 (TS leaf of *Erica*), from Bracegirdle and Miles (1973) used by kind permission of Mrs P.H. Bracegirdle. (The drawing was made, as usual, at twice its reproduced scale, and this present illustration is shown at twice the reproduced scale.)

the 1960s. A certain experience was needed to make the two images appear to coincide, and some dexterity to arrange the plane of the drawing board to be in line with that of the microscope.

Projection prisms (fitting over the eyepiece) could be used to project the image down on to a sheet of paper, from the horizontal stand, provided there was bright enough illumination, to allow the outlines to be drawn around very simply.

A squared graticule in the eyepiece could be used, in conjunction with squares of suitable size ruled faintly on the paper, to allow for reasonably accurate outlines to be generated by the pencil.

All of these have been superseded by the drawing tube (see *Figure 4.4*). This is a system of lenses and prisms which allows an image of the drawing board/pencil to be seen in the primary image plane in the microscope tube. The relative scales can be varied at will, as can the relative intensities of illumination. All that is needed is to trace whatever outlines are required, and very little skill is required at this stage. The tubes work with all magnifications of objective, and all kinds of illumination and, although they are not cheap, as they are only occasionally in use, one to suit a particular type of stand will be all that will be needed for a whole department.

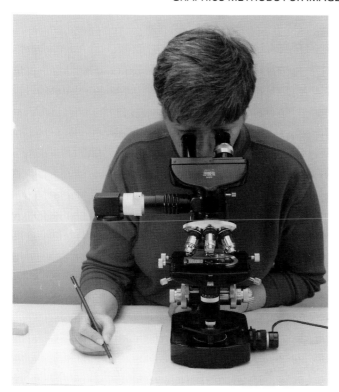

Figure 4.4: Drawing tube in use.
 The Wild drawing tube is shown in use on a Wild M20 microscope. The table lamp shown is given the approximate brightness needed, either by running it through a variable transformer, or by using more or less powerful bulbs in it, and by varying its distance from the paper. The brightness of the field in the microscope is then varied so as to balance the brightness of the image of the pencil point. The size of the pencil image can be varied by the sliding sleeve on the tube, and its sharpness by the collar. Low-power objectives are needed to cover a wide field for outlining in pencil, before filling in the detail with higher powers in ink. Photograph made with the kind co-operation of Mrs P.H. Bracegirdle.

For stereo microscopes, similar attachments are now available, but if one is not available an arm carrying a good quality mirror can be angled well above an eyepiece to project the image on to a card mounted vertically, perhaps on the wall. This is entirely adequate for occasional use.

4.4 Reflected-light drawing for active subjects

Most of the specimens drawn using the camera lucida or drawing tube will be static, and this is a requirement for such work. The system of making a faint print can also apply to flash pictures of active living organisms by reflected light, for example. This is one of only two effective means of securing accurate outlines of such specimens. The other is simply to put the original transparency or negative in the enlarger, and trace the outlines directly on to card on the baseboard. Care must be taken not to overheat the original transparency (especially if it is irreplaceable), but most modern enlargers are relatively cool in use. The transparency is then viewed directly in a hand viewer to add to the outline whatever other details are necessary, and a sequence of transparencies can be used to make a synthesized composite drawing, or one showing several stages of movement, for example.

References

Bracegirdle B and Miles PH. (1973) *An Atlas of Plant Structure*, Volume 2. Heinemann, London.

Hill TG. (1915) *The Essentials of Illustration*. Wesley, London.

Jacobson RE, Ray SF, Attridge GG. (1988) *The Manual of Photography* (8th edn). Focal Press, London.

Lamb L. (1962) *Drawing for Illustration*. Oxford University Press, London.

Staniland LN. (1952) *The Principles of Line Illustration*. Burke, London.

5 Recording the Image in Monochrome

5.1 Black and white photography

Although colour illustrations are far more commonly used in scientific work than was the case only 10 years ago, black and white pictures will probably remain preponderant for some further years. Modern photographic materials are excellent in quality and, although the usual advice in photomicrography has been to find a suitable film and then stick with it, nowadays some experimenting is to be advocated. General advice on photography is provided authoritatively and understandably by Langford (1986), but the specialist photomicrographer will benefit from a knowledge of what is revealed by the characteristic curve for a particular material/developer combination, and of a few other purely photographic matters, so they are discussed here.

5.2 The characteristic curve

Following the receipt of a number of photons by a tiny crystal of silver bromide, the latent image so formed can be developed; this amplifies it about a million times, making tiny threads and clusters of silver metal. The kind of development provided affects the contrast and some other characteristics of the image quite markedly. The response of the emulsion to light may be represented graphically by plotting the optical density of the silver produced on development against the logarithm of the relative exposure. To provide the data, the even exposure of successive parts of the negative is done at constant aperture and intensity, but with a doubling of each successive exposure time, giving a range of perhaps 1024:1, followed by rigorously controlled standardized processing. If the optical density of each area is measured with a transmission densitometer, and the values plotted against log exposure, a characteristic curve is obtained (see *Figure 5.1*). This represents the behaviour of the particular emulsion

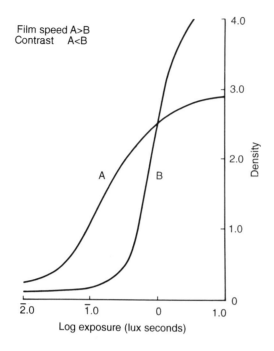

Film speed A>B
Contrast   A<B

A   B

Log exposure (lux seconds)

Density

Figure 5.1:   Characteristic curves.
   The characteristic curve of two different films given the same development. Film A is for general purpose use and has a medium contrast. Film B has a much steeper curve and, with this development, would give a high-contrast negative with restricted grey tones. Film A would be faster than film B and would have more latitude in exposure.

processed in a particular developer at a particular temperature for a particular time. The curve is the shape of a flattened S, with a toe (at low levels of exposure) followed by a straight line portion leading to a shoulder (at the highest levels of exposure).

   Where there has been no exposure at all, there is still some density, which is that of the base itself plus that fog which is produced as the result of the developer making some silver even from grains not having a latent image. If this base + fog level is higher than a small minimum, it indicates that stale film, or too energetic a developer, or fogged film, or too high a developing temperature, or more than one of these, have affected the result.

   The slope of the curve ('gamma') indicates the contrast of the negative, and this is one of the most important factors to be considered in choosing a film for a particular purpose. The development given exerts an effect on contrast, although the main determinant of contrast is the nature of the emulsion as formulated by the maker. The greater the contrast, the smaller the number of grey tones produced. When exposing the negative, the darkest shadow area of the original should be put deliberately on the straight line part of the curve, just above the toe. This allows the tones to be recorded accurately, whereas if this tone was on the toe (underexposed) or on the shoulder (overexposed), details would be lost. Such a placing for photomicrography is determined by actual calibration of the equipment with a particular film/developer combination, as described below (Section 5.6).

5.3 Contrast index

An alternative measure of the contrast is the concept of contrast index (CI), which is the slope of a line joining a point on the characteristic curve where the image density exceeds the base fog level by 0.1 or 0.2 density units, to a point on the curve at a density of 2 units above the lower level (see *Figure 5.2*). This concept mirrors more closely than gamma the behaviour of a film in actual use. The main point to understand about either is that modifying the development modifies the contrast, and this is most useful in photomicrography (see Section 5.6). The concept is further explored in the very useful Kodak publication F-5 (Anon., 1990).

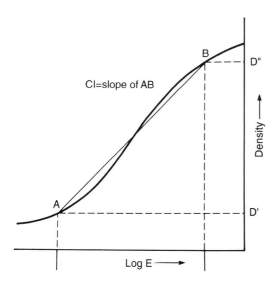

Figure 5.2: The definition of contrast index.
The characteristic curve of a film to show the concept of contrast index (CI). CI is the average value of the slope of that part of the curve between point A (0.2 density units above base fog) and point B which is 2.0 density units higher than A. The ordinate of the plot represents optical density, whilst the abscissa is the log (relative) exposure. Curves redrawn from Thomson and Bradbury (1987) with permission from the Royal Microscopical Society.

5.4 Sensitivity of emulsions

The sensitivity, or spectral response, of films is also a matter of great importance in scientific work. All basic photographic emulsions are blue sensitive, and have long been described as 'ordinary' if this is so. Their response to ultraviolet and blue extends to about 500 nm (and can thus be processed in an amber safelight); the older photographic papers had emulsions of this kind, and, as they are often of inherently high contrast, negatives having ordinary emulsions are sometimes used in metallographic work, where the specimens lack colour and contrast.

Where dyes are added to the emulsion to make it respond as far as yellow (to about 600 nm), the emulsion is described as orthochromatic. These can be processed in a red safelight, and usually offer inherent high contrast. In photomicrography, such an emulsion will greatly enhance the contrast of small red features in a mainly blue or green specimen.

Further dyes will extend the sensitivity to about 680 nm, giving panchromatic emulsions sensitive to all visible light (as well as the ultraviolet). These need total darkness for their handling, and some of them have an exaggerated red sensitivity, giving them apparent extra speed in artificial light. This can have the effect of giving a blue contrast filter a very high factor in photomicrography! (see *Figure 5.3*).

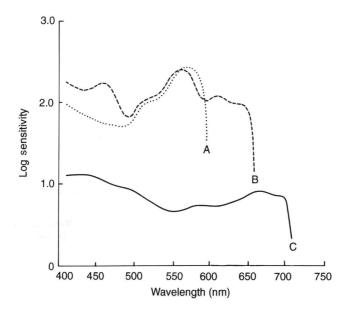

Figure 5.3: Spectral response curves.
   The spectral response curves of orthochromatic, panchromatic and extended-red sensitive emulsions (A,B and C, respectively). The height of the curve at any point gives an indication of the relative sensitivity of the film at that wavelength.

Emulsions can also be made sensitive to infrared (but often only to about 850 nm). Special precautions have to be taken in using such films (see Section 5.7), and they are expensive.

5.5 Film speed

Emulsions vary widely in the amount of exposure required to produce a negative of the same density from the same scene. Films requiring less exposure are said to be faster, and a speed is usually given by the manufacturer, either as an ASA speed (American Standards Association) or, more recently, as an ISO speed (International Organization for Standardization). The two are identical in practice, both being arithmetical systems, so that an increase of one stop is indicated by a doubling of the quoted speed. The extremes of the speeds range are between about ISO6 and about ISO2000 nowadays, but it is essential to calibrate one's own equipment and procedures to establish one particular speed known to be correct for a particular film (see Section 7.3).

5.6 Practical choice of films

Once a proper image has been formed in the image plane, as set out in Chapter 2, for almost all work in monochrome, using both transmitted and reflected illumination and various contrast techniques with the microscope, only two films (Kodak T-Max 100 and Kodak Technical Pan) used with two developers (Kodak HC-110 and any PQ Universal) will record most subjects. These recommendations are based on the authors' own specific trials, of course, but many other products are available for those interested in conducting their own experiments for particular jobs.

A few subjects, often in materials work, require higher contrast, and are satisfactorily dealt with by Agfa Ortho 25 film in the PQ developer. The two Kodak films with the two developers provide six distinct and repeatable contrast indexes. The intention is to provide a negative which will print on normal contrast paper, and this is important. If a negative was to print only on an extreme-grade paper, there would be no leeway in producing a proper range of tones, and the negative itself would be a poor one. A poor negative cannot produce a good print, and is not acceptable for communication in science.

Where reflected-light work is undertaken, strong contrasts are often produced by the lighting employed, and a trial should be made with a CI of about 0.5 or 0.7. For transmitted-light work with subjects of high inherent contrast, such as preparations viewed by dark ground, a CI of 0.7 or 1.0 may prove correct to contain the range of tones.

For stained histological slides, an index of 1.5 will usually be suitable, unless contrast filters are in use, when 1.0 might be preferable. Phase contrast and differential interference contrast (DIC) work is also suited by an index of 1.0. For flash photographs of living organisms, an index of 2.0 might be best and, for reflected-light photomicrographs of low-contrast specimens such as polished metal surfaces, an index of 2.5 is often right.

This is summarized in *Table 5.1*, where the speed quoted is the *starting point for calibration of the equipment with trial exposures* (see Section 7.3 – calibration).

Table 5.1:   Variable contrast indexes

Contrast index	Film	Developer at 20°C	Development time (min)	Speed (ISO)
0.5	T-Max 100	HC-110 (B)	7	80
0.7	T-Max 100	HC-110 (B)	11	100
1.0	Tech.Pan	HC-110 (F)	13	64
1.5	Tech.Pan	HC-110 (D)	6	100
2.0	Tech.Pan	HC-110 (B)	10	150
2.5	Tech.Pan	PQ Univ (1:6)	3	150

The films are available in 35 mm, roll and sheet sizes (but Technical Pan films have different type numbers according to their size). Kodak HC-110 developer is sold in two sizes; the larger is much more viscous and in consequence less easy to use. The bottles give instructions on making up the various lettered strengths; those in *Table 5.1* are dilutions B, D and F only. Any PQ universal paper developer may be used with Technical Pan films but, if used with T-Max 100, high fog levels and staining are produced, and thus this combination is not recommended. (See *Figures 5.4* and *5.5*.)

Where still higher contrast is occasionally required, Agfa Ortho 25 (actually intended for copying line drawings) is used with any PQ universal paper developer, 1:6 at 20°C for 3 min, to give a CI of 3.2 and a starting speed for calibration of ISO20.

When only part of a bottle of monochrome or colour developer has been used, the rest can be preserved for a long time by squirting into it a generous blast of a dust-off aerosol, with the tube close to the surface of the liquid, before replacing the cap. This displaces the air and minimizes later oxidation.

When processing films, the authors use continuous agitation in a rotating tube processor (the Jobo; see Tinsley, 1992); all are treated alike and thus results are comparable between films. If a rotary processor is not available, and ordinary tank development is used, the agitation is, of course, done by inverting the tank. The authors recommend continuous inversion for the first 30 sec of the developing time, and then six separate

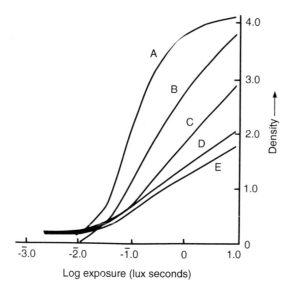

Figure 5.4: Characteristic curves of a film.
 Characteristic curves of the same film (Kodak Technical Pan 2415) after differing developments showing the differing values of contrast index (CI) which are possible following
different development procedures. (A) developed in PQ Univ, 1:6, 3 min, CI = 2.5; (B)
developed in HC110 (dilution D) 8 min, CI = 2.0; (C) developed in HC110 (dilution D) 6 min;
(D) developed in Technidol liquid developer 11 min, CI = 1.0; (E) developed in Technidol
liquid developer 7 min, CI = 0.5.

double inversions during each minute thereafter. This schedule must be
adhered to rigorously, and this is important whatever procedure is used.
Do *not* be tempted to exceed the stated processing temperature. Do *not* be
tempted to exceed the stated processing time. Do *not* make up the
developer in a more concentrated form than that stated. What is needed
to control contrast is accuracy and repeatability in processing. Use an acid
stop bath with plenty of agitation, and fix thoroughly in a *fresh* hardening
rapid fixer with plenty of inversion before inspecting. After washing, which
need not be unduly prolonged, add a *tiny* amount of rinse agent to the final
wash water in the tank, shake off excess water with the film still in the
reel, and hang up to dry without squeegeeing.

5.7 UV and infrared monochrome films

Ultraviolet sensitivity is universal in silver halide emulsions, and thus the
film can be chosen to provide the contrast required. The source must

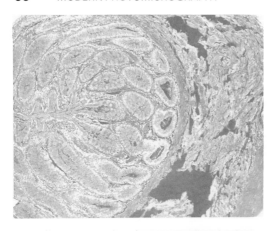

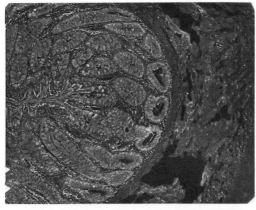

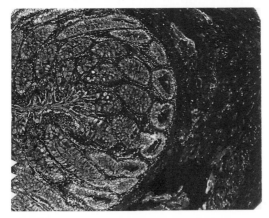

Figure 5.5: Negatives of contrast indexes 0.5, 1.5 and 2.5.
Three camera-original 4 × 5 in negatives are reproduced, produced with the specified contrast indexes, as described in the text, of a histological section. The negative with one notch has a CI of = 0.5, that with two notches has a CI of = 1.5, whilst three notches is of CI = 2.5. The ability to provide repeatable contrast indexes, precisely to suit the nature of the subject, is a vital part of modern photomicrography. That of index 1.5 is correct for a stained section.

provide plenty of the required wavelengths (which cannot be very short if glass lenses are in use). Focusing through a deep blue filter is usual, to minimize differences in focus between visible and UV. Processing is normal, but exposure trials are recommended compared with white light use, as many emulsions have an exaggerated red response, and may well appear slow to the blue in consequence.

Infrared films must be specially purchased, from a limited range. In 35 mm and in 4×5 sheet-film, Kodak High-Speed Infrared emulsion is available; in roll-film only Konica 750 nm. Both are noticeably more expensive than ordinary monochrome films, and both should be stored in a freezer to maintain their infrared sensitivity. Basic exposure indexes are ISO64 for the Kodak films, and ISO25 for the Konica, when processed in HC-110 (B) for 7 min at 20°C. Use of a powerful tungsten–halogen source run at full voltage is recommended to ensure the presence of enough longer wavelengths in the illumination. The exposure is measured in white light, then a deep red filter is inserted for focusing, and then a visually opaque red filter for the actual exposure, to cut out all the shorter wavelengths to some of which the emulsion is also sensitive. Thus the image is formed from the infrared only, with sharpness of focus. Initial calibration for exposure is, of course, a vital requirement. See Kodak publication M-28 (Anon, 1977) for further details of infrared work.

5.8 Instant films for monochrome work

Polaroid make a wide range of monochrome films for various cameras, including their SLR66 (see Section 2.6). For large format, their type 65 provides medium contrast and a permanent negative as well as an instant print, but it does require compensation to its nominal speed for exposure times longer than 1 sec. For 35 mm cameras, using a dedicated Polaroid Autoprocessor, Polapan CT has similar uses. The financial penalty of using such instant materials may be justified by instant access, especially when recording difficult reflected-light subjects.

5.9 Darkroom work in monochrome

The darkroom is often the weak link in the photographic chain. No matter how good the microscope, how skilled its operator, and perfect the specimen, much is often lost in processing the negative and making the print.

Darkroom equipment is often outmoded, while technique may have become sloppy, and chemicals be chronically overused. If this is indeed the case, the result is to throw away all the work which has gone into obtaining the image, and also to fail effectively to communicate at the end of the whole process.

The basic division in the darkroom as between the wet bench and the dry, should be rigorously maintained. It must be a matter of personal technique always to rinse and dry the fingers when leaving the wet bench to return to the dry, and this avoids many stains and spoiled results. The wet bench is a sink of ample size, set at a height at which the operator can lean on its edge while manipulating its contents, thus avoiding much backache and fatigue; the back and sides should have built-in splash guards. Much could be said of personal technique in the darkroom, but it is not peculiar to photomicrography, and it must suffice here to say that there is no substitute for a year or more spent in a well-run busy commercial darkroom to learn all the many tricks of the trade and to acquire a rigorous approach while learning to recognize a good print and to have the confidence to reject poor ones. (Some details of darkroom work in monochrome are given by Coote, 1982.)

It is well to avoid mixing chemicals in the darkroom, especially if they are in powder form. The dust which inevitably escapes cannot all be swept up even if an occasional attempt is made, and *will* affect negatives and prints in due course.

Proper processing equipment is an individual choice, but the weak link is usually the enlarger, and especially its lenses. In the dark, such equipment is rarely carefully inspected for wear and tear, even if it was good enough when new. It is manifestly pointless to buy an expensive microscope and camera, and a cheap enlarger and lens. The authors use Durst enlargers and El-Nikkor lenses in all formats from 35 mm to half-plate, and the considerable outlay has proved well spent. The use of exposure aids can be recommended, as they save materials of value greater than their cost in the longer run, as well as much time should it be an unfamiliar subject being printed. Proper safelighting is also necessary; that is safelighting of ample intensity but proven safety relative to the emulsions exposed to it. It is elementary, if infrared materials are in use, to check the darkroom for infrared safety on a bright sunny day, and not a dull one in winter.

The enlarger and all its surfaces should be kept clean with a dust-off aerosol applied frequently, while a suitable paper handkerchief lightly wetted with isopropanol should be used to wipe negative carriers (and spectacles) and the like, to leave them clean and static-free.

A white light used for inspecting prints should be well shaded, with its switch high on the wall and set sideways; it may be marked with a piece of luminous tape. The proper quality of a final print is judged only after much experience, and in the light of its intended use. If it is being made for a particular printer, he should be shown an early specimen for depth and range of tones before the whole series is made. A large number of poor half-tones still appears in the literature; they cost just as much as good ones, and detract from the quality of the author's text into the bargain. What is usually needed is fairly high contrast but without the blacks being totally dense (see also Chapter 8).

5.10 Silver halide motion pictures in monochrome

Relatively little such work is now undertaken, but if it is necessary there is a fairly wide range of emulsions still available in 35 mm and in 16 mm formats. Processing to negative and the subsequent printing is usually carried out by specialist laboratories, at some expense. The advantage of conventional motion pictures is their ability to alter the time dimension, by shooting faster than the projection speed (high-speed cine, to slow down rapid motion, perhaps for analysis), or slower than projection speed (time-lapse, to speed up very slow movements). Such use still produces very much better quality than the equivalent techniques in video.

5.11 Monochrome video recording

This is now easy and cheap to carry out, with the great advantages of instant replay and the ability to operate at much lower light levels than those required by silver halide systems. The camera equipment nowadays is small in size and light in weight, both being considerable advantages; many closed-circuit TV (CCTV) cameras are smaller than a 35 mm camera, and can be added to a suitable port with little difficulty, as they require no extra support. The professional models with C-mount lenses are the only ones seriously to be considered, as addition to the microscope of a suitable relay lens (a coated negative achromatic doublet of correct focal length) makes placing the image on the sensor very easy. For experimental purposes, ex-security cameras are suitable, although perhaps larger, and can be obtained very cheaply. Surprisingly little intensity of illumination is usually required for the microscope system, and setting up is made easy by viewing the results in real time on the monitor. Of course, the microscope is adjusted for the normal visual focus, and then the relay lens adjusted to place the image in sharp focus (see Chapter 1). Such records will normally be in analogue form with older equipment, giving the usual playback quality from the usual video cassette recorders.

More modern (and more expensive) equipment may record the image in digitized form using a CCD chip, although this is usually restricted to colour systems. The results appear the same on replay, but such images can be manipulated electronically, stored on disc and can also be transmitted electronically, instantly and without loss of quality (see also Chapter 5).

References

Anon. (1977) *Applied Infrared Photography*. Kodak Publication M-28, Rochester, NY.
Anon. (1990) *Professional Black-and-White Films*. Kodak Publication F-5, Rochester, NY
Coote JH. (1982) *Monochrome Darkroom Practice*. Focal Press, London.
Langford M. (1986) *Basic Photography* (5th edn). Focal Press, London.
Thomson DJ. and Bradbury S. (1987) *An Introduction to Photomicrography* (RMS Handbook no. 13). Oxford University Press, Oxford.
Tinsley J. (1992) *The Rotary Processor Manual*. R. Morgan, Chislehurst.

6 Recording the Image in Colour

For recording in colour, much the same considerations apply as to monochrome, but with two important differences. The first is that the colour temperature of the film must match that of the source, and the second is that contrast can be controlled to only a small extent. Elementary points, such as using neutral density filters and not a voltage control to vary the intensity of a lamp, must be taken for granted in colour work. Despite these points, working with colour transparency materials is often easier in practice than with monochrome, for they have the high inherent contrast needed for most photomicrography. Modern tungsten materials are a good match for tungsten–halogen sources (although ordinary tungsten sources require filtering), while daylight materials match electronic flash perfectly. If both monochrome and colour originals are required, it is rarely completely satisfactory, as well as being rather tedious, to try to make monochrome copies from colour transparencies. The authors strongly advise making two separate exposures from the original once set up, one on each type of film, even though this may mean having two different 35 mm camera backs in use. General remarks on colour photography are provided by Langford (1989), but the effects of reciprocity failure must be mentioned here.

6.1 Reciprocity failure

In general, doubling the exposure time requires a lens aperture one stop smaller to maintain correct exposure of the film. This reciprocal relationship, in fact, works only for exposures of moderate lengths of time; very long or very short exposures exert less than the expected effects, and this is a function of the duration of exposure only. When using flash, which may be controlled by the light reflected off-the-film (OTF) and quenched well before its full normal duration has been reached, a very short exposure time (perhaps 1/2500 sec) may be given to the film, which will not, as a consequence, be exposed as fully as was intended. Similarly, if long exposures (say, 5 sec or more) have to be given with low levels of illumination, the same effect may be produced. As the exposure time becomes even shorter or even longer, so the effect becomes more pronounced; this is reciprocity failure. In monochrome work this is serious enough, leading to under-exposed negatives, but it may be compensated for by using a wider aperture or greater intensity or a much longer exposure time, than that calculated as correct. Each film has different reciprocity failure characteristics, which are noted on the sheet packed with it; it is quite usual for failure to commence at durations of only a few seconds. With colour materials, which are essentially three different films coated on top of each other, the reciprocity failure thresholds and characteristics might well differ between each layer (see *Figure 6.1*). In normal conditions, the three characteristic curves lie parallel but, for very long or very short exposures, they may cross over (see *Figure 6.2*). This introduces a colour cast which is impossible to remove, and is one reason why tungsten-balanced materials are made to have longer exposure times than daylight-balanced films.

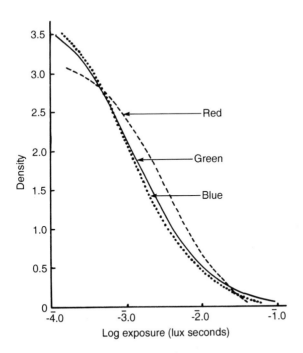

Figure 6.1:   Characteristic curves of colour reversal material.
   This diagram shows the characteristic curves of the the three emulsions in the coating of a processed reversal colour film emulsion. Note that for the majority of their length the curves for the red, green and blue emulsions run alongside one another (i.e. the image would appear visually neutral).

6.2 Colour transparency work

As with monochrome materials, the authors have tested and calibrated for their own purposes a range of films from several manufacturers. Others should try their own experiments with the large number of emulsions available, taking into account that the range of films tends to vary rapidly these days, as makers often produce special products suited to particular commercial needs. All must be matched fairly closely to the colour temperature of the source in use and, although these are restricted in range in modern microscopy, some further consideration of this is required.

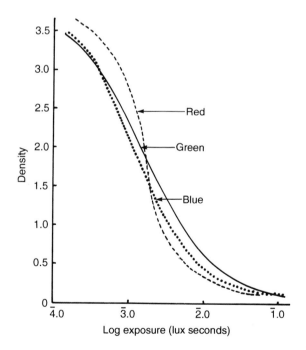

Figure 6.2:   Characteristic curves of colour reversal material.
  Here the curves representing the three spectral colours 'cross'. The curve for the red image is significantly higher in the shoulder region of the curve than those for the other colours and crosses them so that at the toe of the curve it lies below the other two. The image thus would not be neutral. The shadows would appear to have a cyan cast (since the red curve is here above the other two) but the highlights would have a reddish tinge (the red curve here is below the other two).

6.3 Colour temperature

Colour temperature is a measure of the blueness or redness of a source, with its theoretical basis in its equivalence to that radiation emitted by a physicist's black body raised to a particular temperature, measured in kelvins. The higher the temperature, the bluer the light. In photographic practice, the main actual use of this concept is to allow sources to be balanced among themselves, and also to be matched to a particular emulsion. For this reason, the values are given not in degrees above absolute zero, but as mireds (micro-reciprocal degrees, where 10 000 K = 100 mireds, 4000 K = 250 mireds, 2500 K = 400 mireds, and so on). Filters using such values have a constant effect on the blueness or redness of a source. *Figure 6.3* shows, for example, that a 6 V tungsten lamp has to be run at no less than 9 V to raise its colour temperature to match a tungsten-balanced colour emulsion, while the same effect could be obtained (with much longer lamp life and production of much less heat) by using a bluish 50 mired colour-balancing filter in front of the lamp.

Various makes of colour-balancing filters with definite mired values are made by several companies, in gelatin, resin or glass; all are widely available and interchangeable. Brownish filters (to lower the colour temperature) might have a plus sign in front of their value, while bluish ones (to increase the colour temperature) might have a minus sign. In general, it is best practice to choose an emulsion for a particular job which needs either no filtration, or the least possible. It is possible to use very dense colour-balancing filters to allow a tungsten-balanced film to be used in daylight, and vice versa; this is rarely satisfactory (it seems often to introduce a colour cast). If used for long periods of time with intense sources, it is sensible to check especially the less dense colour-balancing filters for freedom from fading, perhaps by simple comparison with a new one of the same value.

6.4 Choice and processing of colour transparency films

The authors recommend, from their own personal experience, films such as Kodak Ektachrome 64 (available in 35 mm, roll and sheet formats) for flash; it gives sharp images in use and has a calibration starting film speed of ISO64. When slightly more speed is required with flash (as in reflected-light work), Kodak Ektachrome 100 Plus (in the same formats) has excellent colour saturation, and a calibration starting point of ISO100. For

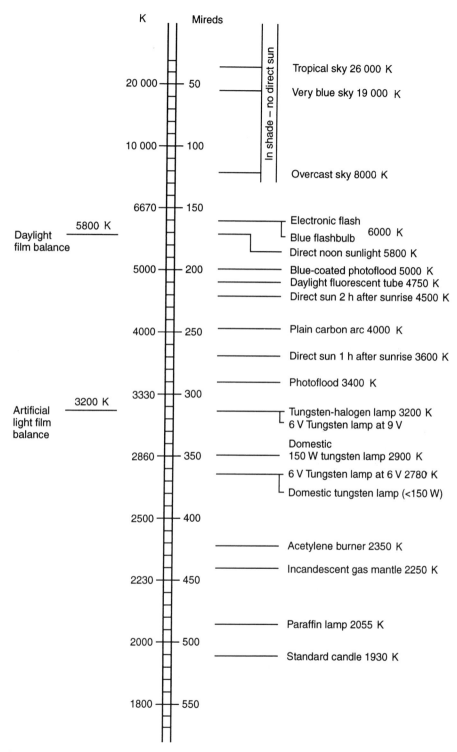

Figure 6.3: Mired values.
A diagram showing the mired values of some common light sources.

tungsten sources, Kodak Ektachrome 64T and Ektachrome 160T have proved satisfactory; both are available in the same formats already described, and have calibration starting points of ISO64 and ISO160 respectively. Fujichrome 64T is another excellent tungsten emulsion, in sheet- and roll-film sizes and 35 mm, with a calibration starting point of ISO64.

In processing these films, either the E6 process is used, or a more modern modification using fewer baths. When necessary, all of the above can be push-processed to double their effective speeds with very little loss of quality, but very careful control of temperature is required for accurate and repeatable processing. The authors use Chrome Six one-shot chemicals supplied by Photo Technology Ltd in Jobo processors (Tinsley, 1992), to achieve excellent results consistently. The process is rapid in use, and costs much less for the chemicals used than the cost of sending a film to be processed in a laboratory, with the additional advantage that the results of a shot which may have been especially difficult to set up are seen within an hour. Colour transparencies of transmitted-light originals can be evaluated very easily once thoroughly dry, as the background should be one shade of density darker than pure transparent, and without colour cast of any kind.

If transparencies must be trade-processed, it may be found that a wide variation in results occurs between some trade laboratories, and also within a particular laboratory over time. In this context it may be worth reporting that the Agfa processing centre will accept all makes of E6, and that the authors have found their work impeccable over many years. All that is needed is to buy a pre-paid envelope from a dealer and send off the 120 or 35 mm film in it by post (Agfachrome Service, see Appendix).

6.5 Colour prints from colour transparencies

It is not difficult to make Ilfochrome (original name Cibachrome) prints from colour transparencies, especially if they happen to be transmitted-light photomicrographs (Anon., 1987). Such a transparency is *known* to be satisfactory from simple inspection when it is being chosen for printing, by its mere appearance to the eye. The process requires very little filtration in the enlarger, beyond that specified on the initial pack for the particular batch of paper in use. Ilford supply sets of chemicals, and the processing is not too demanding. The resulting print is easy to evaluate (when fully dry); it must have a cast-free background one shade darker than pure white. A daylight-blue spotlamp (of the kind widely sold in embroidery shops) ceiling-mounted in a fitting with integral switch is ideal for evaluating such prints in uniform conditions. Similar prints on a transparent base can be made for back-lighting for display, and the results (using the dye–bleach process) are much more light-fast than other colour prints. If it is necessary to have Ilfochrome prints of photomicrographs made commercially (and the service is widely and nowadays relatively inexpensively available), there can be no argument possible on delivery as to their correctness, of course!

6.6 Colour negative films

Although many photographers may use colour negative films such as Kodak Gold 200 for casual holiday snaps, and more than 90% of films sold worldwide are of this kind, their use in photomicrography is unusual. Perhaps multiple copies of a micrograph may be required for illustrating an internal report, and in such a case the quality will be adequate, but such prints are not suitable as originals for illustrating books and papers. If used, colour negative films require generous exposure in all circumstances (even for holiday snaps); at least half a stop more exposure should be given than the nominal speed of the film would suggest. In photomicrographic work, of course, proper calibration will have been carried out in advance to provide an acceptable speed value for the equipment in use.

If a tungsten source is used with an ordinary colour negative film, a daylight-blue correcting filter should always be interposed, as it will make the final selection of the filter pack for printing very much easier. If this kind of work is done very often, a film balanced for longer exposures (rather than the usual shorter) should be selected; Fujicolour 160L has proved very suited to such work, as it avoids any difficulties with reciprocity failure with exposures in the >1 sec range. It should be noted that this has nothing to do with considerations of colour temperature as such, which needs correcting for separately, as already mentioned.

Printing colour negative films is slightly more difficult than printing positive films, in that choice of filter pack and exposure time are less obvious. Some aid to negative evaluation is helpful, and there are many to choose from, and the actual processing can be carried out in a variety of machines. For small-scale use, the Jobo has proved excellent in the hands of the present authors, used with the Photocolor FP two-bath kits supplied by Photo Technology Ltd, which processes both C41 and RA4 materials very successfully. General remarks on darkroom work are offered by Ray and Taylor (1985).

6.7 Infrared colour films

Kodak produce a 35 mm infrared colour film (Ektachrome Infrared Film Type 2236), in 36-exposure cassettes, which has occasional application in photomicrography. The emulsion is also available (but only in large quantity) as 70 mm Aerochrome Infrared Type 2443 film (intended for aerial photography, especially for detecting camouflage). The emulsion is processed, unfortunately, in E4 chemicals, rarely called for (although there are a few commercial laboratories which will process this film, and a kit called Speedibrews E-4 is available from Silver Print Ltd, see Appendix). The film produces 'false-colour' results, having an infrared-sensitive, cyan image-forming layer instead of the usual blue-sensitive layer. There is no yellow filter layer in this daylight-balanced film, and thus a yellow filter must be used somewhere in the system, in front of the film. It has about twice the effective speed of Kodak High-speed infrared film, but equipment and lighting must be calibrated for speeds and also to determine the colour translation of the particular subjects being recorded. It is essential to store this film at a temperature no higher than $-20°C$, to avoid loss of infrared sensitivity. The film produces interesting results obtainable in no other way, the usual stained sections revealing sometimes surprising details, especially if metallic impregnation procedures have been applied. See Kodak Publication M-28 (Anon., 1977) for further details.

6.8 Instant films for colour work

Polaroid supply several colour print instant films, including Polacolor 64 Tungsten which may be of interest in some photomicrography, as it gives rich and saturated colours with exposures in the range of 2–8 sec. Their Polachrome CS and HC films are quick-access 35 mm reversal films (daylight-balanced), intended specifically for projection, and thus valuable for preparing lecture material in small quantities at short notice. The HC version, having more contrast, is usually best for transmitted-light micrographs.

6.9 Recording motion: analogue colour movie films

The application of the cine camera loaded with colour film to the microscope still thrives. Even in 35 mm format the cost still compares favourably with broadcast-quality CCTV recording, and the relatively easy availability of time-lapse and slow-motion techniques with cine is a further powerful argument in its favour. Most of the technique of using the camera (see Baddeley, 1979; Reisz and Miller, 1994) is secondary to setting up the microscope and choice of specimen, and the actual coupling and use of a reflex cine camera of 16 mm or 35 mm format (C-mount, but lensless or with a purpose-made relay lens) is easy. No other type would be considered by the professional but, if needs must, any ordinary 16 mm or even 8 mm camera could be used with its (fixed) lens in apposition to the microscope eyepiece, with alignment by simple inspection.

Use of really heavy stands is an initial requirement, with avoidance of vibration and rigorous setting up. A good range of film stock is available to cover most requirements, and many processing houses provide excellent service. Much of the success of motion picture work resides in the final editing, and a ratio of 10:1 between film shot and that used is excellent. Some modification of the final image is possible, but tedious, and the medium is essentially for straightforward scientific recording.

6.10 Recording motion: analogue video recording

Many large modern microscopes have video ports built in (perhaps for use simultaneously with various formats of film), but attaching modern colour video cameras to less advanced or older stands is not difficult (*Figure 6.4*). Video cameras fitted with C-mount lenses are fitted directly, and without lens of course, with a projection eyepiece with (negative) relay lens if required to focus the image on the sensor in the usual way. Modern cameras are light enough to require no separate stand. If an older photomicrographic apparatus with bellows is in use, a darkslide can easily be modified to carry a C-mount adapter to carry the video camera; a shorter than usual extension will be required, but the apparatus is easy to set up.

For cameras (including camcorders) with fixed lenses (which may be very sophisticated models otherwise) attachment is less straightforward but still possible. The camera will have to be supported independently over the microscope, with its lens set at longest focus and infinity. Instead of

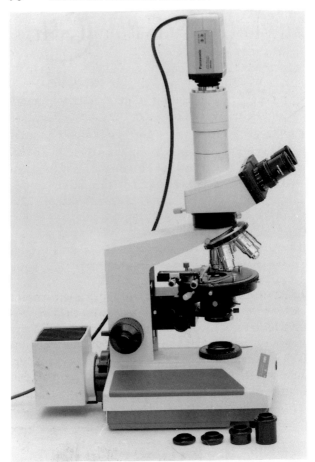

Figure 6.4:   CCTV camera on microscope stand.
A modern Olympus BHS stand is fitted with the trinocular head, which carries a Panasonic CCTV camera. This small camera has the usual C-mount lens threads, and the adapter shown below it carries a negative relay lens to put the image from the projection eyepiece on to the sensor. Four different powers of eyepiece are available and, in addition, the C-mount extension tubes shown in the plate can be interposed to provide effectively higher magnifications – but with some loss of quality at higher powers if the microscope is defocused to put the image on to the sensor at a greater extension.

the eyepiece of the microscope, an extension tube (carrying a large-diameter projection lens) of such length that it projects an image to infinity (determined by experiment) is used. The microscope is set up with its eyepiece in the normal way, eyepiece removed, and projection lens attached below the camera, leaving a gap of about 20 mm. This gap is then adjusted to focus the image, by inspection of the monitor, when the various zoom settings can be used to place more or less of the whole image circle on the screen (Thomson, 1991).

The results are usually of good quality, and are produced in real time with cheap and easy recording on any domestic-type video cassette recorder (or more sophisticated versions of course), giving instant replay. Contrast is dramatically increased at will, low levels of illumination only are required and images from wavelengths not normally visible are easily recorded. Such attributes have been of particular interest to those recording the behaviour of small and active organisms with the microscope. [The standard basic text is Inoué (1986) and an introduction to modern video in general is provided by Cheshire (1990).]

6.11 Recording motion: digital video recording

As opposed to storage of analogue video signals, the much more recent advent of digitized images, however generated, allows them to be stored and retrieved without degradation, to be manipulated in ways which are astonishing and to be transmitted instantly at the speed of light also without degradation. Larish (1991) provides a survey of digital imaging, and a note of some of the possibilities is all that can usefully be provided in this present volume, with a word of caution appended on the use of image manipulation in scientific work. No descriptions of hardware and software are included, as their design and availability currently change almost on a weekly basis.

The actual use of a digital video camera is entirely the same as that of an analogue video camera: it is simply attached to a suitable port and switched on. An existing photomicrograph, print or transparency, colour or monochrome, can also be scanned into digitized storage in binary form. The equipment for recording digital images is still expensive (although built in to some modern electron microscopes and the like), and the sampling intervals (the resolution) vary: the higher the d.p.i. (dots per inch) the more the quality begins to compare with normal film. The signals are recorded on WORM (write once, read many) discs, and equipment for amateur level digitally stored picture making is already a consumer product. The professional standard is somewhat higher, and produces files as large as 100 megabytes from formats as large as 4×5 in.

The stored image, a series of points (picture-elements or pixels), shows on screen as a series of tiny squares filled with one hue of colour or one shade of grey. Once captured in this way, the picture can be copied electronically and transferred instantly by wire or satellite with no loss of quality. More importantly, it can be enhanced, or cleaned up, or modified, entirely without detection, until it resembles the original only slightly or not at all. All this is accomplished at the computer screen, and needs skill and purpose on the part of the operator. In a non-scientific situation, artistic ability of a high order can produce quite stunning images, perhaps seamlessly put together from several sources. Once the desired image is obtained, it is output to a suitable printer, some of which can produce dye-sublimation A0 prints of superb quality.

In the scientific context, digitized images generated, for example, by the most modern electron microscope may hardly ever be printed in the normal way, but stored for future comparison and used as required and entirely without degradation. It has long been the case in this context that such stored images have been analysed (at some considerable expense) to extract data rapidly and accurately; image analysis is a very important development in scientific work, with established procedures (Bradbury, 1987; Russ, 1990). Now that image manipulation (a very different matter) is also becoming established, with processing platforms possessing very powerful and sophisticated software, and hard-copy output devices producing superb results, those supplying scientific photographs which have been digitized at any stage will, in the future, have to declare exactly how and to what extent the final image has been manipulated – whether only reduced signal-to-noise ratio, or enhanced colour, or rather more.

References

Anon. (1977) *Applied Infrared Photography*. Kodak Publication M-28, Rochester, NY.

Anon. (1987) *Ilford Cibachrome-A*. Ilford, London.

Baddeley WH. (1979) *The Technique of Documentary Film Production*. Focal Press, London.

Bradbury S. (1987) Processing and analysis of the microscope image. *Quekett J. Microsc.* **36**, 23–39.

Cheshire D. (1990) *The Complete Book of Video*. Doring Kindersley, London.

Inoué S. (1986) *Video Microscopy*. Plenum Press, New York.

Langford M. (1989) *Advanced Photography*. Focal Press, London.

Larish, J. (1992) *Digital Photography: Pictures of Tomorrow*. Micro Publishing Press, Torrance.

Ray SF, Taylor J. (1985) *Photographic Enlarging in Practice*. David & Charles, Newton Abbot.

Reisz K, Millar G. (1994) *The Technique of Film Editing*. Focal Press, London.

Russ JC. (1990) *Computer-assisted Microscopy*. Plenum Press, New York.

Thomson DJ. (1991) Video microscopy using a TV camera fitted with a zoom lens. *Microsc. Bull. Newslett. Quekett Microsc. Club* **17**, 12–13.

Tinsley J. (1992) *The Rotary Processor Manual*. R. Morgan, Chislehurst.

7 Special Problems and Techniques

7.1 Exposure determination

In the older days of photomicrography, with long horizontal cameras to accommodate objectives often used without eyepieces, and with intensities of illumination which might be low, exposures were often measured in tens of minutes, were estimated on the basis of long experience with particular objectives and were checked immediately afterwards, as it was the norm to develop the plate in a dish as soon as the exposure was completed. This method undoubtedly worked, especially as the image was inspected as it appeared, and 1 or 2 minutes less or more in the exposure time would not be critical.

With more modern equipment, using shorter bellows lengths (or the equivalent) and much brighter illumination, the duration of exposure is not often more than a few seconds at most, and shorter durations require more precise control, which requires more precise estimation of exposure. For those using equipment made up from separate camera and microscope, a range of exposure-estimating devices is available and will be considered first. Those with fully automated equipment will be considered second and, for both groups, the overriding importance of initial calibration will be stressed.

Of course, if equipment using integrated exposure estimation or any other kind of measurement is already satisfactorily in use (which means that only one exposure of a subject is ever required), then this usage need not be altered!

7.2 Estimating exposure with non-automated 35 mm cameras

The widespread adoption of through-the-lens (TTL) metering as standard for SLR 35 mm cameras, from the 1960s on, simplified exposure control in photomicrography, as well as in general photography. In early models, the illumination was bounced off part of the shutter, after setting the diaphragm, to a metering element, and the shutter speed set accordingly. Later models bounce the light off the film surface while the exposure is actually happening (off-the-film, OTF) and alter the duration accordingly (see Ray, 1983). This is a very satisfactory method, and the only one worthy of adoption for use in scientific work. Most modern 35 mm cameras offer a choice of full-frame metering, or spot metering. It should be noted that if the spot-metering mode is used (measuring the brightness of perhaps 5% of the total image area), the exposure as measured by some models of camera can be affected markedly by the brightness of an adjacent area not itself in the spot area. Be that as it may, shutter speeds of as long as several minutes can be controlled accurately by TTL metering, as can speeds as short as a few 10 000ths of a second when flash is being used, the flash being quenched when enough light has passed. Some roll-film cameras can have similar devices built into particular viewfinders, although this sophistication does not come cheaply.

7.3 Calibration

All TTL/OTF exposure estimation is automatic, requiring only the setting of the speed of the film in use. In some cameras this also is done automatically, from markings on the cassette itself. This will not do for scientific work.

It is absolutely essential, in order to avoid later frustration and poor results, to calibrate particular equipment with a particular film/developer combination, before routine work is carried on. This is, of course, tedious. It also takes valuable time (and money). Nonetheless, in the long run, it will save a lot of tedium, time and money, as it will guarantee future excellent results in minimum time with minimum materials.

The basis is to obtain proven perfectly exposed negatives/transparencies by guided trial and error. The very first detail to be considered is that of taking the brightness reading initially, and it is here that the first precaution in securing repeatability is required. With standard photomicrography of stained histological sections, or any other brightfield work (including DIC and phase), the brightness reading is to be made from the background *only*. If spot metering is in use, the spot must be reading background only. If metering of the whole frame has to be used, the preparation must be moved aside so as to have in the field only the background mountant/slide/cover.

The reasoning behind this is that the background brightness will then be the level selected as establishing the part of the characteristic curve to which the exposure is pegged, and the reasons for doing this are that it will always be bright enough to obtain a reading in the middle of the metering range (which will thus be more accurate than one taken at the low end), and that it contains essentially white light so that any colour bias in the metering system will never matter. The brightness range of such images is easily contained by all the monochrome and colour films available, so the mere act of putting the background brightness at the right and repeatable point on the characteristic curve will guarantee precise exposure: it will never again be necessary to make bracketed exposures. All this presupposes accurate and repeatable processing, as already outlined in Chapters 5 and 6, of course.

If colour contrast filters are to be used, a white-light reading is taken, the filter inserted, and the exposure increased by the calibrated filter factor (which may be considerable).

The sole drawback with the method of reading only the brightness of the background is the necessity of remembering to return the preparation to the field if it has had to be moved for measuring the brightness!

When such a method of measuring the background brightness is used, calibration is begun by making a series of exposures round a central film speed. In monochrome work, a film/developer combination is chosen according to the contrast index required for the particular subject being photographed (as advised by the listing in Chapter 5). The quoted median speed from that list is used as the central point for seven exposures, at half-stop intervals. If using a camera with an exposure-compensating dial, the film speed is set to the value suggested, and the dial used to introduce half-stop differences in exposure time, three each side of the unmodified time. If such a dial is not fitted to the camera, the speed setting dial is moved round to give different speeds to correspond. Naturally, if the camera has automatic reading of the film speed (DX coding), this must be disabled (and can well be left so for serious work). It is easily done by covering with black tape the squares printed along the side of the cassette, so that the camera will revert to manual speed selection. More than one bellows extension (and then more than one objective) should be used, so as to create a range of exposures set by the camera (those used must be carefully noted of course). The negative strip is processed rigorously according to time and temperature, with standard agitation, and allowed to dry. Whichever negative *of median to low overall density* gives a perfect print was the one exposed for the correct time, and this is correlated with the apparent speed of the film for that duration. Several such readings should produce one definite value for the film speed to be set, applicable to all magnifications, and this is used for all future work to give one exposure for one required picture. What is wanted in the final print is one level of density above pure white as the background, and similarly in a colour transparency.

Working with colour film, exactly the same procedure is followed, with constant processing. The resulting 35 mm colour transparencies are judged *by projection*, and not merely by eye direct, although 6 × 7 cm and

4×5 in transparencies may be so judged. Again, one film speed setting will produce the best results for all magnifications.

With modern TTL readings, the effects of bellows extension (which used to loom so large in the old days) are automatically accounted for in the readings, and if TTL/OTF flash readings are also the norm, then a similar series of exposures (using daylight film if working in colour) will establish the correct settings for flash also.

When dark ground illumination is used, and with some fluorescence images, or those with crossed polarizers in use, a reading of the background is likely to be too dim (although the same procedure should be followed if the background happens to be bright enough to be readable with any accuracy). In such cases, a spot metering system is used to read only the brightest highlight as the basis of the calibration procedure, which is otherwise the same. Precisely the same considerations apply if a compound microscope is used to make pictures of solid objects by reflected light.

For fluorescence images, a fast (ISO400 or ISO1000) daylight colour transparency film is required, which may be push-processed one stop in addition. This is to avoid problems with reciprocity failure with the often very dim images, and to minimize the time that the specimen is exposed to the exciting radiation which inevitably causes fading of the fluorophore.

With roll-film cameras fitted with TTL/OTF metering, precisely the same procedures are followed. If the camera in use is not so fitted, it should be metered as for large format cameras.

It cannot be overstressed that keeping full records, *made at the time*, of the several variables both in calibration and in routine work will repay over and over again the tedious writing up required. Sooner or later a difficulty will be encountered which may well be solvable by referring to proper records of what has already been done at some time in the past. Having to hand a studio record book, and a pen to use with it, are prerequisites.

7.4 Calibrating large format cameras

If a larger camera does not have TTL metering, the brightness of the background at the focusing screen may be measurable by placing a fibre-optic probe light meter against it (such as the Profi-flex attached to a Gossen meter such as the Mastersix). This measures a circle 5 mm in diameter and, even with a small screen, can usually be accommodated. The end of the probe must be in contact with, and normal to, the screen surface, of course, and there should not be a high level of ambient light behind the operator's hand. Similarly, a spot meter (with an acceptance angle of $1°$) may be used to measure one definite background area of the screen; again, the meter should be in line with the optical axis of the system. Such a reading will have to be made at some distance from the screen, unless a powerful (4-dioptre) supplementary lens is used over the spot meter. If such a supplementary lens is used, it must be used for every such reading made from the screen, as the extra lens might alter the absolute value of the readings, but it will not alter their relative values. As examples, the Pentax spot meter (using a silicon photo-diode) has a 20-stop measuring range, accurate to one-third of a stop, while the Minolta Spotmeter F (with a range of 22.5 stops) has flash-measuring capability also. The classic SEI Photometer, often found cheaply secondhand, is also totally serviceable for such use; it has a range of 1 000 000:1, and an acceptance angle of 0.5°. It also can be fitted with a small supplementary lens (see *Figure 7.1*).

For large-format cameras or backs (4 × 5 in–10 × 8 in), the Sinarsix meter is used. This carries a small area measuring spot on a probe which can be placed anywhere in the picture area. This actually measures the intensity of illumination in the film plane itself, and does not merely take a reading off the ground glass, which is displaced backwards during the reading.

All such devices are used to calibrate the equipment as described for 35 mm cameras. In the case of these instruments, however, definite brightness readings are obtained (as opposed to the setting of exposure

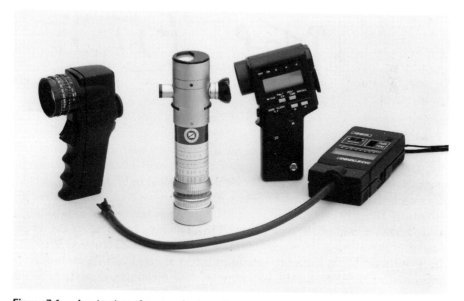

Figure 7.1:   A selection of meters for focusing-screen readings.
On the left is the Pentax digital spot meter, and second right is the Minolta digital spot meter with flash capability also. The Gossen Mastersix meter with fibre-optic probe is on the right, while second left is the classic SEI Photometer, still to be found reasonably priced on the secondhand market.

times). Such definite readings can have definite exposure durations applied to them during calibration, of course, so that a future background reading (or highlight reading in the case of dark ground or crossed polarizers) will allow setting of one definite exposure time, and this will be correct. When making trial exposures with sheet-film, it is a mistake to put too many on one sheet, by progressive withdrawal of the darkslide in the usual manner. Too small an area thus exposed prevents proper final evaluation, and it is recommended to place no more than three such areas on a sheet of 4×5 film.

7.5 Calibrating automated equipment

Modern large research stands always provide integrated automated photography, perhaps with ports carrying two different 35 mm backs, a 4×5 back, perhaps a drawing tube and almost certainly at least one TV outlet (perhaps with analogue as well as digital output) in addition. Slightly older or slightly less advanced equipment tended to provide automatic exposure on a 35 mm and/or 4×5 back, using a separate control box and separate beam-splitter giving viewing and exposure estimating ports.

The personal preferences of the authors in photomicrography incline to having as few surfaces as possible in the optical train between eyepiece and film but, with integrated stands, this might be difficult to achieve in view of the complexity and multiplicity of their arrangements. Their manufacturers, of course, have been at some pains to provide images of exquisite quality in whatever conjugate planes they are to be found, and exhibit a tendency to prevent the mere user from interfering with any part of the system; however, it must be possible to keep the various surfaces perfectly clean if the images are not to degrade with time. It remains possible to set and reset the film speed, and it is still desirable to calibrate even the most expensive and advanced equipment to be sure that it is in tune with the particular user's needs. By using whatever aids to exposure determination are provided in any particular case, a series of exposures is made as described in Section 7.3, and the results evaluated in the same way. It may well turn out to be the case that entering a film speed different from that printed on the box may produce superior results from a film processed acccording to your own standard conditions, and so this should always be done. When using quite ordinary monochrome films in general photography, it is surprisingly often the case that the maker's quoted speed is a stop higher than proves best in practice.

Further treatment of exposure in photography is provided by Dunn and Wakefield (1981).

References

Dunn JF, Wakefield GL. (1981) *Exposure Manual* (4th edn). Fountain Press, London.
Ray SF. (1983) *Camera Systems*. Focal Press, London.

8 Publishing the Results

8.1 Criteria of excellence in prints and transparencies

When an excellent image suited to its intended purpose (which will thus have been defined in advance for maximum effectiveness) has been obtained, an excellent monochrome print or colour transparency must be made of it. The criteria for defining excellence of a monochrome print in this context are that a full range of tones is present, with the whitest white just one degree of density less than pure white, and the blackest black several degrees of density lighter than pure black, and the whole is of correct, perhaps fairly high, contrast. For a colour transparency the whitest white (often the background) should again be one degree of density darker than pure transparent, but the blackest black can be as dense as the transparency will make it.

If very many pictures are being produced to illustrate a long article or a book, it is a very good idea to send a specimen print to the publisher right at the beginning, so that he can get his printer to acknowledge their suitability for the way he works with his particular machinery. It may, of course, still be that the eventual printing of your excellent monochromes will leave a lot to be desired (especially as to contrast, as muddiness is one of the most common faults in printed half-tones), but the ball will then very definitely be in the printer's court and not yours.

Fewer faults tend to occur when printing colour transparencies, the most usual being a background colour cast where that on the original was pure white. This also is a fault of the printer, and you are entitled to insist that it be put right. A great deal of cash must still be invested to produce a page of colour plates, which is why they are much more likely to be used in a journal (on the back of colour advertisements) than in a book.

This situation might change dramatically in the next few years. It is even now possible, with the very latest printing technology, to store all the text and pictures, monochrome and/or colour, for even a long book, in digital form, digitizing from the usual kind of originals. These files are then simply fed into the machine, and a book emerges as sheets ready for binding. This is possible even for one single copy, although some economies of scale will always be secured with greater numbers. However, now that books with colour illustrations do not all have to be machined at one time, thus tying up a lot of capital, more such books might be available in future; a publisher might print only 100 copies, and get his outlay and profit back, before printing another 100, and so forth!

When sending monochrome prints to a publisher, it is well to include *wide* white margins on them. The edges will always be damaged between publisher and printer, and this safeguards the actual picture area quite adequately. When sending in colour transparencies, 35 mm frames are well enough protected in the mounts as returned by the processor, but should be held in separate pockets of a larger sheet of some kind (of the kind used for vertical filing of slides, for example). Larger transparencies should at least be put in the special, correct size, envelopes available for the purpose, or even in card mounts with borders which are then enclosed in such a transparent envelope.

8.2 Inserting scales and lettering

This is best done by the publisher. Modern practice requires insertion of a scale bar in a picture, rather than a statement of the magnification in the caption alone. The actual length of the scale bar to be inserted should be shown on an attached label, and it will usually be placed in the same position on each picture, as this looks very much better on publication than such bars being put apparently at random in a series of half-tones. All labels to be put into a picture area are printed to secure high quality, and are then attached. You need to show *exactly* where a leading line should end in your half-tone, and this is best done by a firmly attached overlay in tracing paper, showing only the outlines to be labelled, the label itself if more than one, and the end of the lead line. A separate typewritten list of labels must be provided, for printing from.

8.3 Mounting, for presentation and for poster sessions

If a presentation for a possible book is being made to a potential publisher, the appearance of the manuscript and its illustrations may well exert some influence on the outcome. Needless to say, with the advent of word

processors and laser printers, there is no excuse for sending in a manuscript which is less than *perfect*. Accompanying illustrations must also be
impeccable – not dog-eared and bent. Only a few specimens will be needed
for such a purpose, and they are best sent to the publisher as perhaps
slightly larger prints than will have to be provided finally (10×8 in is
about right), in a transparent pocket in a not too elaborate A4 ring binder,
and *each with its matching caption secured below it in the same pocket*.
Transparencies should be sent in as a size larger than 35 mm if possible,
no matter if that is the size which will be used for the actual illustrations.
If a few 4×5 in transparencies can be made specially, and mounted in
similar pockets in correctly sized card mounts, with captions, so much the
better for your chances!

For poster sessions, dry mounting remains an excellent means of
attaching text and pictures to the backing sheet, if facilities are to hand.
If not, one of the spray mounts widely available can be used. A good
alternative is the new roll-on applicator (the Rollataq, see Appendix) which
applies a thin and even layer of a PVA-based adhesive, which allows
repositioning for 10 min or so before giving a final permanent bond.

The backing sheet should be *dry*, as should pictures and sheets of
captions/text. A thinnish covering of adhesive is then given to cover the
whole of the rear of each sheet to be attached, in turn, with a little more
at the edges. It is strongly recommended to roll the sheets into firm and
total contact with the backing by use of a wide rubber roller. The effect of
a poster is ruined if bubbles show up behind pictures. Do not fix any sheet
too close to any edge – these *will* be damaged in transit or when being
attached to the display board.

Attention to a particular poster is best secured by a compelling picture,
rather than by use of coloured backgrounds or those unusual typefaces so
easily generated nowadays with a word processor.

8.4 Captions for books, journals and posters

The nature of the captions intended for these three categories of communication necessarily differ from each other, as each has a different
potential readership.

In all captions, clarity of expression is paramount, while the avoidance
of grammatical error will avoid engendering irritation in those reading
what is written. In a paper in a learned journal, however, it may be
assumed that the audience has specialized knowledge, and therefore the
captions to the illustrations may use a specialized vocabulary without
much additional explanation. In general, such captions should not be too
long. Do not forget to include a value for any scale bar in the illustration.

Even in a specialist book, some at least of the readership may be expected to have a less specialized knowledge, and the nature of the captions must reflect this. Too technical a caption, with too specialized a vocabulary, is to be avoided, although slightly longer captions might be useful. Many illustrations are also provided for more general books, and the captions for these must not be intimidating, or they will never be read at all. Short words in a few short sentences must be the rule if communication is to be established and the illustration is not to be mere adornment.

On posters, technical details and a specialized vocabulary are often required, but a more generally understandable introduction is also a requirement. It is as well to keep to one basic typeface, varying the effect if need be by using bold on occasion, and a few different sizes as necessary. It is only too easy to create a mere jumble of styles if the considerable capabilities of word processors and laser printers are exploited, and this actually detracts from the message it is intended to convey.

8.5 Protecting illustrations

Small illustrations, graphic or photographic, should have *ample* margins. When being posted they should be enclosed in a *strong* envelope, with a rigid backing board which may or may not be built in to the heavyweight envelope. It is prudent to use two such boards, one on each side of the pictures; lightweight boards of corrugated plastic are available, and are economical in postage costs compared with ordinary boards. If only one board is used, the pictures should be to the rear of the board in the envelope. It is also prudent to seal each seam of the envelope with parcel tape or cellulose tape.

When posting transparencies, similar considerations apply to their enclosure in suitable strong and rigid envelopes. In addition, if a number of transparencies is being sent, each should be in a separate glassine or similar envelope of suitable size; it invites damage to enclose a loose assortment of transparencies rubbing together in an envelope.

When posting large illustrations, posters and the like, they should be sent in a heavyweight postal tube. They are rolled up with the illustrations to the *outside* of the roll, and not to the inside (which admittedly seems more natural). The reason is that the stretching which ensues from being rolled backwards is easier for the print/adhesive to cope with than the compression which ensues if rolled forwards. The outermost surface is covered with plain paper to minimize damage when the whole is being inserted or removed from the tube. The edges of the poster should be kept a few centimetres from the ends of the tube containing it, and these should be well sealed with parcel tape.

8.6 Preserving illustrations

Graphics should be kept flat and horizontal in shallow boxes or trays. If made on proper quality card with indian ink they have a long life, and if kept in the dark most colours will survive for 50 years at least – provided that the card is acid-free and in contact only with other acid-free card.

For monochrome photographic prints, permanence is not assured unless the image is on a well-washed base, and is gold-toned after initial printing. Only in extreme cases will such expensive treatment be justified, and for more ordinary pictures it must suffice to ensure that each print is *thoroughly* washed, and then kept in the dark only in contact with acid-free paper specially supplied for the purpose (by a supplier such as Conservation Resources, see Appendix). That is, a mere pile of prints in a drawer is not recommended for archival preservation. When archival standards of preservation are required, very special air conditioning of a special room is needed but, for anything not extraordinary, such extraordinary conditions would be inappropriate.

If a negative turns out to be very special for one reason or another, it should be rewashed thoroughly but not excessively, with three final soaks in changes of de-ionized water, air dried, put into a special conservation envelope, and kept at lowish temperatures in the dark, at moderate humidity, in an unpolluted atmosphere.

Colour transparencies are best kept unmounted in separate conservation-quality negative bags, in a coolish room, in the dark at moderate humidity, in an unpolluted atmosphere. It is recommended to make a transparency on similar material of a standard colour chart, such as that by Macbeth, and keep that with the others. This may allow future estimation of the extent of any fading (by comparing the transparency of the chart with a new actual colour chart), which *will* occur.

Colour prints are not suited for archival storage, unless they are made on Ilfochrome/Cibachrome. These latter are treated as colour transparencies.

Digitized stored images are, to all intents and purposes, permanent. However, in future years the hardware required to read them may no longer be available; already, very few present-day computers can read data stored on the old 8-in floppy discs.

More details are provided by Kodak Publication F-40 (Anon., 1985), Keefe and Inch (1994) and Martin (1988).

References

Anon. (1985) *Conservation of Photographs*. Publication F-40, Eastman Kodak Company, Rochester, NY.

Keefe LE, Inch D. (1994) *The Life of a Photograph* (2nd edn). Focal Press, London.

Martin E. (1988) *Collecting and Preserving Old Photographs*. Collins, London.

Appendix

Manufacturers and suppliers

Agfachrome Service, PO Box 32, Bury, Lancs, BL9 0AD, UK.

Conservation Resources (UK) Ltd, Unit 1 Pony Road, Horspath Industrial Estate, Cowley, Oxford, OX4 2RD, UK. Suppliers of archival storage products, conservation adhesives and other conservation and restoration materials.

Rollataq 300 is made by Daige Inc., 1 Albertson Avenue, Albertson, NY 11507, USA, and is widely available through photographic and other suppliers. A wide range of other adhesives is sold through the same outlets and various graphics suppliers, who also offer a range of pens and other drawing aids.

Silver Print Ltd, 12 Valentine Place, London SE1 5QH, UK. Suppliers of Speedibrews E-4. (Processing of E-4 films is offered by Argentum, 1 Wimpole Street, London W1M 8AE, UK.)

Index of names

Index

ORDERING DETAILS

Main address for orders

BIOS Scientific Publishers Ltd
9 Newtec Place, Magdalen Road,
Oxford OX4 1RE, UK
Tel: +44 1865 726286
Fax: +44 1865 246823

Australia and New Zealand
DA Information Services
648 Whitehorse Road, Mitcham, Victoria 3132, Australia
Tel: (03) 873 4411
Fax: (03) 873 5679

India
Viva Books Private Ltd
4346/4C Ansari Road, New Delhi 110 002, India
Tel: 11 3283121
Fax: 11 3267224

Singapore and South East Asia
(Brunei, Hong Kong, Indonesia, Korea, Malaysia, the Philippines,
Singapore, Taiwan, and Thailand)
Toppan Company (S) PTE Ltd
38 Liu Fang Road, Jurong, Singapore 2262
Tel: (265) 6666
Fax: (261) 7875

USA and Canada
Books International Inc
PO Box 605, Herndon, VA 22070, USA
Tel: (703) 435 7064
Fax: (703) 689 0660

Payment can be made by cheque or credit card (Visa/Mastercard, quoting number and expiry date). Alternatively, a *pro forma* invoice can be sent.

Prepaid orders must include £2.50/US$5.00 to cover postage and packing
(two or more books sent post free)

Desktop DVD Auth

Contents at a Glance

Desktop DVD Authoring

Douglas Dixon

with Jim Matey

New
Riders

201 West 103rd Street, Indianapolis, Indiana 46290
An Imprint of Pearson Education
Boston • Indianapolis • London • Munich • New York • San Francisco

Desktop DVD Authoring

International Standard Book Number: 0-7897-2752-8

Library of Congress Catalog Card Number: 2002101445

Printed in the United States of America

First edition: October 2002

06 05 04 03 02 7 6 5 4 3 2 1

Interpretation of the printing code: The rightmost double-digit number is the year of the book's printing; the rightmost single-digit number is the number of the book's printing. For example, the printing code 02-1 shows that the first printing of the book occurred in 2002.

Trademarks

Warning and Disclaimer

PUBLISHER
David Dwyer

ASSOCIATE PUBLISHER
Stephanie Wall

PRODUCTION MANAGER
Gina Kanouse

ACQUISITIONS EDITOR
Elise Walter

SENIOR MARKETING MANAGER
Tammy Detrich

PUBLICITY MANAGER
Susan Nixon

DEVELOPMENT EDITOR
Clint McCarty

COPY EDITOR
Nancy Sixsmith

INDEXER
Chris Morris

COMPOSITION
Ron Wise

MANUFACTURING COORDINATOR
Jim Conway

BOOK DESIGNER
Barb Kordesh

COVER DESIGNER
Aren Howell

MEDIA DEVELOPER
Jay Payne

To my mother and father, who helped start me on the journey, and to my family, Connie, Karin, and Brian, who make the trip so fascinating.

Table of Contents

About the Author

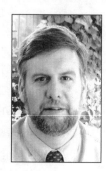

Douglas Dixon is a technologist and author who has worked in the "Video Valley" of Princeton, N.J. for more than 20 years, at the bleeding edge where advanced consumer video applications meet personal computers. He recently authored *How to Use Adobe Premiere 6.5*, and also writes regularly on technology and business for *Camcorder and Computer Video* magazine and the *U.S. I Newspaper* in Princeton.

As a technology leader at Sarnoff Corp., and previously as a software product manager at Intel Corp., Doug has gained extensive experience developing multimedia and web technology into consumer products.

As a technology writer, Doug is a contributing editor for *Camcorder and Computer Video* and *Digital Photographer* magazines, covering video-editing and streaming-media technology and tools, from DV to DVD, desktop to handhelds, consumer to professional.

Doug has published technical articles related to his projects in publications ranging from *ACM* and *IEEE* journals to *Computer Graphics World*. He also is active in professional activities; and has spoken at local, regional, and national meetings, from user groups to PC Expo, Comdex and the ACM SIGGRAPH Conference.

Although he writes about new and cutting-edge technology, Doug's focus is on making technology understandable and useful for real people. For more on these topics, see his Manifest Technology web site at www.manifest-tech.com.

About the Contributing Author

Jim Matey is a Senior Member of Technical Staff for Sarnoff Corporation, Princeton NJ and an adjunct professor at Rider University in Lawrenceville, NJ. He received a BS from Carnegie-Mellon University and an MS/Ph.D. from the University of Illinois.

Dr. Matey has been programming (and building) computers and computer-based systems since the late 60s and has participated in the development of consumer electronics equipment at Sarnoff and in the development of image and video-processing systems for both commercial and government clients.

Jim was an editor for *Computers in Physics* magazine, chair of the Instrumentation and Measurement Science Topical Group for the AIP, held various offices in the Princeton chapter of the ACM, is a member of the American Physical Society, and a Senior Member of the IEEE. He has 15 U.S. patents and more than 50 professional publications.

About the Technical Reviewers

These reviewers contributed their considerable hands-on expertise to the entire development process for *Desktop DVD Authoring*. As the book was being written, these dedicated professionals reviewed all the material for technical content, organization, and flow. Their feedback was critical to ensuring that *Desktop DVD Authoring* fits our reader's need for the highest-quality technical information.

Philip De Lancie is a freelance writer covering technology and market developments for production professionals in fields such as video, film, audio, interactive multimedia, and the Internet. He has written extensively on topics including DVD, surround sound, streaming media, and high-definition video. Since 1985, De Lancie has been published regularly in *Mix*, where he is the New Technologies editor. He is also a contributing writer for *Millimeter*, and a frequent contributor to magazines, including *EMedia*, *Video Systems*, *NetMedia*, and *Digital Video (DV)*. His work has also been published in *NewMedia*, *Post*, *Electronic Musician*, and *WEBTechniques*. De Lancie's writing draws on his own professional experience in audio engineering, including 13 years in CD premastering, as well as in multimedia production for the web and CD-ROM.

Bruce Nazarian is an Apple Solutions Expert, a recognized DVD consultant, a factory certified DVD trainer for Sonic Solutions, and an award-winning DVD producer. He is also a member of the DVD Association—Americas Advisory Board, where he sits on the Training and Careers Working Group. Bruce specializes in digital media production for video, broadcast, DVD, and the web. Bruce is the owner of Gnome Digital Media, an award-winning DVD production company in Burbank, CA. He has created the DVD Companion for Macintosh, and the popular Pro-Pack products. You can visit his DVD web site at www.recipe4DVD.com to learn more about how to make DVD authoring easier.

Irwin Eberhart has continuously contributed his multi-faceted skills to the communications industry in various ways. While studying broadcast production at Chicago's Columbia College, he helped pioneer Chicago's own brand of music called "House Music." Under the stage name of Chip E. he produced and recorded many "House Music" classics. Many of his recordings, including "Like This," "Godfather of House Music," and "If You Only Knew," became hits in cities throughout the U. S. as well as in Europe—where Chip E. made many personal appearances. Irwin always had a keen interest in technology, and he became a key player in the Internet industry—managing web development staffs for several top communications corporations. As digital video began to play an important role in the industry, Irwin began to hone his skills as a film, video, and DVD guru. Irwin has been a featured speaker on DVD technology at events, such as MacWorld Expo, teaches video editing and DVD authoring at Chicago's Mac University, and has authored hundreds of DVDs for corporate museum and film clients. He is currently producing his first film, a documentary about the immersion of "House Music" focusing on the unusual suspects or the unsung heroes who contributed to that style of music—and, of course, it will be distributed on DVD.

Rob Pinniger, after leaving Corpus Christi College, Oxford in 1994 quickly became involved in new media and has since held a number of senior positions at post-production facilities, new media companies and recording studios throughout London. He has also been a freelance consultant and record producer and has written training courses for a variety of major software packages. Rob encoded and authored some of the first DVDs created in the UK and recently passed his three hundredth DVD project. He is currently Technical Manager at Abbey Road Interactive, the new media division of EMI's famous recording studios. In this role he has been involved in the creation of award-winning web-sites and DVDs for a variety of national and international clients. More information can be found at `www.abbeyroadinteractive.com.`

Acknowledgments

It has been a real pleasure working in and writing about the PC and multimedia industries over the years, from computer and video equipment manufacturers to system and application software developers. The great thing about this field is that people tend to enjoy their work, and that spirit comes through in their products. I would particularly like to thank all the companies I worked with on this book for their continued help in staying up-to-date with technology and product developments. I would like to specially acknowledge Andy Marken and Tony Jasionowski of the RDVDC for their continued support throughout this process.

I am greatly appreciative of the help of my friend and colleague, Jim Matey, in contributing to four chapters of this book.

Thanks are also due to the team at New Riders Publishing who helped make this book: Jeff Schultz, who helped conceive this project, Lloyd Black, who started it rolling, Stacia Mellinger and Gina Kanouse, who kept it on track, and most of all Clint McCarty, who drove it from end to end. Thanks also to Philip De Lancie, Irwin Eberhardt, Bruce Nazarian, and Rob Pinniger for their suggestions for improving the book. And thanks to Neil Salkind and Studio B for their support in developing these writing opportunities.

I would like to thank Bob Wolenik, Tony Gomez, and Mark Shapiro for the continuing opportunity to cover these developments for *Miller Magazines*, and Rich Rein and Barbara Fox for the great learning experience of writing for the *U.S. 1 Newspaper* in Princeton. Thanks also to Andy van Dam and my compatriots at the Computer Science program at Brown University for making writing a natural part of technology education.

Tell Us What You Think

As the reader of this book, you are the most important critic and commentator. We value your opinion and want to know what we're doing right, what we could do better, what areas you'd like to see us publish in, and any other words of wisdom you're willing to pass our way.

As the Associate Publisher for New Riders Publishing, I welcome your comments. You can fax, email, or write me directly to let me know what you did or didn't like about this book—as well as what we can do to make our books stronger. When you write, please be sure to include this book's title, ISBN, and author, as well as your name and phone or fax number. I will carefully review your comments and share them with the author and editors who worked on the book.

Please note that I cannot help you with technical problems related to the topic of this book, and that due to the high volume of email I receive, I might not be able to reply to every message.

Fax: 317-581-4663

Email: stephanie.wall@newriders.com

Mail: Stephanie Wall
           Associate Publisher
           New Riders Publishing
           201 West 103rd Street
           Indianapolis, IN 46290 USA

Introduction

Desktop DVD Authoring opens up the world of DVD at your desktop—for playing movies, archiving data, and authoring video productions. Whether for business presentations or family events, the new medium of DVD offers an exciting new way to create and distribute video material as high-quality interactive presentations.

Just as the use of CDs for creating personalized music has exploded in the past decade, DVDs are now becoming available for desktop video authoring. This is the next revolution in personal computers, with full-quality digital video and DVD on the desktop.

With a DVD-ROM drive on your computer, you can watch movies on DVD, and explore them to find hidden special features. With a DVD recordable drive, you can use DVD as a bigger and faster CD to store more data and larger files. But most of all, you now can author video productions to DVD.

With this book, you can easily create and share great-looking productions on DVD and even CD, with real, full-quality digital video and audio, complete with professional-style menus. Even better, the DVD discs that you burn at your desktop can be played almost anywhere—not only on computer DVD drives but also on consumer set-top DVD players.

But what about all the different DVD formats? And what are all these different DVD products: consumer and computer, players and recorders? How might DVD make sense for you, for your particular needs? This book will answer these questions by helping you make sense of DVD—discs and formats, consumer and computer products, computer systems and peripherals, for playback and authoring, across both the Windows and Macintosh platforms.

This book takes a broad approach because there is no single answer with DVDs. This book shows you the range of possibilities for desktop DVD authoring, whether you are starting out by just transferring some videotapes to DVD as easily and simply as possible, or stepping up to designing your own interactive presentations.

Desktop DVD Authoring introduces a wide range of DVD authoring tools, for both Windows and Macintosh, progressing from personal applications to more professional tools. It explains the different categories of tools, and shows how to use the tools step-by-step, highlighting differences and special features. Appendix D, "DVD Authoring Software Gallery," at the end of the book then provides a visual overview of a wide range of available tools for DVD authoring and video editing.

You even can try out the software applications used in the book and work along with the text by downloading trial versions of these products from the company web sites listed in Appendix B, "DVD References."

From CD to DVD

The tremendous interest in CDs for digital audio was of course driven by the enjoyment of music, but it was enabled by technology, standards, and declining prices. As computers became faster, and CD-ROM playback drives became standard equipment, it became feasible to record or rip music from a CD to your hard disk. With growing hard disk capacity and the standardization of the MP3 audio compression format to squeeze down the file sizes, it became quite reasonable to store your music collection on disk for convenient playback. But the final breakthrough was the growing availability of CD-R/RW drives and the decline in CD media prices to under $1, making it possible for you to burn your own music mixes to take along with you.

And now, the same excitement is being repeated with DVD and digital video. In the first two years of the new millennium, DVD-ROM drives have become common equipment on personal computers as processor performance has increased so much that you can play DVD movies on your computer, at full rate and full-screen resolution, along with surround-sound audio. Meanwhile, the growth of digital DV camcorders and adoption of the FireWire/IEEE 1394 interface has brought full-quality digital video to the desktop, so you can capture, edit, and record video with no compromises.

Which brings us to the last component: DVD recording. Just as with CDs, DVD recording drives and recordable media are moving down the price reduction curve as manufacturing volumes ramp up. The year 2001 saw the introduction of bundled desktop computer systems; external DVD burner drives; and lower-cost, general-purpose DVD media, all supported by a wide range of DVD authoring tools. And as DVD burners fall under $500, and recordable DVD discs fall to around $1, the last cost barriers to DVD are being swept away.

Who Should Use This Book?

Desktop DVD Authoring is for anyone who has some interest and experience with working with video on computers, particularly digital video, and is interested in the possibilities for using DVD to create, share, and archive video material. You may already have some experience using photo-, audio-, or video-editing tools; and with playing and burning CDs. And now you would like to explore DVD authoring.

If you are just starting out with video on computers, you can use this book to learn how to use the "automated" DVD tools to quickly transfer video to DVD with a minimum of fuss, complete with professional-looking titles and back-grounds. And even if you do not have a DVD recordable drive, you can use this book to create and share DVD productions on CD.

If you want to make an interactive production, this book will show you how to use the personal DVD authoring tools, organize your clips into nested menus, and provide more customization of the menus and navigation.

And to create more complete productions, this book demonstrates the professional DVD authoring tools, with advanced DVD features, such as multiple video, audio, and subtitle tracks.

With this book, you can make sense of all the different options for DVD, and pick the right solution for your needs. If a simpler personal tool does what you need for the moment, then you can start out quickly and inexpensively. And even if you need the features in a more professional tool, you still may find it handy to use a more automated tool to quickly transfer some video with a minimum of fuss.

How to Use This Book

This book is organized into six parts, covering DVD consumer products and formats; DVD on computers; and three parts on DVD authoring tools, from automated to personal to professional. (The final part is a set of references for your use.) Trial versions of many of the software applications used in this book are available for downloading. See the author's web site www.manifest-tech.com.

For help in getting started with DVD, start with Chapter 1, "Making Sense of DVD," for a quick summary of the different aspects of DVD; and see Chapter 2, "Consumer DVD Players: DVD Video and Audio," for an overview of DVD on the set-top for movies and music. Then see the second half of Part I to find out about recording to DVD for consumer products and on Macintosh and Windows computers.

Use Part II to learn how to play back DVD movies on your computers, and to explore how DVD discs are organized when they are authored.

Then see Parts III through V to dive in to authoring your own DVDs. By understanding the different types of tools, and exploring how they are designed, you can decide which tools are best for you. And by working along with the book, you can create your own first DVD productions, or step up to a more advanced tool to create more customized DVD designs.

Part I, "Understanding DVD: Consumer and Computer," introduces you to the broad dimensions of DVD, as it was designed as a convergence medium that spanned Hollywood movies to computer data storage. It explores DVD formats for different types of content, video and audio, and the competing disc formats for recordable media. It then discusses how this wide range of DVD applications and formats is being used in both consumer and computer products.

Part II, "Exploring DVDs on Your Computer," shows how to take advantage of a computer DVD-ROM drive to play movies on DVD, using popular Macintosh and Windows DVD player software. On your computer, you can go beyond the front-panel control of a set-top DVD player to examine and understand the contents of a DVD movie, and find the "hidden" extra features on the disc. This part also discusses web DVD movies, with both DVD video and computer and Internet applications.

Part III, "Automated DVD Authoring," shows you how to jump right in to creating simple DVD productions, and record them on a DVD recordable drive or even on a CD. It walks you step-by-step through selecting a collection of clips or even recording directly from a tape, automatically generating DVD menus with thumbnails of your clips, and then burning the result to a disc. These are quick one-stop tools; just pick the clips, burn, and play them back.

Part IV, "Personal DVD Authoring," introduces DVD tools that provide more flexibility customizing the design of your production. It shows you how to use these tools for importing media clips, laying out menus, linking menus and clips, changing the graphical design, and then creating a DVD recording. These applications assume that you have already edited your video content, whether one long production or a collection of clips, and now are ready to design a DVD production for them.

Part V, "Professional DVD Authoring," opens the full potential of DVD with more advanced authoring tools. These applications let you create multiple video, audio, and subtitle tracks, give precise control over interactive graphics effects, and provide access to DVD scripting and programming. They also support advanced DVD features, such as encryption, region coding, widescreen, and Dolby Digital audio.

Finally, Appendix A provides a technical summary of DVD formats for content and discs.

Appendix B provides a list of references and web links to more information, including DVD information and hardware and software products.

Appendix C is an extensive Glossary of terms and concepts used in DVD authoring and video and audio editing.

Appendix D is a DVD Authoring Software Gallery that provides a visual overview of these and other tools for DVD authoring and video editing.

Part I

Understanding DVD: Consumer and Computer

Before diving into desktop DVD authoring, it is helpful to understand the many different perspectives of DVD. As a collection of formats, DVD encompasses both physical media formats for optical discs, and logical file formats for movies, music, and data storage. And as products, DVD players and recorders are available both as consumer electronics products for the set-top and as computer disc drives.

Chapter 1, "Making Sense of DVD," provides a broad overview of the many dimensions of DVD—why it was created, disc formats, consumer electronics products, and computer hardware and software.

Chapter 2, "Consumer DVD Players: DVD Video and Audio," describes how to hook up a DVD player. It introduces the DVD-Video format for movies and discusses related formats, including DVD-Audio and Video CD. It also explores the capabilities of set-top DVD players, and steps through navigating movies on DVD.

Chapter 3, "Consumer DVD Recorders: Recordable Formats," then introduces set-top DVD recorders, including DVD-based digital VCRs, and digital camcorders that record on mini DVD discs. It also walks through three examples of current recorder products, for DVD-RW, DVD+RW, and DVD-RAM.

Chapter 4, "Digital Media and DVD on the Macintosh," covers OS X on the Macintosh. Apple provides full-integrated systems that include a bundled DVD drive, plus built-in software support for DVD access, playback, and authoring.

Chapter 5, "Digital Media and DVD on Windows," covers Windows XP on the PC platform. As usual, you have a much more diverse situation with PC systems, with full bundled PCs from some manufacturers, a wide variety of add-on drives, and many options for software tools across a broad range of capabilities and cost.

chapter 1

Making Sense of DVD

So, WHAT IS DVD, and why is it interesting for desktop computer users? The letters in DVD can stand for "Digital Versatile Disc," or "Digital Video Disc", and *versatile* sums up DVD quite accurately. DVD is an optical disc format that was designed as a "convergence" media, bridging from computer to consumer, from data storage to multimedia playback. DVD spans the needs of Hollywood to computers, from the entertainment industry to the consumer electronics industry to computer manufacturers, and from consumers to business. And DVD has lived up to that original promise, first becoming a huge success as a product for watching movies, and now rolling into personal computers.

This chapter provides an overview of these different dimensions of DVD, and how it is becoming a useful and cost-effective tool for desktop video and data storage. It begins by discussing the motivation for the DVD format, and how it has exploded as a consumer product. It then explores DVD consumer formats and products for playing movies and even recording video. It then discusses the development of DVD on the desktop, including recordable formats, DVD burner drives, and authoring tools.

DVD has been a runaway success as a consumer product for watching movies, and now all the elements are in place for DVD on the desktop, with declining hardware and media prices and the availability of a wide variety of authoring tools.

See Appendix A, "DVD Technical Summary," for a more in-depth discussion of the technical details of the DVD formats.

The Dimensions of DVD

DVD can be thought of in several dimensions—as a concept, a disc, the basis for a whole new category of consumer products, and a really interesting new capability for digital video on computers (see Table 1.1).

TABLE 1.1   The Different Facets of DVD

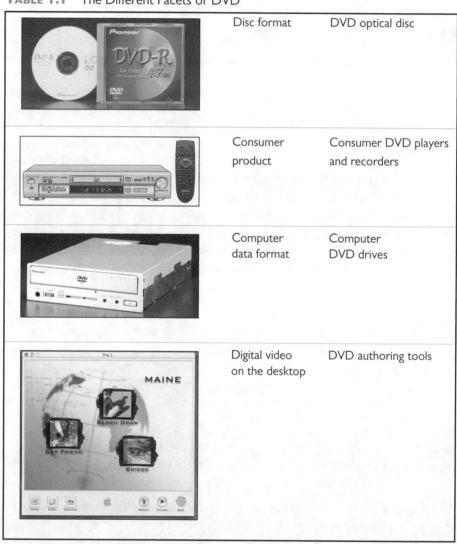

	Disc format	DVD optical disc
	Consumer product	Consumer DVD players and recorders
	Computer data format	Computer DVD drives
	Digital video on the desktop	DVD authoring tools

DVD is many things, and its scope is expanding:

First, DVD is an optical disc format.

- DVD is the next step beyond CD, using the same size disc to provide a bigger and better format. The DVD disc format not only is capable of fitting seven times more data on the same size disc, but also is suitable for everything from data to audio and video.

The DVD format is the basis of several new lines of consumer electronics products.

- DVD consumer electronics products range from DVD movie players with high-quality picture and surround sound, to digital video recorders that record to removable digital DVD discs, and even to digital camcorders that record on miniature DVD discs.

DVD is also a computer data format.

- DVD provides 4.7 billion bytes of removable storage (and more) with read and write speeds much faster than CD. As products, such as multimedia encyclopedias grow larger than will fit on even a few CD discs, and as more desktop users work with large multimedia files, the larger storage capacity of DVD becomes even more important for sharing and backing up files.

Finally, DVD is the fulfillment of the promise of digital media on the desktop.

- With a broad range of affordable DVD hardware burners and software-authoring tools, all these aspects combine to make DVD the last piece of the puzzle for digital video on computers. It is now feasible for individual users, from business professionals to consumer hobbyists, to process digital video directly from camcorder to DVD on the desktop. You can capture full-quality video from a DV camcorder on your computer, edit it with inexpensive tools, author video clips into professional-looking DVD productions including interactive menus, and then burn the productions to DVD discs—all with full digital video and audio quality.

The Origins of DVD: Convergence Media

The DVD format has been primarily driven by the DVD Forum (www.dvdforum.com), which is an industry consortium of hardware manufacturers, software firms, and other users of DVD formats that has about 230 participating companies. In cooperation with Hollywood and computer industry organizations, the DVD Forum developed the initial standards for the DVD-Video digital video format for movies and the DVD-ROM format for computer data storage (see Table 1.2).

Hollywood's needs were for a movie experience with high-quality video supporting widescreen theater *aspect ratios*, multichannel *surround-sound* audio, and *content protection* technology to prevent wholesale copying. The computer industry's needs were for a family of data storage and recording solutions, compatible for both data and video. The resulting DVD formats available today have fairly successfully satisfied these needs, although, as we will see, there is still too much confusion with competing formats for different applications.

TABLE 1.2   Hollywood and Computer Industry Needs for DVD as a
Convergence Media

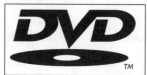

Hollywood Wanted
High picture quality, better than laser disc
5.1 channel high-quality sound
135 minutes (2+ hours) of recording
3–5 language capabilities plus subtitles
Multiaspect ratio
Copy protection
Parental lock features
Low cost drives and media
Computer Industry Wanted
Unified format for AV and PC
Backward CD read compatibility
Write-once (WORM) and rewritable compatibility

| Single file system for all content, disc types |
| Random-access, high reliability |
| No mandatory cartridge |
| High online capacity |
| High performance for both sequential and nonsequential data |
| Future capacity expandability |
| Low cost |

Logos used with the permission of the DVD Format/Logo Licensing Corporation.

DVD Success as a Consumer Product

In the past few years, the market has judged how successfully these goals for DVD have been achieved—in a convincing fashion. The Consumer Electronics Association (CEA) has declared DVD to be "the fastest-selling consumer electronics product of all time," and DVD unit sales actually surpassed VCRs for the first time in September 2001 (see Figure 1.1).

Compared to VHS videotapes, movies on DVD discs are great for consumers for several reasons. DVD offers higher quality than VHS, of course, with higher-resolution video and a sharper picture, plus multichannel surround-sound audio with higher *sampling rates*, and more bits per sample. DVD also offers interactive access, with no more waiting to rewind or to fast-forward through a long tape, so you can jump directly to a chapter to pick up the story, or skip through the movie to see your favorite parts again.

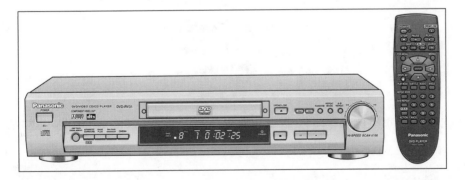

FIGURE 1.1

DVD players like this Panasonic DVD-RV31S DVD/Video CD/CD Player have become the fastest-selling consumer electronics product of all time.

Another important advantage of DVD over videotapes is that the discs can be played over and over again without degrading the quality. As parents with young children know, kids like to watch their favorite movie over and over again, but repeatedly playing a tape eventually starts to damage it. Videotapes will wear out as the tape head spins over the metallic surface of the tape. Over time and multiple viewings, the quality of the video signal will be reduced, and eventually will start having dropouts. With optical discs, such as DVD, however, there is no physical contact. Light from a laser is used to "read" pits in the surface of the disc to extract the digital data, so the data does not wear off, and the digital value is exactly the same each time you read it. In addition, videotapes degrade over time as the metallic particles flake off the tape, so videotapes can become unreadable in 15 years or less, depending on how carefully you store them. By comparison, different formats of CD and DVD discs are predicted to last more than 25 years, and may last up to 100 years.

At the same time, the digital DVD format fits well into similar trends with the adoption of digital (DV) camcorders and the growth of CD recording on personal computers. DV provides high-quality video input so desktop machines can become video workstations, and DVD goes beyond CDs to provide the capability to burn video productions to a removable disc, which can be played on both consumer and computer equipment.

Consumer DVD Movies: DVD-Video

The first consumer DVD products were DVD video players: set-top units that play DVD movies on your television. These products are based on the DVD-Video format, which was designed specifically for showing Hollywood movies that last more than two hours, with high-quality picture and sound (see Table 1.3).

TABLE 1.3   Features of the DVD-Video Format for Movies

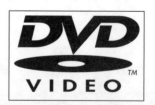

Full-Quality Digital Video and Audio
MPEG-2 video
Dolby Digital (AC-3) surround audio
Interactive Navigation
Menus, chapters, seamless branching

Alternate Tracks
Alternate video camera angles
Multiple audio language tracks
Subtitle tracks
Content Protection
Parental controls
Region coding
Macrovision analog and CSS encryption

Logos used with the permission of the DVD Format/Logo Licensing Corporation.

Besides high-quality digital video and sound, and interactive menus, the DVD-Video format also provides advanced features to enhance your viewing experience with multiple tracks of video, audio, and subtitles.

For example, with multiple video tracks, you can watch a music performance, and switch between different camera angles to see individual performers and their different instruments.

With multiple audio tracks, you can watch the same movie dubbed in different languages, or listen to a director's commentary discussing how the movie was made.

And by combining multiple audio and subtitle tracks, you can practice your language skills by watching a movie dubbed in one language with the corresponding subtitles in the same or even a different language. Or you can turn a movie video into a karaoke experience, listening to the music while watching the subtitles to sing along with the lyrics.

Like audio CDs, DVD-Video movies are *mastered*; the disc contents are designed and authored at a production house, and the final disc image is then sent to a mastering facility so that the disc can be manufactured in large quantities. Unlike videotape, which needs to be recorded from beginning to end, CD and DVD discs can be manufactured—essentially "stamped out" at the factory, which lowers the manufacturing cost.

The definition of the DVD-Video format includes both the physical structure of the disc, in terms of how the data is stored on it, and the logical organization of the audio and video material and control information found on the disc. A set-top DVD player product, or a computer DVD player software application, can then read the raw data off the DVD disc, search through the disc file structure to find the menus, jump to the chapter points, and play the audio and video streams from the disc.

Movies are converted to DVD by first *digitizing* the frames of film and associated channels of sound into digital format. The digital data is then compressed, typically into MPEG-2 video format and Dolby Digital (AC-3) or linear PCM audio format (see Chapter 2, "Consumer DVD Players: DVD Video and Audio"). The movie is then authored into DVD format by adding alternate tracks and subtitles; and then building in the navigational structure to the movie with chapters, menus, and links. Finally, all the DVD material, content and navigation, is combined and *multiplexed* together into the final DVD *image*, the exact data that will be written to the DVD. For making single copies of a DVD, the disc image can be burned to the DVD using a DVD recordable drive.

Consumer DVD on CD: Video CD/SVCD

Although DVD is thought of in the United States as the disc format for video, the CD format is also used for premastered material (especially CD-Audio discs), and there is nothing preventing the distribution of video on CD as well. In fact, the Video CD (VCD) and Super Video CD (SVCD) formats have become very popular, especially in Asia, as an inexpensive medium for distributing shorts, such as music videos and even full-length movies (see Table 1.4). Many current set-top DVD players, and most DVD player software applications, will play discs in VCD format, and sometimes the SVCD format as well.

VCD uses the older MPEG-1 compression format, and has lower video resolution than DVD, but it can fit 74 minutes of "VHS-quality" video on a CD disc. The newer SVCD format uses the same MPEG-2 video compression format as DVD, although at a lower resolution, to fit around 35 minutes of "near-DVD" quality material on a CD. SVCD also supports interactive menu navigation like DVD. See the VCD Help web site (www.vcdhelp.com) for more information on VCD and SVCD.

Another approach to sharing DVD content on CD discs is to simply do exactly that: Author DVD productions that are short enough to fit onto a CD (around 18 minutes at reasonable quality). These discs typically do not play on set-top DVD players, but they can be played on a computer with DVD player software. To make these discs more universally playable on any computer, some DVD authoring-software tools provide the option to include a DVD player software application on the CD disc.

TABLE 1.4   Consumer DVD on CD—Video CD and SVCD Formats

VCD—Video CD
74 minutes, VHS-quality
MPEG-1 video, 352×240 resolution

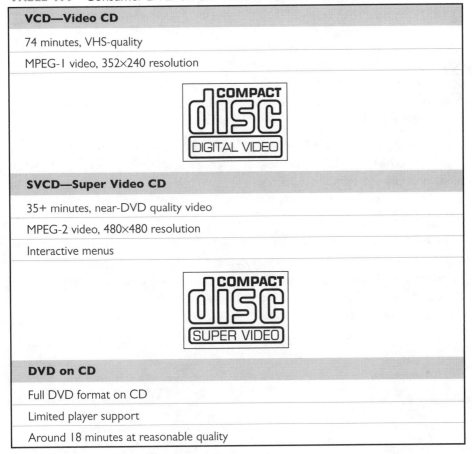

SVCD—Super Video CD
35+ minutes, near-DVD quality video
MPEG-2 video, 480×480 resolution
Interactive menus

DVD on CD
Full DVD format on CD
Limited player support
Around 18 minutes at reasonable quality

Logos used with the permission of Philips Electronics.

DVD Video Camcorders and Recorders

DVD-Video can be used for more than just video playback. Just like CDs, DVD discs are available in both DVD-R recordable (write-one) and DVD-RW rerecordable (rewritable) formats. As a result, it is feasible to use DVD media to replace tape or hard disks in digital video recorders and videotape in digital camcorders.

DVD discs can be used in digital video recorders to provide digital recording on removable discs. You can use DVD recorders like a VCR to record TV shows. Unlike digital recorders that use built-in hard discs, DVD is a removable medium, so you do not have to worry about running out of disc space—and you can save lots of shows to watch later. In addition, you can use a DVD recorder to transfer analog video sources directly to DVD. You can connect your 8mm camcorder or VHS VCR to convert old videotapes to DVD format so that they are saved in digital format (and are much more accessible and convenient to watch).

A roughly half-size mini DVD format (80mm versus 120mm for full-size DVD and CD discs) is being used for small devices, such as camcorders. Replacing tape with DVD provides the capability to easily review the material that you have recorded on your camcorder, as well as the instant gratification of popping the disc into a set-top DVD player to watch it on a TV.

Unfortunately, there are several different, and incompatible, recordable DVD formats currently available—and some recordable formats may not play reliably on standard DVD-Video step-top players or computers. See Chapter 2 and Chapter 3, "Consumer DVD Recorders: Recordable Formats," for more on compatibility issues between different DVD formats.

D I S C S   A N D   D I S K S

Have you noticed that those flat round things that we use in CD and DVD players are called "discs" (with a "c"), whereas floppies and even the big spinning storage devices in your computer are called "disks" (with a "k")?

You can look it up: A "disk" is round and flat, a thin circular plate, but the word is often also spelled "disc." When you throw a pie plate with a spinning action, it becomes a "flying disc." And in athletics, at a track meet, you throw a "discus."

The convention in the computer industry is to use disk with a "k" for magnetic storage, including hard disks built into your computer and removable floppy disks, and to use disc with a "c" for optical storage, including CD (Compact Disc) and DVD (Digital Versatile Disc).

Consumer DVD Music: DVD-Audio

More recently, the DVD Forum has defined a digital audio format, DVD-Audio, which was designed as a higher-quality upgrade from CDs. Like DVD-Video, the audio format supports multichannel surround sound, with higher quality than CD-Audio (see Table 1.5). Some higher-end or "universal" DVD players now support playback of DVD-Audio format discs, but the market for audio-only DVD-Audio players is still developing.

TABLE I.5   DVD-Audio Features

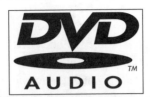

Higher-quality audio
Multi-channel surround sound
Navigation
Track information
Menus
Multimedia
Menus, art, slide-show graphics, video

Logos used with the permission of the DVD Format/Logo Licensing Corporation.

The DVD-Audio format supports menus and navigation, much like DVD-Video. However, DVD-Audio is designed to support a wide range of player devices and capabilities. DVD-Audio discs can be used even in a simple CD-like car player that can simply jump from track to track, or on a smarter player with a text display that can display track information, or on a universal DVD player with a full graphical display on a TV screen with menus, slide-show graphics, and even video.

The DVD-Audio format was defined only recently (in 2000), so the market for the format is still developing. Many consumers are happy with CD-Audio, and even with compressed MP3 audio on their computers and portable audio players. Audiophiles are interested in CD-Audio for the higher quality and surround-sound experience, and the record companies like it because it provides the kind of content-protection and copy-prevention features that are totally missing from CD. The CD-Audio format is becoming more accessible as CD-Audio playback capability is built in to some set-top DVD players and DVD player software. However, the audiophile market is also fragmented by a competitive format: Super Audio CD (SACD), developed by Sony and Philips.

DVD on the Desktop

With the success of DVD as a consumer electronics product for watching movies, DVD-ROM drives for computers also have been catching on as standard equipment on new machines. DVD on computers provide a fun way to explore movies on your desktop, or, even better, to watch the movie of your choice on your laptop during a long airplane trip. DVD player software applications can make the experience of watching a movie even more interesting because they provide more control than set-top players—with features including direct access to the navigational structure of the disc, the capability to display multiple subtitles at the same time, fast scanning while still being able to listen to the audio, and Dolby Headphone processing to hear surround-sound effects from standard headphones.

Just this popularity of watching DVD movies has been enough to drive the sales of DVD drives on computers, DVD is also becoming a common option on desktop and laptop computers, especially with new combination DVD-ROM readers and CD-R/RW read/write drives. However, the goal of being able to write DVDs on the desktop really became achievable only in 2001, with the breakout success of DVD-Video—plus the convergence of stable formats, affordable burners, and usable software.

DVD Discs: Size and Capacity

The basic DVD disc formats, and even the storage capacity, has taken several years to settle down. Even at the end of 2001, there was a surprising variety of formats for different uses (that is, write-once versus rewritable; data versus multimedia) and an ongoing marketing battle between two different formats designed for the same purposes. But the good news is that the market has settled on a standard basic capacity, and it is now feasible to burn DVD discs on your desktop and expect them to reliably play back on the vast majority of set-top DVD players.

The basic physical design decision for DVD discs was to use the same form factor as CD, a 12cm (120mm) diameter disc. Through advances in lasers and disc materials, however, DVD discs can cram more information onto the same surface area, or 4.7GB (billion bytes), versus 650 to 700 million bytes on a CD disc.

DVD MATHEMATICS: "BILLIONS OF BYTES"

Be careful if you are trying to precisely measure DVD storage capacity, for example, when squeezing as much data as possible onto a DVD disc. For no good reason, the capacity of optical media, such as CD and DVD, are typically specified differently than magnetic media, such as hard disks (see Table 1.6).

The capacity of optical discs, such as DVD, is measured in billions of bytes, in the conventional decimal meaning of a billion (1000 cubed, or 10 to the 9th power). However, most other computer-related measurements, including memory size and magnetic disk capacity, are measured in binary powers of two. Hard disk capacity is commonly measured in gigabytes (GB), with the meaning of the closest power of two near a billion (1024 cubed, or 2 to the 30th power).

As a result, even though DVD disc capacity is commonly advertised as "4.7GB," this is not the same as 4.7GB of hard disk space. The "4.7GB" number is actually billions of bytes, or actually only 4.377GB in computer storage, or 93% of the expected size. And a difference like that can add up: If you simply try to copy 4.7GB of data (over 5 billion bytes) from hard disk to DVD, it will not fit because the DVD is actually 347MB smaller than you expect.

This use of "GB" for DVD capacity is unfortunate and confusing, although it does produce the result that a larger number can be used in advertisements. Although there has been an attempt to introduce new standard international terminology for decimal versus binary units, it has not caught on. Instead, in this book, we will use the technically incorrect "GB" as it is used in the industry, and refer to "billions of bytes" when being precise about storage capacity.

TABLE 1.6   Terms and Abbreviations for Storage Capacity

Abbreviation	Measurement	Actual Size	Thousands Power	Binary / Decimal Power
BB	Billion bytes (decimal)	1,000,000,000	1000^3	10^9
GB	Gigabytes (binary billion)	1,073,741,824	1024^3	2^{30}
MB	Megabytes (binary million)	1,048,576	1024^2	2^{20}
KB	Kilobytes (binary thousand)	1024	1024	2^{10}

Unlike CDs, prerecorded DVD discs are available in double-sided formats, with twice the storage capacity (9.4GB) on a single disc. Some movies on DVD take advantage of this format to provide two copies of the same movie, *widescreen* on one side and cropped for television displays on the other; or to provide additional material, such as promotional trailers and "making of" documentaries, on the second side.

DVD discs also can be manufactured with two layers on the same side. By refocusing the laser beam, DVD players can "see through" the top layer of a dual-layer disc, to read the data on the second layer. Dual-layer discs (but single-sided) provide somewhat less than twice the storage capacity (8.5GB). Dual-layer discs are particularly useful for storing longer movies on a single side because the disc does not need to be turned over to access the additional capacity. However, there is a slight glitch when refocusing between layers, so the DVD needs to be designed to disguise the transition (for example, during a scene change in the movie with a fade to black).

In another example of fuzzy mathematics in the industry, single-sized 4.7GB discs are called "DVD-5," dual-layer 8.5GB discs are called "DVD-9," and double-sided 9.4GB discs are called "DVD-10,"—all through creative rounding up.

In addition, like CDs, DVD discs can be manufactured at a smaller size. Smaller CD discs are particularly useful as computer-readable business cards and promotional items because they can contain contact information, and even product demos and brochures. The smaller DVD disc was designed for use in portable consumer electronics devices, such as digital camcorders. These "mini DVD" discs provide convenient and quick access for recording, viewing, and editing video right on the camcorder. They can then be removed and played back in a set-top DVD player, or read directly on a PC to view and edit. These smaller DVD discs are roughly half-size, or 8cm (80mm), and can store 1.4GB (or 2.8GB on both sides).

DVD Formats: Physical and Logical Discs

Defining a DVD disc format includes two aspects: the physical composition of the disc and the logical structure of the data stored on the disc. The physical disc format includes the surface material, the cylindrical groove structure and pits used to store data around the surface, and the type and wavelength of the laser used to read the data. The logical data format includes disc header information used to identify the type of disc, file structure, and data layout information used to find the different types of data on the disc (that is, audio and video, and chapter points), and the actual data formats (such as MPEG-2 video).

The physical disc format and surface composition also determine whether the disc can be modified to record new data, that is, by having the laser "burn" new data pits onto the disc, or even "melt" the material to erase data and then burn new information. The disc format may be prerecorded and manufactured with permanent read-only information; recordable—a blank surface than can be written to once; or rewritable—with a surface that can be written and then erased and rewritten.

As with CDs, various logical data formats can be stored on different physical disc formats. You can buy software on prerecorded CD-ROM data discs, or burn your own data files and directories to CD-R (*Recordable, or write-one*) (see Figure 1.2) or CD-RW (*ReWritable, or re-recordable*) physical discs. You can also buy music on a prerecorded CD, or burn your own music in CD-Audio logical format to CD-R or CD-RW discs.

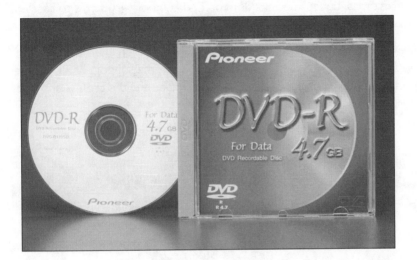

FIGURE 1.2

DVD recordable media is available in a variety of formats, including write-once Recordable (R) and ReWritable (RW).

The DVD Forum originally defined the basic formats for prerecorded discs, starting with DVD-Video for movies and DVD-ROM for computer data, and then recently adding DVD-Audio for music.

The DVD Forum also defined three recordable formats: DVD-R, DVD-RW, and DVD-RAM (see Table 1.7). The DVD-R/RW formats are recordable/write-once and rewritable/re-recordable formats, in the same spirit as the now-familiar CD-R/RW formats.

The DVD-RAM format, championed especially by Panasonic, was designed for data storage applications, with the capability to read and write randomly (instead of writing in long streams and bulk erasing), and with built-in error correction and defect management. Although DVD-RW discs can be overwritten 1000 times, DVD-RAM is designed to be written more than 100,000 times. For archival purposes, these kinds of DVD discs also can be expected to last 30 to 50 years.

In addition, the DVD-R format was split into two versions in early 2001 to help bring down prices for non-professional uses. The original format, now called DVD-R for authoring, still provides the capability to make full DVD-Video discs, including the content protection and copy-protection features. Drives for professional use also continue to support the old 3.95GB authoring format as well. A new lower-cost format, called DVD-R for General, was introduced without the content-protection features, but still permits desktop DVD authoring systems to create DVD-Video discs that play back on most set-top DVD players.

However, the DVD Forum is an industry coalition, not an international standards body, so the success of these formats depends on the support of its members in creating products, and ultimately on their acceptance in the professional and consumer markets.

TABLE 1.7　DVD Forum Recordable Formats

Format	Properties	Description
DVD-ROM	Read-Only	Prerecorded, PC data, reference
DVD-R	Recordable	Write once, best compatibility, set-top players
DVD-R General		Business and consumer
DVD-R Authoring		Professional, content protection

Format	Properties	Description
DVD-RW	ReWritable	Re-recordable
DVD-RAM	Random Access	Read and write like hard disk

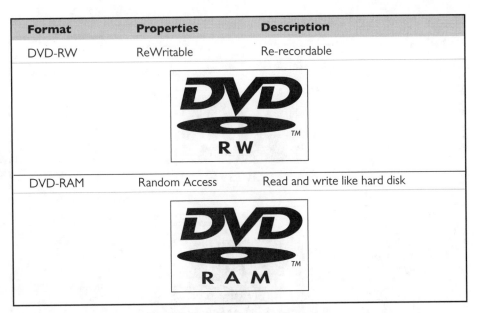

Logos used with the permission of the DVD Format/Logo Licensing Corporation.

Meanwhile, a second industry group, the DVD+RW Alliance (www.dvdrw.org), developed an alternate rewritable format, DVD+RW, ("plus RW"). The DVD+RW format was intended to provide many of the advantages of DVD-RW and DVD-RAM, and also to be more compatible with existing set-top DVD players. After a long development period, products based on DVD+RW started to be released in the second half of 2001. A second related format, DVD+R, was also defined to compete with the DVD-R recordable format (see Table 1.8).

DVD+RW is backed by a core group of companies, including Hewlett-Packard, Mitsubishi/Verbatim, Philips, Ricoh, Sony, and Yamaha; and has received support from Dell and Thomson/RCA.

TABLE 1.8   DVD+RW Alliance Recordable Formats

Format	Properties	Description
DVD+R	Recordable	Write once
DVD+RW	ReWritable	Re-recordable

DVD+RW logo used with the permission of Philips Electronics.

Unfortunately, these competing formats will result in continued confusion in the marketplace and frustration with incompatibilities. The competition between them is based on technical, usability, and marketing factors, including competing claims of compatibility, consumer preferences for using rewritable media, and corporate partnerships to introduce broad ranges of products that support these formats. The result for consumers, we can hope, will include rapid reductions in hardware and media prices, and better compatibility with set-top players, if not between different PC drives. The results for the companies defining these formats will be better market share and a share of the income from the patent licensing pool.

DVD Formats: Compatibility

Given all these different formats and the ongoing marketing battle that may mean some of them may become obsolete, how can we choose which formats to use? Or is it better to delay getting into DVD in the hopes that things will get clearer in the near future?

The answer is actually pretty clear: If you are ready to use DVD on your desktop, then go ahead and get started now. You can use DVD as a large data disc to archive and share your computer files. You can use DVD to burn video productions that can be played on set-top players and PCs. You also can use DVD to create digital archives of your home recordings.

In particular, the DVD-R format is very well-established, so DVD-R discs that you burn at the desktop can be expected to play on almost all recent set-top DVD players and computer DVD-ROM drives. The DVD-RW format is physically similar, but some older drives were not designed to recognize the format, and may reject the discs. The new DVD+RW and DVD+R formats were designed to provide good compatibility, but they are still being established in the market, and will be verified over time. Finally, the DVD-RAM format is physically quite different from the DVD-R baseline, and can be used only in players and drives that are explicitly designed to support it.

But no matter the format, the DVD discs that you burn today will be just as compatible tomorrow, no matter what happens with the popularity of that specific medium for recording in the future. In fact, the whole competition over rewritable (RW) formats may become somewhat moot, at least for desktop uses. After all, write-once recordable (R) formats will always be popular for burning permanent copies of material to share and archive. In addition, as seen with the dramatic drop in CD-R media prices, if the price of recordable media is low enough, it is cheaper and more convenient to just use the same recordable media for everything, even if you expect that you could reuse the disc later.

However, with DVD, unlike CD, there is an additional large potential market for rewritable media in consumer electronics products, such as digital video recorders and digital camcorders. This is the key area of competition between the different rewritable formats, to provide a removable digital medium that provides the capability to quickly record, rerecord, edit, and play back video in recorders and camcorders. But the trade-off with these formats is that the discs they create may be less compatible with existing set-top players and PC drives.

DVD for Computers: Affordable Equipment and Media

Another major breakthrough in DVD for the desktop in 2001 was the dramatic drop in prices for both hardware and media, along with the increase in companies selling DVD equipment—from set-top players to PC drives to consumer electronics, such as video recorders and camcorders.

Pioneer has been a driving force behind DVD-R, building the first professional drives and then helping to lower prices with the release of consumer drives in 2001. In 1997–1998, creating DVDs on PC workstations required a SCSI DVD-R burner for $17,000, DVD media for around $50 each (and with a smaller 3.95GB capacity), and professional authoring tools costing tens of thousands of dollars. In the middle of 1999, Pioneer introduced a second-generation burner for only $5,400, and the media price had dropped to around $35. Although this was a significant improvement, it still was not mass-market pricing. Interestingly, however, a broad market in DVD authoring tools had developed anyway, with quite powerful tools under $1,000 and consumer tools under $150.

The big breakthrough came early in 2001, with Pioneer's introduction of the first combination recordable DVD/CD drive for consumer PC use. The Pioneer DVR-103 / DVR-A03 was an internal DVD drive for $1,000 that could record to DVD-R/RW, and even included CD-R/RW burning capability so it could replace a CD burner (see Figure 1.3). The DVD-R for General media also was introduced with this drive at significantly lower pricing, so the professional drive was still required for creating professional productions on DVD-R for Authoring media.

Also early in 2001, Apple and Compaq introduced new DVD authoring systems bundled with the new Pioneer drive. Apple included the new Pioneer drive on its new Power Mac G4 systems as the combination CD-RW/DVD-R SuperDrive. Apple also introduced two DVD authoring tools, iDVD for consumers and DVD Studio Pro for professionals. The Compaq Presario 7000 PC system included the Pioneer drive, along with a video-editing software bundle. Along with these systems came new aggressive pricing for the DVD-R for General media, dropping the price to around $10.

The second half of 2001 then saw an explosion of new options for DVD recordable drives, including DVD-R/RW, DVD-RAM, and DVD+R/RW. Pioneer reduced the DVR-A03 price to $649, and DVD-R media to $15.99. Third-party manufacturers also repackaged internal drives as external drives, moving from the SCSI interface to the more convenient *FireWire* or *IEEE 1394* interface (also called *iLINK* by Sony). With 1394, external DVD drives could become truly plug-and-play, and use the same interface that was becoming popular for use with DV digital video camcorders. With all this activity, DVD recordable drive prices dropped rapidly down to around $500.

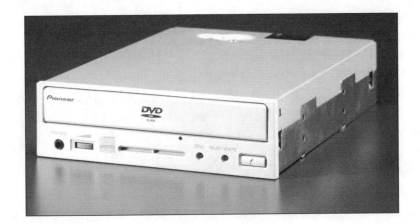

FIGURE 1.3

The Pioneer DVR-A03 combination recordable drive writes to both DVD-R/RW media and CD-R/RW.

DVD Software Applications

Perhaps the most exciting development in the growth of DVD on the desktop in 2001 was the availability of a broad range of DVD software applications. Using DVD on the desktop requires several types of software: operating system support to access the disc drives, player software to view movies on DVD-Video disks, data burning software to write computer data files to DVD discs, and DVD authoring software to create your own video productions on DVD.

The first step in supporting DVD on PCs is to provide the necessary operating system support for DVD drives, including removable media and plug-and-play. Like CD drives, the media are removable and can be changed at will. And with external drives, the drive itself can be powered on and plugged in or removed, all while the computer is running. All this was in good shape on the Windows and Macintosh platforms by the end of 2001 because these systems already supported other kinds of removable media and plug-and-play drives, and had added support for 1394/FireWire interfaces to support DV camcorders.

DVD Player Software

The next type of software, needed even with DVD-ROM read-only drives, is DVD player software to read, decode, and play back DVD-Video movies on your desktop—and even let you watch a movie full-screen on your laptop system. With the rapid advances in computer processing power and data bandwidth, these players can now read the compressed data off the DVD, decode the MPEG-2 video and Dolby Digital (AC3) audio, and play it back in real-time on your computer.

On the Macintosh platform, the Apple DVD Player is bundled on DVD-equipped systems. On Windows, player applications, such as CyberLink PowerDVD and InterVideo WinDVD, are now widely available, with trial downloads on the web and Windows XP upgrades, and are often bundled with DVD hardware.

Besides the standard set-top DVD playback functions, these software players also offer other useful features, especially direct access to all the data on the DVD, including alternate audio tracks, multiple subtitles, and "hidden" video features. Some players also can zoom around in the video picture, fast-scan through the video while still playing intelligible audio, and provide surround-sound audio through earphones with Dolby Headphone technology.

Some commercial DVDs also contain special features for computer use, included on the same discs with the movie. These Enhanced DVDs contain both a DVD-Video section with the movie content, and a DVD-ROM section with files that can be used only on a computer. The enhanced features can include computer applications or games, web pages with links to online content, and even material that combines viewing the local DVD video and accessing related online content. These kinds of web DVD features can also include DVD menu links that automatically launch a web browser to display a web page.

DVD Data-Burning Software

When you step up from a read-only DVD-ROM drive to a recordable DVD burner, the next type of software you need is for burning data files to the DVD to archive and share. This support for burning data to DVD as well as CD is finally being built into the operating systems, especially Macintosh OS X and Windows XP.

You can write data to DVD discs in two ways, much the same as when dealing with CD-R/RW discs. You can use a stand-alone DVD data-burning tool to specify a collection of directories and files, and then burn them to DVD. And especially important for rewritable formats, such as DVD-RAM, you can access a DVD like a hard disk, and just drag and drop files to write them to disc.

DVD Authoring Software

However, creating movies as DVD-Video discs is not as easy as we have grown accustomed to with burning audio CDs. The directory and data format of CD Audio discs is very simple, with just a single list of files—each containing uncompressed audio data. As a result, CD-burning tools typically offer the option to burn both data discs and audio discs from the same application. But DVD-Video discs have a much more complex format, with multiple channels of compressed video and audio data, menu and subtitle graphics, plus navigation information. As a result, creating DVD-Video discs requires specialized authoring tools.

The DVD authoring software market developed rapidly through 2001, with consumer tools available for under $50 and professional tools under $1,000. The variety of tools also blurred the lines between DVD layout and authoring tools (which added video-editing features), and video editors (which added DVD capability).

Apple introduced two stand-alone DVD authoring tools in early 2001. The consumer iDVD tool was bundled with the Power Macintosh G4, and was designed as an easy-to-use tool in the spirit of Apple's iMovie video editor (see Figure 1.4). The professional DVD Studio Pro tool provided full-featured DVD authoring for $999, again in the spirit of Apple's Final Cut Pro video-editing application.

On the Windows platform, Sonic Solutions has developed a wide product family of DVD authoring tools, starting with the consumer MyDVD product for automated layout at $99; and the more professional DVDit!, which dropped in price at the end of 2001 to $299 for the SE (standard edition) and $599 for the PE (professional edition). By July 2001, Sonic had shipped more than one million units of these desktop DVD publishing applications. The Sonic product line also includes a broad range of professional DVD production tools and systems for Windows and Macintosh, including ReelDVD (around $1,500), DVD Producer (from $4,000 for software to a $13,000 system), DVD Fusion, DVD Creator, and Scenarist (from $10,000 to around $30,000).

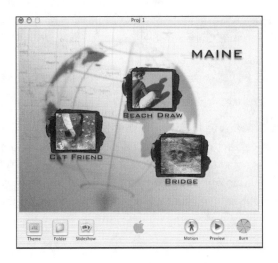

FIGURE 1.4

Apple's iDVD is an entry-level DVD authoring tool bundled with Macintosh systems that include DVD burners.

Meanwhile, video-editing tool companies expanded their product lines to include DVD authoring tools. Pinnacle Systems has a broad range of consumer and professional video software and hardware, including the Pinnacle Studio 7 video editor at around $130. In 2001, Pinnacle released the separate Pinnacle Express product for basic DVD authoring at around $50, as well as the higher-end Impression DVD-Pro at around $1,000.

These inexpensive consumer video-editing tools were evolving rapidly. Near the end of 2001, new releases of several tools provided built-in DVD authoring for around $130, including MGI VideoWave 5 and Ulead VideoStudio 6. Ulead also introduced a stand-alone simple DVD authoring tool, DVD MovieFactory, for around $50.

The capabilities that are built in to some of these low-end tools are amazing. You can capture video directly from a DV camcorder, or import video clips from files on your hard disk in a variety of formats. The tools then provide wizards and built-in template designs to automatically lay out your clips onto menus, complete with the DVD navigational structure. When capturing video, these tools can even automatically segment it into separate clips, based on visible scene cuts in the video, or (even better) on the time stamp on DV tapes that show when you started and stopped recording each segment.

Some of these tools even provide automated transfer from videotape to DVD. They capture incoming video and audio from a DV camcorder, transcode the DV compressed material to MPEG and DVD audio, create the necessary DVD menus and data structures, and burn the result to DVD disc. Some tools, such as MedioStream NeoDVD, even can perform end-to-end DV to DVD conversion in real time as the input DV tape is playing. And all this can be done on a consumer machine, although you may want a higher-end machine—around 1.2GHz or higher.

The Future of DVD

The future of DVD seems to look bright and shiny. As a consumer product, DVD player sales continue to set new records. As a computer peripheral, DVD-ROM readers are becoming standard on new computers—and even DVD burners are becoming more common options. The history of consumer electronics and the computer industry tell us that prices will continue to decline, as they have with CD-based products.

On the compatibility front, newer players are designed to read a wider range of formats, and to do so more reliably. You should be confident that your investment in making permanent recording on Recordable (R) discs will not be obsolete, but for the immediate future you will still need to check the compatibility of specific burners, players, and disc media just in case.

The situation with the competing ReWritable (RW, RAM) formats is less clear. You can certainly use this type of media for specific applications, such as daily data backups, video check discs, and set-top video recorders. However, you need to be more aware of compatibility issues if you want to use these discs in other systems and at other sites.

Meanwhile, technology continues to improve, and the 4.7GB capacity of a DVD begins to seem smaller, just as floppy disks and now CD discs seem to no longer be big enough for our needs.

Several new technical approaches are being pursued to increase DVD capacity for the future, especially for recording and storing material in high-definition (HD) video format.

In early 2002, the DVD Forum decided to pursue the use of more aggressive, low bit-rate compression for storing high-definition material. The intent is to stay within the existing DVD technology by using a newer compression format, such as MPEG-4.

At the same time a second consortium of nine companies, who are also members of the DVD Forum, announced a new large-capacity optical disc video-recording format called Blu-Ray Disc. Blu-Ray can store up to up to 27GB per single-sided disc, or up two hours of high-definition video, or more than 13 hours of standard definition video (at 3.8Mbps). Table 1.9 further outlines the Blu-Ray Disc format.

The Blu-Ray format replaces the red laser used for DVD with a shorter wavelength blue laser, squeezing the tracking pitch in half and permitting higher-density recording. With the increased capacity, Blu-Ray can continue to use the same MPEG-2 format used in DVD and high-definition television.

This group also aims to develop even large capacity formats, such as over 30GB on a single-sided disc and over 50GB on a single-sided double-layer disc.

TABLE 1.9   Blu-Ray Disc Format Specifications

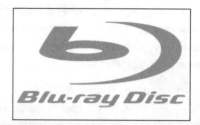

Short Wavelength Blue-Violet Laser
Large recording capacity up to 27BB per side
High-speed data transfer rate 36Mbps
MPEG-2 video format
Uses optical disc cartridge

The desire for these new formats is being driven by the development of high-definition television around the world. The DVD Forum approach provides the capability to use more advanced compression to squeeze HD programs onto red-laser DVDs—at least for premastered videos. The Blu-Ray approach sticks with MPEG-2 to provide the possibility of real-time home recording of HD material, but this requires new technology and increased costs for new equipment.

Although the pace of new technology development, and the corresponding threat of quick obsolesce, can make buying into a new technology a sometimes uncomfortable prospect. The tremendous success of DVD says that it is here to stay, with its widespread adoption within the consumer electronics and computers industries, and across the consumer and professional markets.

Summary

Although set-top DVD players have already become a blowout success as a consumer electronics product, 2001 was a watershed year for DVD on the desktop, with the convergence of lower hardware prices and consumer-friendly DVD authoring tools. DVD became accessible as the final link for desktop digital video processing.

These days, on a standard desktop machine, you can now process full-quality video end to end: capture from DV camcorder, process with video editors and DVD authoring tools, and then burned to DVD disc, to play not only on other computers, but also on set-top DVD players.

As the result of the tremendous activity and competition in DVD software, you can get started with DVD authoring for under $150. Some of these all-in-one tools can work fine for both simple editing and automated DVD authoring, and the basic DVD tools are great for quickly banging out a collection of clips or a copy of a videotape onto DVD with minimal fuss. But as you get familiar with these tools, you will probably want to step up to some of the more professional dedicated DVD authoring tools, to give you more flexibility and control to make a more polished and customized presentation.

chapter 2

Consumer DVD Players: DVD Video and Audio

DVD HAS BECOME TREMENDOUSLY POPULAR in the past few years, as discussed in Chapter 1, "Making Sense of DVD." And with that popularity has come tremendous price reductions: By early 2002, it was possible to purchase an entry-level set-top DVD player for under $100, a feature-rich single disc player for under $300, and even a multidisc changer for under $300.

DVD players are available in many forms: set-top DVD players to connect to your TV and audio system, portable DVD players to watch on the airplane, TV/DVD combo units, DVD recorders (see Chapter 3, "Consumer DVD Recorders: Recordable Formats"), and even built in to video games, such as the Sony PS/2 and Microsoft Xbox. Of course, you can also watch DVDs on your PC, as discussed in Part II, "Exploring DVDs on Your Computer."

The advantages of DVD for watching movies include the improved picture and sound quality over VHS videotape, and the convenience of interactive access to jump directly to your favorite part of the movie.

DVD also promises an even better viewing experience. DVD players can display video on systems ranging from a 50-year-old television (using an inexpensive RF converter), a new television (using video and audio cables to auxiliary input connectors), and the fanciest home theater system (with full widescreen display and multichannel surround sound). With all these capabilities, however, come complexity and potential confusion. If you are shopping for a DVD player, you will see an impressive collection of logos for different disc and audio formats on the front panel, a stunning array of 10 or more different connectors on the back panel, and remote controls with 20 or more closely packed buttons with obscure names.

This chapter will help clarify matters by taking you through DVD formats, video and audio connections, and player menus and controls.

If you just *have* to run out and buy a player today, or even have already bought a player, this chapter begins with two quick-start sections with checklists of what to look for when buying a new player and diagrams for hooking up a DVD player.

If you already are familiar with DVD players, this chapter lays out the wide range of formats and capabilities of the DVD standard, and shows how they are used for typical players and commercial movies on DVD. Part II then shows how you can view DVD discs on a computer to understand more of their structure.

With this background, you can understand the design and terminology used in the DVD authoring tools discussed in the remainder of the book, from introductory tools that automatically create a menu structure to professional tools that provide complete control over almost every aspect of the DVD design and navigation.

If you already own a home theater system, or if you are a videophile or audio-phile, you may find that this chapter does not go deeply into the nitty-gritty of progressive display on widescreen displays or optical digital audio bitstream and cable formats. But because you already understand all this, hooking up a DVD player can simply consist of setting up the player to know what kinds of devices it is connected to and then running the proper cables between them.

Quick Start: Buying a DVD Player

Or, forget the details, I'm going to the electronics store this afternoon…

If you are in a hurry to rush out and buy a DVD player, and do not want to spend the time to read this chapter first, then you can use this section as a summary and checklist of issues to think about when buying a new DVD player, whether it's a set-top DVD player to connect to your television or a portable player so that you can watch movies on trips.

Buying a Set-Top DVD Player

Set-top DVD players (see Figure 2.1) are designed to connect to your living room television for watching movies, or you can use them as part of a home theater system with a widescreen monitor.

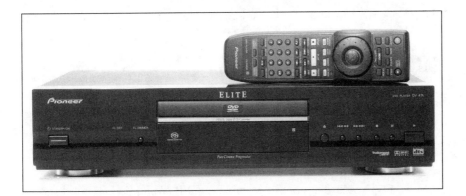

FIGURE 2.1

Sample set-top DVD player: The Pioneer Elite DV-47A DVD Video Player supports playback of formats including DVD Audio, Multi-Channel SACD, Audio CD, and MP3 CD.

The first issue to consider when buying a set-top DVD player is to make sure that you can connect your new player to your existing video—and audio—equipment. As shown in the diagrams in the following section, with most recent television sets you can hook the DVD player directly to a second set of connectors on the TV (in addition to the existing video recorder or cable/antenna connection). But with older TV sets that have only one set of inputs, you may need to get a switch box to switch between the existing input (VCR or cable/antenna) and the new DVD player. Be warned that you cannot hook up the DVD to inputs on your existing VCR—the video signal from the DVD is altered to prevent copying DVD movies onto videotapes, so you cannot view the signal from most DVD players when it is passed through a VCR.

Your best course is to take the owners' manuals for your existing video and audio systems with you to the store. You or a sales person can then check for players that are compatible with your systems, and make sure you have the type of cables you will need to connect the DVD player to your video and audio systems when you get home.

If you don't have the manuals, make a sketch of the connectors on your audio and video systems to take to the store. List the make and model of your video and audio systems, and label the sketch with the names that are printed or embossed on the case next to the connectors. Use Table 2.3 to identify the types of connectors, and indicate the connector types on your sketch.

In both cases, this should be enough for a salesperson to help you select a player, if all you plan to do is play prerecorded DVDs. However, if you plan to play other types of discs in your DVD player, or play DVDs or CDs that you have recorded using a computer or a DVD recorder, you probably need to read the rest of the chapter—and maybe the rest of the book.

The following is a checklist of some important topics to consider when purchasing a set-top DVD player:

- What types of discs will it play?

    - DVD movies (DVD-Video)

    - CD albums (CD-Audio) and recordings on CD-R and CD-RW discs

    - VideoCD movies/clips (VCD) on CD discs

    - DVD recordings on Recordable DVD-R and DVD+R discs

    - DVD recordings on ReWritable DVD-RW and DVD+RW discs

    - MP3 audio on CD discs

- Is it compatible with your audio and video systems?

    - Do you need to upgrade your video or audio systems?

    - Do you need a switcher (for example, between a VCR and DVD)?

- What types of video output formats are supported?

    - Do you want progressive scan output to a widescreen or high-end TV?

- What types of audio output are supported?

    - Does it support Dolby Digital/dts to connect to a surround-sound system?

- Are the remote control and front panel controls convenient and easy to use?

    - Are the controls arranged logically? Is the remote backlit, or does it have buttons with different shapes, so it can be used in a darkened room?

- How does it look and sound when demonstrated through a video and audio system similar in quality to your own?

- What high-end video and audio enhancement features do you want?

    - Do you have high-end equipment so that these features make a detectable difference?

- What advanced controls do you want?

    - How important are controls such as high-speed smooth motion scan, single-frame advance, chapter preview, and audio CD navigation?

Buying a Portable DVD Player

Portable DVD players (see Figure 2.2) let you have movies to go, so you can watch them on a trip, or just away from the living room. The key issue with portable DVD players is trading off the size of the player (smaller is more portable) against the size of the display screen, battery life, and additional features.

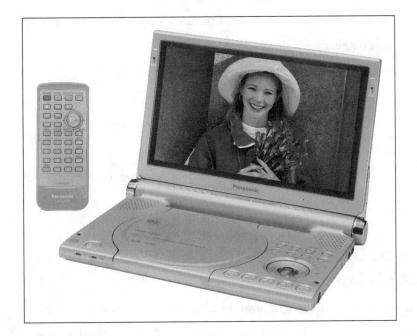

FIGURE 2.2

Sample portable DVD player: The Panasonic DVD-LA95 PalmTheater Portable DVD-Audio/Video Player has a 9-inch LCD monitor and supports playback of formats including DVD-Audio, DVD-RAM, CD, and Video CD.

But although small and light portable DVD players were born to travel, like laptop computers they also may have an important use at home or in the office. If you intend to use a portable as a table-top player, then screen size and built-in stereo speakers are important features. You even can use a portable as a stand-in set-top player, and plug the audio outputs into your stereo or surround-sound system.

In addition the previous list for set-top DVD players, the following is a checklist of some additional topics to consider when purchasing a portable DVD player:

- How heavy is the player? How long does the battery last?
  - Is the battery rechargeable? Can you carry a spare?

- How large and visible is the display?

  - Is the display large enough for your intended use?

  - Is the display widescreen?

  - Is the display brightness adjustable for different viewing conditions?

  - Can the display be viewed from a wide angle for watching in a group?

- What outputs are supported?

  - Does it have good stereo headphones for traveling?

  - Does it have stereo speakers for watching in a group?

  - Does it have external connectors for use as a set-top player?

- Are the front panel controls complete enough?

  - Can you operate the system without requiring a separate remote control?

Quick Start: Setting Up a DVD Set-Top Player

Or, forget the details, I already bought the player and I want to watch a movie.

Even though you are eager to set up your new DVD player, these devices and their connections are complex enough that you really might want to read the manual. An investment in reading the manual will likely save you both time and frustration. With luck (or good planning), you will find that the signal types and connectors on your DVD player and your audio and video systems are compatible, and that the DVD player comes with the cables that you need.

If the connections do not appear compatible, please don't force the connectors, and don't connect signals that are not compatible. Take the manuals for the DVD player and your audio and video systems to the store where you bought the player, and ask for help. If you don't have the manuals for the audio and video systems, make the sketch described in the previous section, and take it with you.

The following diagrams illustrate two typical setups that can be used to connect most DVD players with recent televisions and audio systems. See Figure 2.5 for a diagram of the back panel connectors on a set-top DVD player.

Connect Directly to a TV

The easiest way to hook up a DVD player is to connect it directly to the television. Most recent televisions have an extra set of auxiliary inputs designed for just this purpose, in addition to the main connector used for an antenna, a cable, or a VCR. (As discussed previously, you cannot expect to be able to hook up your DVD player through your VCR because the copy protection designed into DVD players will degrade the signal.) If your television does not have an extra set of inputs, then you will need to get a video switch box to switch between your existing connection and the DVD player.

You can connect the DVD player to your television using standard RCA-type phono jacks with simple push-in connectors that are familiar from audio equipment (see more on connectors in the following sections). Just connect the three Output jacks on the DVD player to the corresponding Input jacks on the TV (see Figure 2.3). Use the labeling on the chassis and the color coding to make the connections: analog baseband Video (typically yellow) and stereo Audio Left and Right (white and red).

Then, to view the DVD display, you need to select the auxiliary input on your television. Depending on your set, this may be done by selecting a special channel, or by pressing a dedicated Video input button.

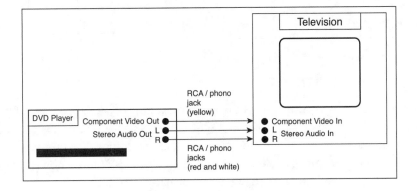

FIGURE 2.3

The simplest setup: Connect your DVD player directly to the auxiliary video and audio inputs on your TV.

Connect to a TV and a Stereo Audio System

Although the best way to experience DVD is in a home theater environment with multichannel surround sound, you can still enjoy DVDs and good audio in a much simpler environment. The easiest upgrade from simply hooking your DVD player up to your television is to connect the stereo audio outputs from your DVD player into your home audio system. Because your home audio system typically has much better speakers than those built in to a television, your DVDs will sound a lot better when played though your audio system.

Most audio systems have an auxiliary input available in addition to inputs for a receiver, CD player, and tape system. Just unplug the stereo Audio Left and Right (white and red) cables from your TV, and connect the DVD player directly to your audio system (see Figure 2.4).

Just remember that to watch a DVD, you now need to both switch the TV to its auxiliary input and turn on your audio system and switch it as well.

FIGURE 2.4

For better sound: Connect the stereo audio outputs from your DVD player to your audio system.

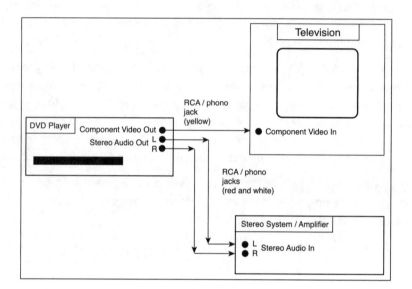

DVD Disc Formats

The first issue with DVD players is the kind of discs they play. Of course, a DVD player will play commercial movies on DVD, but what about music CDs or the new audio formats, such as DVD-Audio? And, besides commercial prerecorded discs, can the player also handle computer CD-R or CD-RW format discs that you have burned yourself, and recordable DVD formats, such as DVD-R?

This section describes a variety of DVD and CD disc formats for video and audio. Besides all these formats, you also should be aware of issues with DVD copy protection and region codes as you use a DVD player.

DVD and CD Disc Formats

As described in Chapter 1, the different DVD formats include logical content formats such as DVD-Video and CD-Audio, and physical disc formats, such as CD-RW and DVD-RAM. Different DVD players support different ranges of these formats, such as a wider range of audio formats or recordable disc media, although newer players typically support more formats.

The good news is that all DVD players should play commercial movies on manufactured DVD-Video discs, including single- and double-layer as well as single- and double-sided discs. All players should play single- and double-sided DVD-Video movie discs (you may need to manually flip them over), although you should check to see what a multidisc changer does with double-sided discs. Most players also should play the smaller-size 8cm discs, although you should try one out if this is important to you.

The bad news is that despite efforts by the DVD industry to establish universal standards, the formats are not all compatible. In addition, some DVD players—especially older players—can have problems playing discs recorded on some recordable (R) write-once media, and the rewritable (RW) formats are less compatible with current players. This places a burden on you to understand the types of discs that you want to use, whether for desktop authoring or a DVD recorder, and to check that the player that you purchase can play them.

The formats are summarized as follows, grouped roughly from more to less commonly available. This discussion ignores details such as double-sided/double-layer DVD-Video discs or smaller-diameter 8cm DVD-RAM discs, which typically are supported if the basic format is supported.

Typically, the DVD player will include the following terms or logos to identify that it can play the associated type of disc, as shown in Appendix A, "DVD Technical Summary."

Common Prerecorded Formats

Most DVD players support prerecorded commercial movies on DVD and music on CD.

All DVD players, by definition, should play prerecorded movies on DVD:

> **DVD-Video**—Prerecorded movies on DVD

Many DVD players also can be used as a CD player, to play and skip through the songs, and even set up playlists:

CD-Audio—Prerecorded music on CD

Because CD-R/RW burners are so common on computers these days, DVD players that can play CDs typically also can play music burned to recordable CD:

CD-R/RW (**CD-R** and **CD-RW**)—CD audio burned to recordable discs

Many DVD players also support the VideoCD (VCD) format for short videos on CD. Support for commercial VCD discs also should mean that you can burn your own VCD discs on CD-R/RW:

VideoCD (**VCD**)—Short video (and audio) productions on CD, CD-R/RW

DVD Recordable Formats

Recent DVD players also should play DVD-Video movies recorded on Recordable (R) discs, and newer players should play ReWritable (RW) media as well. Both set-top DVD recorders and desktop computers can record DVD discs in DVD-Video format. Until the industry matures, however, there will be incompatibilities between different player products and different brands of media. The write-once recordable (R) formats are designed to be compatible with most recent DVD players:

DVD-R—Original DVD Forum Recordable write-once format

DVD+R—Competing write-once Recordable format

Most new players should be designed to also accommodate the write-multiple ReWritable (RW) formats:

DVD-RW—Original DVD Forum ReWritable write-multiple format

DVD+RW—Competing write-once Recordable format

The third DVD Forum recordable format, DVD-RAM, can only be played back on DVD players that are explicitly designed to support it. The DVD-Multi logo is used to identify players that support all three DVD Forum formats:

DVD-RAM—DVD Forum random-access format

DVD-Multi—Supports DVD-R, DVD-RW, and DVD-RAM

Additional Audio Formats

Besides audio CDs, some DVD players can play audio in other formats, either to compress more songs onto a CD for longer playing times or to offer higher-quality surround-sound audio for audiophiles. The audiophile formats are typically offered only as special features in higher-end players.

As with many CD players, some DVD players also can play CDs that have been burned with songs compressed in MP3 format. Because MP3 CDs include many more songs than an audio CD, it is helpful if the player can provide onscreen navigation based on the MP3 filenames.

MP3 Audio—MP3 audio files on CD-R/RW

The Microsoft Windows Media Audio (WMA) format is becoming more available for portable players, and offers more compression than MP3. Some DVD players also can play CDs with songs in WMA format:

WMA Audio—Windows Media Audio files on CD-R/RW

Besides DVD-Video for movies on DVD, the DVD-Audio format has been defined for audiophiles who demand high-quality surround-sound audio recordings:

DVD-Audio—Prerecorded surround-sound audio on DVD media

Sony and Philips also have defined a competing SACD format (Super Audio CD) for high-quality audio recordings:

SACD—Super Audio Compact Disc high-quality audio on SACD media

Additional Video Formats

Some DVD players also support alternate video formats. These formats are attractive for authoring short-form DVD productions because they can be burned and distributed on inexpensive CDs instead of DVD discs. They are uncommon formats, and are not supported in most players.

The enhanced SuperVCD (SVCD) format provides higher-quality video on CD, although with an even shorter playing time:

Super VideoCD (SVCD)—Short video (and audio) productions on CD-R/RW

For short productions, you also can record DVD-format data files to CD instead of DVD:

> **DVD on CD/cDVD**—DVD files on CD-R/RW

Again, Microsoft is promoting the use of the Windows Media video format (WMF) as a method of compressing more video onto a CD or even a DVD:

> **Windows Media Video**—WMF compressed video and audio files on CD and DVD discs

Analog Copy Protection

Besides the confusing DVD disc formats, you need to be aware of the ramifications of the copy-protection schemes that are built into prerecorded DVDs and DVD players.

For most commercial DVDs, the analog video output of the DVD player has MacroVision copy protection, which is similar to the copy protection incorporated into VHS tapes. This copy protection introduces distortions to the synchronization signals in the video output so that video recorders cannot synchronize to the signal properly. As a result, if you attempt to copy the movie to a videotape, the picture will be distorted in various ways: The image may appear torn, or it may jitter or flip. Because televisions are just displaying the signal, not trying to record it, they are more tolerant of these kinds of sync distortions, and the DVD video displays correctly on TVs. However, this is a delicate balancing act—in some relatively rare cases, this type of copy protection causes problems with legitimate playback.

Digital Copy Protection and Region Codes

Besides the analog copy protection, prerecorded DVDs also support digital copy protection by encrypting the data on the disc. This encryption is intended to prevent copying of movies in digital form. Coupled with the inclusion of decryption data on a part of the disc that cannot be written to by normal DVD recorders, it is also intended to prevent copying of the discs themselves.

For almost all legitimate playback in set-top players and in software players, this encryption scheme would not be an issue, except that it helps support a DVD feature known as regional management. Motion picture studios release movies at different times in different parts of the world. A movie might already be available on videotape or DVD in the U.S. while it is just being released to theaters in another country. To protect their theater revenue, the studios insisted that the DVD format include provisions to prevent discs sold in one region from being played in another.

Commercial movies or other DVD discs with regional management have a code that identifies which regions they may be played in, typically listed on the back of the disc case, along with the TV format (NTSC or PAL). When you purchase a DVD player, it has a default region code built in for the region in which the player is intended to be sold. This is no problem if you purchase your player and discs in the same region. However, if you try to mix and match discs and players from different regions, the discs may not play. This is also a problem if you often travel between regions, and want to buy and watch DVDs when traveling in both directions.

Some players permit you to change their regions—at least a few times. Software players also assume a default region when you start playing discs, and provide for only a limited number of changes to the region. If you have any intention of playing mix-and-match across regions (see Table 2.1), you should check the regional management capabilities of your player.

TABLE 2.1   General Geographic Regions Defined for DVD Regional Management

Region Number	Description
1	North America
2	Japan, Western Europe, South Africa, Turkey, and the Middle East
3	Southeast Asia
4	Australia, New Zealand, South and Central America, and the South Pacific
5	Northwest Asia, Russia, Indian Subcontinent, and most of Africa
6	China and Tibet
7	Reserved
8	Special nontheatrical venues (airplanes, cruise ships)

For the purposes of personal DVD authoring, you can ignore copy protection and regions, and simply create discs that can play on any player. For professional authoring, some tools permit you to specify encryption and region codes when you create a DVD master to be used for replication.

Hooking Up a DVD Player: Inputs and Outputs

By itself, a set-top DVD player is a useless box. It has no screen to show the video and no speakers to play the audio. A DVD player becomes interesting only when it is connected to other boxes—a video system and an audio system—so that you can see and hear the contents of your DVDs.

The most crucial issues in connecting any set of boxes into a working system are the interfaces between the boxes: what goes in (an *input*) and what comes out (an *output*) of each of the boxes. We must make sure that the outputs of one box match the inputs of the next box.

On a DVD player, there are three general types of inputs and three types of outputs, as shown in Table 2.2.

TABLE 2.2   Types of Inputs and Outputs for a Home DVD Player

Category	Type
Power	In
DVD/CD disc	In
Controls	In
Status display	Out
Video output	Out
Audio output	Out

The DVD and CD disc formats supported by various DVD players were discussed previously, and the input controls and status display are described in the next section.

These video and audio outputs are used for connecting to a wide variety of video displays and audio sound systems, from standard TVs to widescreen digital monitors, and from stereo receivers to multichannel surround sound systems. (See Figure 2.5 for an example of a back panel of a DVD player.)

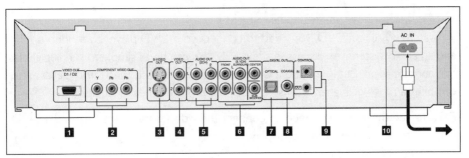

FIGURE 2.5

Sample set-top DVD player back panel from the Pioneer Elite DV-47A DVD-Video Player.

1 D1/D2 VIDEO OUT (D Video connectors)

2 COMPONENT VIDEO OUT: Y, Pb, Pr (RCA jack)

3 S-VIDEO OUT: Y C (S-Video connector)

4 COMPOSITE VIDEO OUT (Yellow RCA/phono jack)

5 STEREO AUDIO OUT: Two-Channel Left and Right (Red and white RCA/phono jacks)

6 SURROUND AUDIO OUT: 5.1-Channel Front and Surround Left and Right, plus Center and Sub-Woofer (RCA jack)

7 OPTICAL DIGITAL VIDEO OUT (Optical digital jack)

8 COAXIAL DIGITAL VIDEO OUT (RCA jack)

9 CONTROL IN/OUT: Chain multiple components to operate with a single remote control (Stereo mini-plug)

10 AC Power In

Power Cable

The most obvious connector on the back panel of a DVD player is the power cord. The players sold in your local stores will conform to the local power; that is, the standard 120-volt AC power in the United States. However, if you plan on traveling with your DVD player, you should verify that it will be compatible with the type of power that you will encounter during your travels.

Hooking Up Video Signals

To watch movies on DVD, you need to connect your DVD player to a video display and an audio system. As discussed previously, this can be as simple as running cables to your television. But if you are a video or audio enthusiast, then DVD players also can offer a range of higher-quality connections to home theater equipment.

First, to see the video, we need to connect the video output signal from the DVD player into some sort of video display.

Video Signals and Connectors

The types of video signals commonly used for DVD players include

- RF
- Composite (baseband)
- S-Video/SVHS
- Component (RGB), (Y, B-Y, R-Y), (Y, Pr, Pb)
- Digital video

Most players offer at least several types of video outputs, and the higher-end players offer additional higher-quality outputs.

To watch a DVD, your television or display system must be compatible with at least one of the video signal types that your DVD player provides. If not, you will need an appropriate signal-conversion box to connect your DVD to your display.

Assuming that your DVD player has a video output that is compatible with a video input on your display, you then need to connect the DVD output to the display input with a cable. Your player may come with a set of cables. If the cables are not compatible with the connectors on your video display, you will need to use cable adapters that convert between different types of connectors or purchase cables with different types of connectors at the ends. Common cable connectors are listed in Table 2.3.

The *F connector* is most often used for RF signals. It is commonly used for the output of set-top cable TV converters and as the antenna connections for VCRs and TVs. The *RCA phono jack* was originally developed for audio, but also is commonly used for composite and component video. The *BNC* connector provides a heavier-duty connector than the RCA phono jack; it is more expensive, and is found on higher-end systems. The *S-Video connector* is a specialized connector used for S-Video signals. The *Firewire connector* is used for digital video signals, such as DV camcorders and other IEEE 1394 digital connections.

TABLE 2.3   Video Cable Connectors

Type	Connector
F connector	
RCA phono jack	
BNC connector	
S-Video connector	
Firewire/IEEE 1394 connector	

RF Video Format

RF video is the simplest and lowest-quality video signal connection. This is the same type of signal that you get from your antenna or your (non-digital) cable TV service. It is also one of the outputs provided by most VCRs and video games.

RF stands for radio frequency; this term is a holdover from the early days of radio. It means that the composite video signal has been modulated onto a high-frequency radio wave that could be transmitted from an antenna tower to your home—provided that the radio wave were strong enough to reach your home. When you tune the TV to the channel corresponding to the frequency of the radio wave, the TV demodulates the composite video signal from the RF, and you get a picture. When connecting a device like a VCR or video game console to a television, the RF signal goes into the antenna input of your TV receiver and is received on Channel 3 or 4. An RF signal also carries an audio signal, so the audio will play back through the receiver as well. It is the only way to get a signal into many older TVs.

RF is the least-desirable video signal because the modulation and demodulation of the video and audio onto the RF carrier reduce the quality of the video and audio signals. As a result, very few DVD players have an RF output and you can expect even fewer in the future as newer televisions come equipped with built-in inputs for higher-quality signal types.

If your DVD player does not have an RF output, and your TV is an older model that only has antenna inputs, you can still connect your DVD player to the TV via an external RF modulator that will pass the DVD signal on to your TV on Channel 3 or 4. If you already have an antenna or VCR hooked up to your TV, you also need a video and audio switcher to select between the antenna/VCR and DVD.

Composite/Baseband Video Format

Composite or *baseband video* is the next step up from RF. Composite video is simply the video that would be modulated onto the RF. By providing the composite video directly to the video display, the composite format skips the modulation/demodulation steps and delivers a better-quality video image.

However, the composite color video standard was designed in the early 1950s. A primary concern at that time was to ensure that the then-new color TV signals would be backward-compatible with the existing black-and-white TVs. The engineers did a remarkable job in 1950 (they developed a standard that survived more than 50 years, in which consumer electronics changed from an analog, discrete component, vacuum tube technology to a digital, integrated circuit, semiconductor technology). However, composite video cannot fully exploit the capabilities of today's DVD technology.

Even so, composite video output played from a good-quality disc on even an entry-level DVD player, and displayed on a good-quality video display, provides a viewing experience better than off-the-air television, VHS tape, or even analog cable.

Composite video does not carry an audio signal. If you use composite video, you need to provide an alternate means for audio, as discussed in the next section.

S-Video Format

S-Video is the next step up from composite video. It is sometimes called Super VHS or SVHS because its first widespread use was in SVHS videotape systems.

In composite video, the brightness (luminance or luma) and color (chrominance or chroma) signals are combined together, but in such a way that a black-and-white TV can separate them to ignore the color image. S-Video keeps the two signals separate and uncompromised. An S-Video cable actually has two smaller cables inside it, one for luma and one for chroma. This is important for DVD because the disc stores the luma and chroma signals separately—with S-Video we skip the steps of combining the chroma and luma in the player and that of separating them in the display. S-Video provides a sharper picture with better color rendition than composite video.

S-Video does not carry an audio signal. If you use S-Video, you need to provide an alternate means for audio.

Component Video Format

Component video is the next step above S-Video. Although S-Video separates luma and chroma, it still combines all the color information into a single chroma signal. Component format separates the video signal into three separate signals (and three separate wires) to avoid any quality loss from mixing signals. This is important for DVD because the disc stores chroma information in a component format—with component video, we skip the steps of combining the chroma information into a single chroma channel and then separating it back out in the display.

The most obvious component format is RGB (red, green, and blue). If you have been creating color images on a computer or have looked closely at the dot pattern on a television screen or computer monitor, you know that you can combine different amounts of red, green, and blue to create all other colors. An alternative form of component video uses signals of the form Y, B-Y, R-Y where Y is intensity or luma; this kind of format is also called YUV, YCbCr, or Y Pr Pb. Most players with a component output can switch between different forms of component output. Just be sure that the player you buy can output in the component form that your display requires.

Component video does not carry an audio signal. If you use component video, you need to provide an alternate means for audio.

Digital Video Format

The final video output, *digital video*, is not yet commercially available for DVD players, although there are DV cameras and other video appliances that can generate digital video and computers equipped with FireWire/IEEE 1394 digital video cards that can accept the output.

The issue with digital video is protecting copyrighted material; how to enforce copyright on a digital video stream coming from a DVD player.

Widescreen Video Display (4:3 and 16:9)

When you have successfully connected the video signal from your DVD player to your display, you still have some choices to make about how the video will be displayed, particularly for movies that were originally prepared for theatrical (rather than video) release.

The standard display format for conventional TV has a 4:3 aspect ratio; the width is one-third longer than the height. However, movies are shot with a widescreen aspect ratio for theatrical distribution, to be displayed on a movie screen that can be around twice as wide as it is high.

When you watch a movie prepared for widescreen on a standard narrow screen, something has to give: You cannot fit a wide rectangular peg (the movie) into a more nearly square hole (the conventional TV screen). The two most common ways of dealing with this are pan and scan, and letterbox. For *pan and scan*, the movie is converted from the widescreen format to a narrow screen format by panning a 4:3 window around in the widescreen frame, and trimming off the ends that are outside the window. For *letterbox*, the movie is converted to a 4:3 aspect ratio by shrinking it to fit within the 4:3 frame and then adding black bands above and below the video content. In letterbox, you see the entire scene, at reduced resolution on the screen. In pan and scan, you see only part of the scene, albeit at full-screen resolution; and you rely on the pan and scan operator to adjust the position of the 4:3 window to show the most important part of the action in the widescreen frame.

Prerecorded videotapes and broadcasts of theatrical movies frequently have a notice similar to the following:

This movie has been formatted to fit your TV screen.

The notice tells you that the movie already has been subjected to pan and scan reformatting to fit a standard 4:3 television screen size.

The preferred format for movies on DVD is the original, full widescreen picture at a 16:9 aspect ratio. Some movies also include a separate pan and scan version, typically manufactured with the two versions on the two sides of a disc, or on separate discs. But DVDs are designed to be displayed more than standard 4:3 television displays; they also can be viewed on the newer widescreen displays.

DVD players then can support multiple display types. For standard 4:3 television displays, DVD players will automatically letterbox a widescreen DVD so it will fit onscreen. For widescreen displays, higher-end DVD players scale the video output to fill the full display screen. Depending on the DVD player and connections, the player can do this automatically, or you may have to select the output video format from the setup menus.

If you are a video enthusiast with a widescreen home theater display, or are interested in becoming one, make sure you get a DVD player that supports the highest-quality video output format to your widescreen display.

Interlaced and Progressive Video Display (3-2 Pull-Down)

A second display issue concerns whether the pictures you are watching on DVD were originally created as television video or came from a movie shot on film. Television and movies actually are displayed at different rates: 30 pictures per second for NTSC video (the U.S. standard), and 24 pictures per second for film.

To avoid a flickering effect, television video is actually drawn onscreen at twice the rate. Television uses an *interlaced* scan: The screen is refreshed 60 times per second (at 60Hz), but only half of the lines in the picture are painted on each refresh. It takes two refresh cycles (two *fields*) to paint all the lines in a full video *frame*. The lines from the first field are interlaced, every other line, with the lines from the second to generate the full frame. Interlace is part of the legacy of the early TV standards—interlace made it possible to provide good quality, low-flicker displays of moving scenes within the bandwidth available in a TV channel.

However, technology has improved over the past 50 years. Your computer monitor most likely uses progressive scan: All of the lines are refreshed 60 times per second or faster. Progressive scan video displays for home entertainment also are available, although they are rather more expensive than interlaced displays. Progressive scan eliminates a number of the artifacts of interlaced displays, especially along moving edges and in narrow lines.

DVD discs are all prepared in an interlaced format for display on standard televisions, even for material that originates from film or from a progressive scan system. When film material is transferred to video, each full frame of film must be converted to interlaced formats, and the different frame rates also need to be adjusted, from 24 to 30 frames per second. The frame rate adjustment is called 3-2 pulldown, and it involves duplicating individual fields in a 3-2 pattern to spread them across the 30 frames/60 fields.

For DVD material that originated from film or a progressive scan system, the disc designer can put hints into the video stream that a properly equipped DVD player can use to convert the interlaced video back into progressive scan video. Because some discs may not contain such hints, or the hints may be incorrect, higher-end DVD players include the capability to automatically detect material with 3-2 pulldown and convert it to the original progressive format. You can see this happening after a cut in a movie to material with a different pulldown pattern, when the interlacing is visible for a moment and then the player snaps back into the correct progressive display.

Higher-end DVD players provide both standard interlaced video outputs and progressive outputs using component formats to widescreen and digital displays.

Hooking Up Audio Signals

None of the video signal types carry any audio signals, with the exception of RF. For all the higher-quality formats, you will need to connect separate cables from your DVD player, either to a television equipped with separate audio inputs or to an audio system for a better stereo or surround-sound experience (refer to Figure 2.5).

The audio signal types in common use are

- RF
- Analog stereo (line level)
- Analog stereo (headphone)
- Multichannel analog
- Digital Audio

If you do not have a separate audio system, and your TV only has antenna inputs, you will need to use an RF video/audio hookup to your TV.

Audio Signals and Connectors

The types of connectors that you are likely to see on the back of your DVD player and audio system include the familiar phono and headphone jacks for analog audio, and a variety of additional connectors for digital audio signals:

- RCA phono: (Analog/Digital)
- Headphone: (Analog)
- SCART: (Analog)
- BNC: (Analog/Digital)
- Firewire/IEEE 1394: (Digital)
- Toslink fiberoptic: (Digital)

Analog audio is most often connected using RCA phono plugs and jacks, although some high-end systems use the more-expensive BNC connectors and some European systems use SCART connectors that combine analog audio and video on one connector. If your audio system and DVD player do not have the same type of connectors, you will need to purchase cables with the appropriate connectors or adapters between different types of connectors.

Popular means for connecting digital audio signals include coaxial cable—the same type used for video connections, IEEE 1394, the digital interface standard also used for DV camcorders, and Toslink (a fiber optic digital interface standard).

If your systems use coaxial cable for digital audio connections, the connectors could be either phono or BNC. If your systems use IEEE-1394 or Toslink, the connectors are standard.

Analog Audio Formats

Most DVD players have Left and Right stereo audio outputs that can be connected to conventional analog stereo systems. These connections are Line level, intended for interconnecting equipment, and without the amplification required to connect to speakers.

In addition, the right and left audio channels can be encoded for Dolby Surround audio. Dolby Surround is a method to achieve surround sound with conventional analog audio signals. It requires Dolby Surround Pro Logic decoder support in the audio amplifier to extract the additional channels. Using clever signal-processing tricks, Dolby Surround encodes two extra channels into the right and left channels, so you still hear two-channel stereo when played back through a conventional stereo system. However, if your audio system is equipped with a Dolby Surround Pro Logic decoder, it will extract the two additional channels: center and surround.

The additional channels go to the Front Center speakers that are between the left and right channels and the Rear speaker behind you to provide an enhanced listening environment: Sound will move more smoothly from right to left and can also move from front to back. However, because there is only one channel in the rear, all sound motion from front to back will seem to originate or terminate at the rear center.

Surround-Sound Audio Formats

The DVD-Video standard supports the use of several different digital audio formats:

- Dolby Digital (AC-3)
- MPEG-2
- Linear PCM (LPCM)
- Digital Theater Systems (DTS)
- Sony Dynamic Digital Sound (SDDS)

Not all players must support all formats, and not all discs must include all formats. NTSC format discs are required to provide at least one audio track in Dolby Digital or PCM. PAL/SECAM discs are required to provide at least one audio track of Dolby Digital, MPEG-2, or PCM. Of course, discs then can include additional audio tracks in alternate formats.

In practice, *Dolby Digital* (also called AC-3) is used for audio tracks on most discs. Dolby Digital supports audio with one to five channels, plus a Sub-Woofer channel for carrying low bass sounds. The five channels are Front Left, Front Center, Front Right, Back Left (or Left Surround), and Back Right (or Right Surround). Full surround-sound Dolby Digital is referred to as *5.1* (for *5* channels plus *.1* for the low-frequency channel). DVD discs typically have stereo or 5.1-channel Dolby Digital audio.

The *DTS* (Digital Theater Systems) surround-sound system is used in many movie theaters around the world, but it is an optional format for DVD. The *SDDS* (Sony Dynamic Digital Sound) format also is supported in the DVD-Video standard, but has not been used in practice.

These digital audio formats stored on DVD discs can then be passed directly to an external surround-sound audio system that can process the encoded audio signal, or they can be converted in the DVD player to analog formats that can be played on conventional audio systems.

Downmixing and Virtual Surround Sound

In a fully equipped home theater environment, you can play surround-sound DVDs through a high-end audio system (see the next section). But even with simpler audio setups, you still can experience higher-quality DVD audio.

If you do not have a surround-sound audio system, DVD players can downmix the DVD soundtrack to two-channel analog stereo, with or without Dolby Surround, so the DVD can be played on a television or stereo system.

Some DVD players, as well as some DVD player software, also offer virtual surround-sound processing. This feature creates a simulated surround-sound effect which can be played on two speakers, and also is especially effective with stereo headphones.

Digital Audio Formats

Some DVD players also include built-in Dolby Digital and DTS decoders, which extract the 5.1 audio channels so they can be output directly as six analog audio signals (typically labeled Front L/R, Center, Surround L/R, and Sub-Woofer). These then can be connected to an external audio amplifier with 5.1-channel inputs.

Many DVD players also provide the option to connect a digital audio signal directly from the DVD player to an external audio system. Depending on the design of the specific DVD disc and the internal settings of your DVD player, the digital audio output of the player is typically PCM, Dolby Digital, or DTS. Formats such as DTS and SDDS are optional for the DVD format, and need not be included on a disc or player. The digital connection can be used for basic stereo audio or Dolby Pro Logic, or for 5.1-channel surround-sound audio.

If you are an audio enthusiast with a surround-sound audio system, then be sure to verify that a new DVD player supports both the audio formats and the external connections used in your audio system.

Playing a DVD: Control and Status Functions

Control and status are the inputs and outputs that let us see what a player is doing and to tell it to do something different. The DVD standards have provisions for many control and navigational features—many of them optional. Although your DVD player may not incorporate all of the features in the standards, you still need to be able to select, control, and monitor those that it does.

Most DVD players have a front panel with a status display and a set of buttons for basic control: Power on/off, Open/Close to load and eject a disc; and basic VCR-type controls including Play, Stop, and Pause. Even more than set-top players, portable DVD players need a full range of controls built in to the player so that they can be operated without requiring a separate remote control (see Figure 2.6).

FIGURE 2.6

Sample built-in controls for a portable DVD player: The Panasonic DVD-LA95 PalmTheater Portable DVD-Audio/Video Player. The controls include buttons for menu, mode, and volume control; a shuttle dial, and menu cursor control; and playback controls.

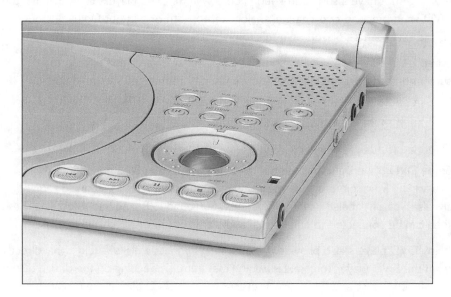

However, the potential feature set of a DVD player is very rich, and a DVD disc can also incorporate disc-specific features. Hence, it is difficult to provide front panel control for all the features in a typical player. Instead, set-top DVD players include a multibutton remote control to access most of the control functions, and use an onscreen display for interaction with most of the status functions using onscreen menus (see Figure 2.7). Portable DVD players typically include smaller remote controls with fewer keys (see Figure 2.8).

T I P

It is important to note that DVD controls are not completely standardized. The control and status functions here are illustrative only; the functions in your player might be organized differently, and the disc you are playing might change the way the functions for your player are accessed.

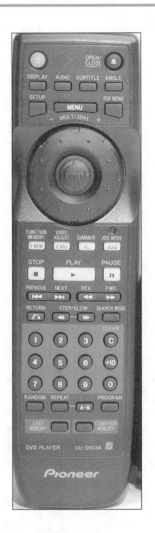

FIGURE 2.7

Sample remote control for set-top DVD player: The Pioneer Elite DV-47A DVD Video Player.

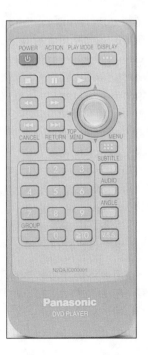

FIGURE 2.8

Sample remote control for a portable DVD player: The Panasonic DVD-LA95 PalmTheater Portable DVD-Audio/Video Player, with basic menu and playback controls.

Basic Player Functions

The first control to use with a DVD player is to press the Power button to turn on the player. You also need to turn on the television to which the DVD player is connected, as well as any external audio system. This also may require switching the TV and audio system to the correct video and audio inputs.

The status display on the front panel of the DVD player typically displays a power-on message, followed by a prompt to load a disc. But even before inserting a disc, your DVD player should display its own startup menu on the TV monitor. This allows you to select various player setup functions, including video and audio configuration, parental locks, and languages (see following). The default setup typically is designed for hooking your player directly to a television set.

To insert a DVD (or CD) disc, press the Open/Close button to slide out the disc tray. Insert the disc, and press the button or tray to close it. The player then starts spinning up the disc to read its contents. When the player recognizes the type of the disc (for example, DVD-Video, Audio CD, or Video CD), and begins to read and play the contents, it typically displays an indication on the status display or as an onscreen text display. It may even display the disc name, which is typically an abbreviation of the movie title.

At this point, the DVD that you inserted takes control of your player. The intent of the DVD specification is that all further interaction is controlled by the contents of the disc, as determined when the disc was designed and authored. The interaction includes navigating the DVD menus, skipping between marked chapter points, and possibly even using buttons overlaid on motion video. For example, to change the language of the soundtrack or turn on the subtitles, you typically need to navigate to an Options menu provided by the DVD author.

The DVD designer can specify the *first play* element on the DVD, the initial clip or menu displayed when the disc is inserted in a player. The first thing you see at the beginning of a commercial DVD is typically not the movie, but legal material, such as the FBI warning. You usually cannot even skip through this material because DVDs can be authored to disable the play controls. Commercial DVDs then may include other promotional materials, such as trailers for other movies.

Finally, the playback will arrive at the main menu of the DVD. This menu typically can be accessed directly from anywhere on the DVD by pressing the Main Menu or Top Menu buttons on the DVD remote control, or often the front panel (this is also often called the Title menu).

To actually play the DVD movie, then, you still need to activate the Play Movie entry on the main menu. This is typically the default menu selection, so you only need to press the Enter button, which is often placed in the center of the navigational controls on the remote control.

The DVD will then jump to the beginning of the movie and start playing it. For widescreen movies, this typically involves changing the display format from standard 4:3 aspect ratio (for the menus) to widescreen format (or letterboxed on a standard TV display).

DVD remote controls typically contain a full complement of buttons, including playback controls, menu navigation, and other DVD player options. The front panels of DVD players usually contain fewer controls, but more players are now including at least the basic playback controls (Skip Forward/Reverse, Pause) and the menu navigation controls so that you can start the DVD playing without requiring the remote control. Of course, for portable players, it is even more important to have a full complement of controls on the player itself, so that a separate remote is not required.

Navigation with DVD Menus

Although the DVD-Video format is fully specified, controls and menus vary widely from player to player; and there is no standard for the layout of the remote control or the onscreen menus. Similarly, although there are common conventions for the layout of the menus for commercial movies on DVD, the final navigational structure, terms used, and graphical design are completely determined by the DVD designer as the disc is authored.

As described in the later chapters on DVD authoring, this navigational structure is a key element of authoring a DVD. With the introductory authoring tools, the navigation can be generated automatically, whereas the more professional tools provide complete control of customizing both the look and the linkage between menus, buttons, and clips.

However, because the basic structure of the disc is visible to the DVD player, it can offer an alternate method of exploring the disc. One of the great advantages of playing a DVD on a computer has been this capability to view the titles, chapters, and tracks on a DVD (see Part II). Set-top DVD players also are adding more of this kind of functionality—to browse the contents of the disc independently of the actual menu structure.

Selecting Buttons

The DVD format is designed to work from a main menu, which is the first thing displayed when you start playing the disc (after some possible introductory material), and can be accessed using the Top Menu/Main Menu button. The disc typically returns to it automatically after it finishes playing back each main section.

The main menu, generated by the kinds of automated authoring tools described in the following chapters, typically is used to access a collection of clips stored on the disc. The main menu then contains a button for each clip, with a thumbnail image of the first frame of the clip. Because a DVD can contain many more than the six or eight clips that can conveniently fit on one TV screen, the main menu can link to additional menus with more clips by using the Next and Previous arrows, or it can contain buttons that act like folders to additional menus of clips organized in a hierarchy.

To navigate this kind of structure, you need a method of selecting individual buttons and then activating them to jump to the associated menu or clip. When playing a DVD on a computer that uses DVD player software, this is as easy as moving the mouse cursor over the button and then clicking. On DVD players and remote controls, you move through the buttons using a navigational pad, with the Up/ Down/Left/Right arrow buttons (see Figure 2.9). Again, even the order in which these buttons move through the buttons on the menu is defined by the DVD author.

FIGURE 2.9

Sample DVD menu navigation controls from the Panasonic DVD-LA95 Palm Theater Portable DVD-Audio/Video Player. Press the edges to move Up/ Down/Left/Right, or the center to activate the current menu selection.

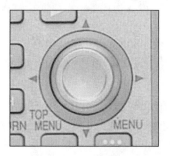

As you cycle through the available buttons on a menu, the currently selected button should highlight in some fashion, typically by changing color or by showing an outline around the button. To activate the button and perform the associated action, press the Enter button on the remote control, which is usually located in the middle of the cursor buttons.

Moving Between Menus

Because DVD menus are typically organized in a nested, hierarchical structure, the DVD format provides for a few special navigational buttons that can be used for moving back up the menu tree (see Figure 2.10).

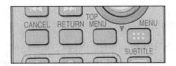

FIGURE 2.10

Sample dedicated DVD menu controls from the Panasonic DVD-LA95 Palm Theater Portable DVD-Audio/Video Player.

Top Menu or *Main Menu* (or *Title*) jumps to the original top-most menu that is displayed when you first play the DVD. It should provide access to all DVD content and features.

Return is intended to return back to the most recent menu from which the current menu was accessed, but may not be implemented in many DVD discs.

Menu (or *Root*) is intended to jump to the main menu of the current section of the disc (such as Special Features). However, this use is totally at the discretion of the DVD designer.

The usefulness of the Return and Menu buttons depend on the organization of the menu structure of each specific DVD, and on whether their uses were defined consistently by the DVD author.

DVD Menus and Alternate Tracks

The DVD menu structure for most commercial movies follows some general conventions. These conventions provide access to not only the movie content, but to playback options such as alternate languages and subtitles.

See Chapter 6, "Playing DVDs on Macintosh OS X," and Chapter 7, "Playing DVDs in Windows XP," for examples of DVD menus and alternate chapters.

The main menu for commercial movies typically contains the following entries:

- **Play Movie** jumps to the movie and begins playing it from the beginning.

- **Scene Index** displays a series of menus with thumbnail buttons for each chapter or key scene in the movie. Much like the menus produced by automated DVD authoring tools, these menus permit you to jump directly to a specific scene, and you can watch the movie from that point to the end.

- **Special Features** links to a menu providing access to ancillary material such as movie trailers, "Making Of" documentaries, and cast biographies. This option sometimes includes the option to watch the movie with an alternate soundtrack, in which the director or other principals provide commentary on the movie.

- **Setup** links to a menu that provides access to alternate tracks of material associated with the movie on the DVD. This option can include alternate audio formats, such as Dolby Digital 5.1 surround sound; alternate audio tracks with different languages; and subtitle text, again in different languages.

These DVD playback options can also be controlled by the DVD player setup menu and by dedicated keys on the remote control.

Movie Playback Controls

DVD playback controls include basic VCR-like controls for moving through the movie like a long sequential tape, plus the capability to skip directly between different chapters and tracks (see Figure 2.11).

The status display on the front panel of the DVD player typically also displays information about the currently playing material, such as the chapter number and elapsed time. Many DVD players also offer additional onscreen menus to display information as you control the disc or skip between chapters and tracks.

FIGURE 2.11

Sample DVD playback controls from the Panasonic DVD-LA95 PalmTheater Portable DVD-Audio/Video Player. These include Play, Scan, and Chapter Skip.

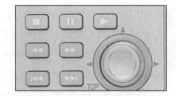

VCR Controls

The basic VCR controls include *Play*, *Pause*, and *Stop*. Pause freezes the playback at the current point; you can then press Play to resume. With DVD, the quality of the frozen image is very high, clear, and crisp without the artifacts that we are accustomed to on a VCR.

Stop cancels playback, and acts like rewinding a VCR tape. When you press Play, the movie playback restarts at the beginning. Because this kind of behavior can be unbelievably irritating if you accidentally stop or eject a disc, more players (and DVD software) are now adding the capability to remember your last playback point, and offer you the option to resume from there.

Also like VCRs, DVD players offer the capability to scan through the disc—moving forward and backward, fast and slow motion, and even stepping frame by frame. Skipping around and moving in reverse though a DVD is somewhat complicated because of the way the MPEG-2 compression used for the video divides the material into groups of frames, but newer players now support a great deal of flexibility with these features.

Scan or *Search Forward* and *Reverse* skip rapidly through the video, typically offering a range of speeds up to 100 times normal speed, or even more. Audio is typically muted, but some players can provide audio as well.

Slow Motion Forward and *Reverse* move slower than normal speed through the video, again typically offering a range of speeds.

When paused, *Step Forward* and *Reverse* move frame-by-frame through the video, so you can examine each still frame.

Some DVD players offer a joystick or circular jog/shuttle control for controlling moving through the video at variable speeds.

DVD Chapter Controls

DVDs, like CDs, are more than just one long sequence of material. On CDs, the audio is organized into individual songs, and on DVDs the content is organized into title sets and chapters—with each title consisting of one or more chapters. Typically, the movie is stored as one title. Other ancillary material, such as movie trailers, are typically stored in separate title sets, which are accessible through the main menu.

Skip Forward and *Reverse* jump directly to the beginning of the previous or next chapter in the current title, so you can jump directly between each major scene.

Some players also have a provision for selecting a particular chapter by entering a number on the remote control keypad.

DVD Display Controls

DVD players are starting to add video and audio effects and enhancements, accessed through the setup menu (see following).

In addition, some players now offer a Zoom function that lets you interactively magnify the image on the screen, which is similar to the digital zoom feature on digital cameras and camcorders. This can be particularly interesting in conjunction with the Pause function: You can pause on a particular frame and then zoom in on a particular part of the image.

Alternate Track Playback Controls

Because the alternate audio and subtitle tracks are well-defined in the DVD format, especially for use in selecting a different language, it is also possible to select the alternate tracks directly from the remote control, instead of needing to use the setup menu provided by the DVD developer (see Figure 2.12). In addition, you can skip between alternate video angles or tracks if they are provided on the DVD.

FIGURE 2.12

Sample alternate DVD track controls from the Panasonic DVD-LA95 Palm Theater Portable DVD-Audio/Video Player.

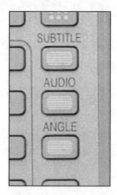

DVD remote controls typically provide dedicated buttons for these three features:

- **Subtitle** alternates between the different text subtitle tracks available on the current section of the DVD. These tracks typically include different languages.

- **Audio** alternates between the different audio tracks available on the current section of the DVD. These tracks can include different languages and other tracks, such as the director's commentary.

- **Angle** alternates between the different video tracks available on the current section of the DVD. This feature was designed for content, such as music performances, in which you can switch between different camera angles to see different views of the performance.

Player Setup Menus

The Setup menu on a DVD player is typically more complex than the setup function on a VCR because the DVD player can do a lot more. The setup function menus include options for selecting the default languages, configuring the video and audio outputs, and enhancing the video and audio (optional). See Chapter 6 for examples of DVD menus.

All of these options are set for the DVD player itself by using its internal setup menu, which is accessed when no DVD disc is inserted in the player, or when the player is stopped.

Output Formats and Connections

If you are connecting your DVD player to home theater equipment, such as a widescreen display or a digital or surround-sound audio system, then you need to use the Setup menus of the DVD player to configure the appropriate audio and video outputs. Although the DVD player may have numerous connectors on the back panel, not all are active at the same time, and different kinds of signals can be generated on the same connector.

For video output, setup options include normal 4:3 or widescreen 16:9 aspect ratio (or pan and scan) output formats.

For audio output, setup options include defining the digital output to your audio system; selecting formats, such as Dolby Digital and DTS; and deciding whether the output is the raw encoded bitstream, or decoded and downconverted by the DVD player to PCM format. The audio setup can also include defining the speaker configuration in your room to balance the sound.

Multilanguage Support

The DVD format has strong support for authoring multilingual titles; with audio tracks, subtitles, and the menus prepared in several different languages. As discussed previously, DVDs are typically authored with a Setup menu that you can use to choose the language for the audio and subtitles, which also is useful for practicing foreign language skills. DVD players and remote controls also offer Audio and Subtitle buttons that can be used to cycle through the available tracks.

Language support in the DVD format goes even deeper, however. The DVD standard specifies unique codes to identify a wide range of specific languages, so the DVD author can explicitly mark material on the disc with its associated language. You can then use the Setup menu in the DVD player itself to select a preferred language. Properly authored DVDs then automatically play with the appropriate language for menus, the audio track, and even subtitles.

Ratings Level Support

The DVD format also supports a parental lock feature to prohibit the DVD player from playing DVD discs with more mature material. This feature is optional, and depends on DVD discs being properly marked with an appropriate ratings level and then using the Setup menu in the DVD player to restrict the playback of movies above a specified level.

Using a password to protect the setting, you can set a level in the player corresponding to a maturity level (that is, G to PG to R to NC-17). Any discs with a classification higher than the level you set will not play in the player, unless you know the password to override the setting. You can also set the level so there is no limit imposed, or to prohibit any disc without a rating (although this prevents viewing discs that you have authored on a computer).

It even is possible to author discs that support multiple classifications: The disc recognizes what the player setting is and then plays back a version of the film that is compatible with the classification. For example, a disc that is nominally rated as R might skip or substitute some scenes or dialog when the disc is played back on a player configured as PG. Even though this ratings feature is part of the DVD standard, the disc classification is voluntary on the part of the disc producer. This feature is not widely used, due in no small part to the complexity of authoring.

Enhanced Video and Audio Features

As DVD players become more sophisticated, they offer additional features for enhancing the video display and audio experience. Many of these features have become common in software players when viewing DVDs on personal computers, and are now appearing in set-top players.

DVD players can provide TV-like controls and image-processing options for improving the video display. These options include individual picture controls (such as brightness, color, contrast, and sharpness), as well as more general enhancements to improve the film image in a living room viewing environment (including enhancing the dark areas to bring out more detail).

DVD players can offer several options for boosting and clarifying movie audio. These include dynamic range adjustment to expand or reduce the range of volume (that is, for late-night viewing); bass boost for subwoofer output, even with two-channel sound; and dialog enhancement to boost the center channel, in which most dialog is located, to make it easier to hear.

For DVD players that can play DVD-Audio discs, the Setup menu can offer an option to play the DVD-Audio content or show the corresponding DVD-Video content that is also usually included on the discs.

Summary

As you have seen, even inexpensive consumer DVD players can support a plethora of disc formats, audio and video connections, and sophisticated controls for interacting with disc content.

Most recent DVD players support prerecorded DVD movies, CD albums, and Video-CD material; as well as recordable CD-R/RW, and at least recordable DVD-R/+R for desktop DVD authoring. New players are adding support for rewritable DVD-RW/+RW formats, and some support DVD-RAM (under the DVD-Multi label). For audio fans, widespread support for MP3 on CD enables storing large libraries on a single CD, as does new support for Windows Media Audio. And for audiophiles, DVD-Audio and SACD offer high-quality surround-sound music.

DVD players also offer a wide range of options for connecting to external displays and audio systems. You can simply connect to the auxiliary input on your television, play audio on your stereo system, or grow into a full home theatre experience with a widescreen television and digital 5.1 surround-sound audio.

After you have your DVD player installed, it is time to play a movie. But beyond just playing a sequential movie, the DVD format provides for interactive menus; random access by chapters; and alternate viewing of video camera angles, audio tracks, and subtitles. All these options are typically controlled by options in the DVD's menu structure, which are created by the DVD designer when the disc is authored. Although DVD remote controls contain dedicated buttons that can be used to move through the menu hierarchy and dynamically change between alternate tracks, some DVD players also offer additional options to view and explore the structure of DVD discs.

Chapter 3 explores set-top units that both play and record to DVD discs. You can use them to replace a VCR for watching off-air programs at a later time, and to transfer your own video to DVD discs to save and archive.

But to really understand the DVD format, the way DVDs are typically designed, and the structure of DVD discs, the best approach is to play and explore DVD movies on a personal computer, as described in Part II.

Using a DVD player software application, you can explore the organization of a disc into title sets and chapters, see the entire navigational structure, and jump directly to any part of the disc. And if you are interested, you also can explore the physical format of the disc to see the folders and data files used for the various formats.

Then, starting in Part III, "Automated DVD Authoring," you can move on to create your own productions on DVD or CD to play on computers and on set-top players.

Consumer DVD Recorders:
Recordable Formats

Set-top DVD-Video players, as described in Chapter 2, "Consumer DVD Players: DVD Video and Audio," have exploded in popularity in the past few years for playing movies, as the DVD player has joined the VCR next to the television in many households. DVD-ROM drives also are becoming common on desktop and laptop computers for playing and exploring movies, as described in Part II, "Exploring DVDs on Your Computer."

Just as CD-R/RW recordable drives have become commonplace, playback-only computer DVD drives are evolving into DVD burners that can be used for authoring DVD productions on the desktop, as described beginning in Part III, "Automated DVD Authoring."

But the DVD format still has more applications in consumer electronics—in DVD video recorders and even DVD camcorders. After all, shuffling videotapes in set-top VCRs is getting old, especially when you accidentally record over a show. And the new all-digital video recorders with hard disks, such as TiVo (www.tivo.com) and SONICblue ReplayTV (www.SONICblue.com), are great for grabbing your favorite shows during the week, but then you have to watch them all soon after or else end up erasing them to make room for the next week's shows.

DVD recorders would seem to promise an unbeatable combination in one box (see Figure 3.1): high-quality recording to digital discs combined with removable media that you can save to watch later—and for prices that have dropped under $1,000. And beyond consolidating a VCR and DVD player into one unit, DVD recorders also offer other possibilities. In addition to recording TV shows off the air, you can record your own home videos to DVD, from analog or digital camcorders, or from your old videotapes. You also can play the discs that you record on other DVD players and on computer DVD drives. Because the video is in digital format, there is even the possibility of editing it on a computer.

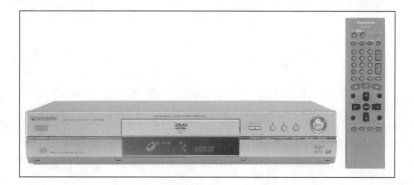

Some newer DVD recorders also include both a hard disk and a DVD burner. This enables you to capture material to the hard disk—even when no DVD media is loaded—and then copy shows or clips to a DVD disc to watch later.

However, the potential of DVD recorders is limited by the continued confusion over different DVD formats, and even different usage modes for individual formats. The different formats impose trade-offs between capability and compatibility because supporting cool random-access recording features limits the ability to play the discs on other DVD systems.

But even with these issues, the current generation of DVD video recorders offers compelling features for time-shifting and saving videos on DVD discs. Just be sure you understand the different capabilities provided by the competing formats, and how they fit with your anticipated needs. Although these products are also new and still developing, they also are beginning to move down the aggressive price-reduction curve that DVD players have followed.

This chapter explores the capabilities of DVD recorders for recording broadcasts, copying existing tapes to disc, and organizing your own collections of clips. If you are eager to buy a recorder, it begins with a quick-start section containing a checklist for what to look for when buying a new DVD recorder. The chapter then describes the common capabilities of DVD recorders for recording, playback, and editing. Finally, it reviews the capabilities and differences between three example recorders based on the different DVD formats.

Quick Start: Buying a DVD Recorder

Or, forget the details; I'm going to the electronics store this afternoon...

If you are in a hurry to get a DVD recorder and do not want to spend the time to read this chapter first, then you can use this section as a summary and checklist of issues to think about when looking at your different options.

The following is a checklist of some important topics to consider when purchasing a set-top DVD recorder:

As a video recorder:

- What types of disc formats will it record?

- Does it record to a recordable write-once (R) media for permanent archiving?

- Does it provide convenient controls for recording broadcast shows (for example, program timers)?

- Does it interface well with your existing television and VCR?

- Does it support recording from different types of external sources (VCR and camcorders)?

- Does it provide high-quality analog and digital connections for audio and video, including DV/IEEE 1394?

- How flexible is the interface for erasing and reusing available space on a disc?

- What range of recording times and quality levels can you select?

- What is the quality in the different recording modes?

As a DVD player (see the preceding chapter):

- What types of discs will it play?

- Is it compatible with my audio and video systems?

- What types of video output formats are supported?

- What types of audio output formats are supported?

- What high-end video- and audio-processing features do you want?

- What advanced playback controls do you want?

As a DVD editor and authoring tool:

- What kind of index menu does it create?

- Does the index menu include thumbnail images of clips?

- What kind of information does it display automatically?

- Can you edit titles, or select the thumbnail images?

- Are the chapter points added automatically, at regular intervals, or manually?

- What is the interface for editing the clip list?

- Can you rearrange the order, hide and unhide, to create playlists?

- Can you delete clips and reuse the space?

- What is the process for using a disc on a regular DVD player?

- Does the disc need to be "finalized" or "adapted" first?

- How long does this take?

- Are there restrictions on the amount of material on the discs?

- What is the process for using discs recorded on other machines?

- Is there some "adaptation" process required to convert the format?

- What are the tradeoffs between editing capabilities and compatibility?

- Do you loose edits when the disc is viewed on regular players?

DVD Recording and Playback

DVD recorders combine the off-air recording capabilities of VCRs with the playback capabilities of DVD players. Besides the differences in disc formats, DVD recorders also are differentiated by the range of features for these basic functions.

Recording Live Broadcasts

Like VCRs, DVD recorders include a built-in television and cable tuner for recording live broadcasts. They include the capability to schedule timed recordings, as well as features, such as VCR Plus+, to simplify timer recording. Also like tape-based recorders, they typically offer a range of recording times, typically ranging from one to six hours, with a corresponding trade-off in image quality due to the reduced data rate.

Unlike videotapes, however, DVD recorders offer "one-touch" recording because they can start recording instantly, without the need to fast-forward or position a tape (as long as there is available unused space on the disc). Even better, the playback can be instant too, without having to wait to rewind a tape. Using DVD menus, you can jump directly to a program on the disc; and using chapter points, you can skip rapidly though clips, without needing to visually scan through a tape to find it.

Recording External Video

Even though DVD recorders work with digital video, they typically provide analog video and audio inputs for recording from analog sources, such as a VCR or an 8mm camcorder. In addition, many recorders provide a FireWire interface (also called i.Link or IEEE 1394) to input digital video from a DV or Digital8 camcorder, or other FireWire source (such as your video-editing computer).

DVD recorders use the same digital media formats as commercial DVDs, including MPEG-2 for video and (often) Dolby Digital AC-3 for stereo audio. They include hardware to convert the input video to these compressed formats in real-time. The range of supported bit rates and quality depends on the specific player. Some use basic CBR (constant bit rate) video compression; others provide VBR (variable bit rate) compression, which can adjust dynamically to the complexity of the video to provide better quality (for example, they use fewer bits in relatively static scenes, and use more bits in segments with fast motion or high detail).

DVD Player Features and Connections

Because DVD recorders also are DVD players, they can play various prerecorded and recordable DVD and CD formats, as described in Chapter 2. Recorders can include the same range of advanced player features, such as progressive scan video output, and built-in Dolby Digital and DTS (Digital Theatre System) audio decoders.

Hooking up a DVD recorder is like hooking up a VCR—with video input signals to record and video outputs to display. But as described in Chapter 2, DVD players and recorders support higher-quality video and audio connections than you may be used to finding on a VCR—and particularly digital signal connections.

The back panel of a typical DVD recorder (see Figure 3.2) typically includes not only traditional RF television connections, but also component video and S-Video connections, and coaxial and optical digital audio connections.

FIGURE 3.2

Rear panel connections for a DVD recorder. Courtesy of Pioneer Corporation.

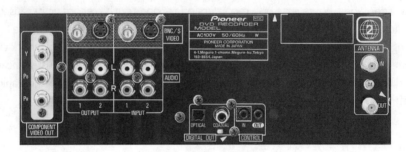

The various connectors for a sample DVD recorder are identified in Figure 3.3.

FIGURE 3.3

Example of rear panel connections for a DVD recorder (Pioneer DVR-7000 recorder).

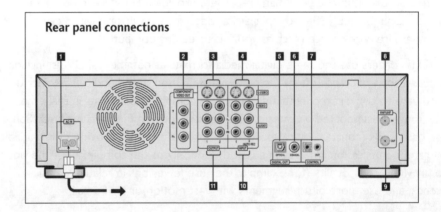

Rear panel connections

1 AC POWER IN

2 COMPONENT VIDEO OUT—Video connection to TV or monitor.

3 S-VIDEO OUTPUT 1, 2—Higher-quality video connection to TV, monitor, or AV receiver.

4 S-VIDEO INPUT 1, 2—For recording from a camcorder, VCR, or other video source with S-Video output.

5 DIGITAL OUT OPTICAL—Digital audio optical connection to an AV receiver or Dolby Digital/DTS decoder.

6 DIGITAL OUT COAXIAL—Digital audio coaxial connection to an AV receiver or Dolby Digital/DTS decoder.

7 CONTROL IN /OUT—For connecting to other A/V components.

8 VHF/UHF IN—Television input from TV antenna.

9 VHF/UHF OUT—Pass through the VHF/UHF television input to TV or monitor.

10 AUDIO/VIDEO INPUT 1, 2/AUTO REC—Additional audio/video input for recording from a camcorder, VCR, satellite receiver, or other equipment.

11 AUDIO/VIDEO OUTPUT 1, 2—Additional audio/video input for connecting to the A/V inputs of a TV, monitor, AV receiver, or other equipment.

DVD recorders also often provide FireWire/IEEE 1394 connectors for connecting to DV digital video camcorders (see Figure 3.4). The FireWire connection permits you to transfer from your DV camcorder and record to DVD, and also to edit clips on DVD and then transfer and record the results back to DV tape.

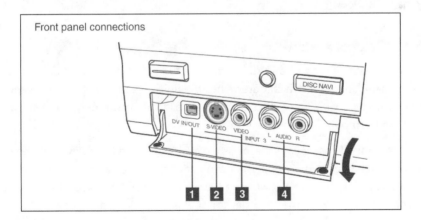

FIGURE 3.4

Example of front panel connections for a DVD recorder (Pioneer DVR-7000 recorder).

1 DV IN/OUT JACK—FireWire/IEEE 1394 interface for connecting a DV digital camcorder.

2 S-VIDEO INPUT (INPUT 3)—Additional S-Video input.

3 VIDEO INPUT (INPUT 3)—Additional composite video input.

4 AUDIO L/R (INPUT 3)—Additional analog stereo audio input.

DVD Menus and Editing

For convenient access to your clips during recording and playback, DVD recorders can create a DVD menu on the discs. Menus can include the channel number and time that a clip was captured, a name or title entered by the user, and any additional information available to the recorder (such as the station identification and program name). Even better, some recorders can automatically create index menus with thumbnail images of each segment on the disc. These menus are also tremendously useful when you take the discs created on these DVD recorders and play them on regular DVD players or computer DVD drives.

When using rewritable discs, DVD recorders can provide editing features for the clips that you record on a disc, depending on the disc and recording format. You can delete a clip, of course, and rearrange the order of the clip in the disc index. With some formats, you can append to a clip, divide a clip, or add additional chapter points within a clip.

You also can create a playlist to play through some of the clips in a specified order. This does not require moving the clips on disc; it just creates a list of clips to play in a specified order.

Some recorders can store the date and time of recorded digital video along with the video as DVD subtitle tracks, so that you can choose to view them when you play back the video.

DVD Compatibility

The fundamental feature of a DVD recorder is the set of recordable DVD disc formats that it supports, which determines the flexibility of the recorder in editing clips and the compatibility of discs that you record with other DVD players, both set-top and computer.

If you are primarily using your player as a digital VCR to temporarily save shows that you watch later in the week, then compatibility with other players is not a big issue. You then should use a rewritable format (RW or RAM—see Figure 3.5), and focus on the flexibility of the recorder for accessing, erasing, and adding shows on a disc.

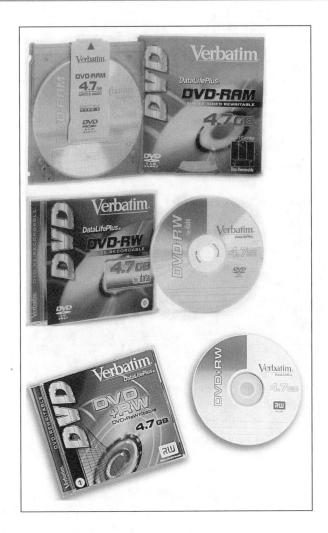

FIGURE 3.5

ReWritable DVD media: DVD-RAM, DVD-RW, and DVD+RAM.

If you also intend to use your recorder to copy existing videotapes to DVD—to have digital copies to save and share—then you want the discs to be playable on other set-top and computer DVD players. In this case, no matter what rewritable format the recorder supports, you should use a write-once recordable format (R—see Figure 3.6) so that your recordings are permanent and the discs cannot be erased accidentally. These formats should be compatible with most DVD players—more than the rewritable formats.

FIGURE 3.6

Recordable DVD
media: DVD-R
and DVD+R.

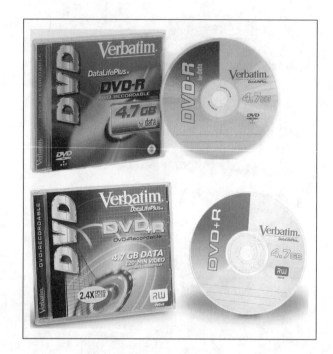

The format issue, then, gets more difficult when you want the best of both worlds: the ability to edit a disc after it is recorded, but with some expectation that it can be played on other regular DVD players. The choice of formats then depends on your needs and preferences, and the intended use of the player.

DVD-R/RW Recorders

Pioneer Electronics (www.pioneerelectronics.com) has been the driving force behind the original DVD-R/RW formats. Pioneer introduced the first DVD-R burners to support professional DVD authoring several years ago, and kick-started desktop DVD authoring with new generations of low-cost burners for general use in 2001 that have been bundled by computer manufacturers, including Apple and Compaq.

Pioneer launched its first DVD-R/RW recorder for the U.S. market, the Pioneer Elite DVR-7000, in fall 2001 (see Figure 3.7). This was a video-enthusiast product—with high-end features including a time base corrector and progressive scan output—at a cost of $2,000 (MSRP). Pioneer also launched a professional DVD-R/RW recorder, the PRV-9000, for $2,050 in November 2001.

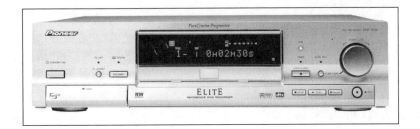

FIGURE 3.7

Pioneer Elite DVR-7000 DVD-RW/DVD-R recorder.

These units support two recording modes: a Video mode for both DVD-R and -RW for best compatibility with DVD players; and a Video Recording (VR) mode that provides more editing flexibility for rewritable DVD-RW discs, but with less compatibility.

When using a DVD-R disc, you can keep recording until the disc is full or until you finalize (close and complete) the disc. When using a DVD-RW disc, you can free up space by erasing the last title recorded on the disc.

Discs include a text-only title list menu, from which you can play, name, and erase clips; and record additional clips. After the disc is finalized, this becomes the main menu for playing the contents of the DVD.

Video Mode—DVD-R/RW

Video mode recordings are playable on regular DVD players (after finalizing), but have limited recording and editing features.

The Video mode recording on the DVR-7000 offers two picture quality/recording time settings: one hour at high quality or two hours at standard quality.

You can erase clips from the disc menu after recording in Video mode. The material is still present on the disc, but it is not accessible from the menu.

Video Recording (VR) Mode—DVD-RW

Video Recording (VR) mode can be used only on DVD-RW discs. The recordings can be extensively edited, but are not playable on most regular DVD players.

VR mode recording offers two recording options: two hours for standard play or a manual setting mode with 32 quality/time settings (between one and six hours).

In VR mode, you can use a visual disc navigation mode to view your clips as thumbnails, create a playlist, rearrange clips, enter titles, erase clips, and add chapter points. You can also view a visual index of chapters within each clip. In Video mode, chapter points can only be inserted automatically at regular intervals.

Compatibility Issues

Much like "closing" a recordable CD, you must finalize the disc to be able to play it on a regular DVD player or computer DVD drive. Finalizing a disc writes all the necessary control information to the disc, and adds a main menu. After a Video mode disc is finalized, you cannot edit it or add more material to it, but VR mode discs can be edited after finalizing.

The amount of time finalization takes depends on the type of disc, the amount of material recorded on the disc, and the number of clips on the disc. Discs recorded in Video mode can take up to 20 minutes to finalize; discs recorded in VR mode can take up to one hour.

DVD+R/RW Recorders

As with CD discs, the basic DVD-R/RW formats were designed for sequential streaming of audio and video, with DVD-RAM for random access. The DVD+RW Alliance designed the newer "plus" format to offer editing features without a separate VR recording mode, and without the need to finalize discs (sometimes).

Philips Consumer Electronics (www.dvdrecorder.philips.com) introduced DVD+RW recorders in 2001 (the DVDR1000 and DVDR1500), but they supported only the +RW format. A new DVDR985 recorder that also supports DVD+R (see Figure 3.8) shipped in mid-2002 for $999 (MSRP).

DVD+RW Recording

The "plus" recorders can automatically create an index menu with thumbnail pictures of each clip on the disc. Each clip is identified with the program name, length of recording, recording mode/speed, and date of recording.

You can edit from this menu; rename clips; or append, divide, and erase the clips. You can hide and unhide individual clips to be skipped when you play the disc.

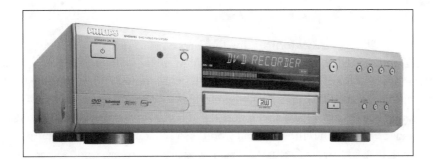

FIGURE 3.8

*Philips DVDR985
DVD+RW/
DVD+R recorder.*

The DVDR985 can record at four rates: one hour at high quality (9.73Mbps), two hours at standard quality (5.07Mbps), and three and four hours for extended recording (3.38Mbps and 2.54Mbps). You can set chapter markers manually during the recording or have chapters inserted automatically at a regular interval.

DVD+R Recording

By adding support for the new write-once DVD+R format, the new recorders permit you to make permanent recordings without the possibility that they can be erased and rewritten. But because the format is not rewritable, there are some limitations in the capability to edit the material on the discs.

For example, you cannot split a clip on a DVD-R disc. You can perform some index screen and chapter marker edits after recording and before finalizing, but they are not available on regular DVD players.

Compatibility Issues

To play on a regular DVD player, the DVD+R/RW discs need to contain at least five to 20 minutes of recorded material (depending on the quality setting).

DVD+R discs must be finalized before they can be played on regular DVD players. The disk then cannot be changed after it is finalized.

Although DVD+RW discs do not need to be finalized, if you have performed edits on a rewritable disc, then you still need to perform a similar process to have the player modify or adapt it to make it compatible with regular players.

If you are having problems with compatibility, the DVDR985 offers three different modification modes that you can try, although this may cause the disc to become incompatible with players that it was previously compatible with. You also may need to use this process if you want to record on a disc that was created on a different brand of recorder.

DVD-RAM Recording

Besides the CD-like R/RW formats, the DVD Forum also defined a third recordable format, DVD-RAM (Random Access Memory), to provide the capability to access a DVD more like a hard disk. However, the DVD-RAM format is significantly different from the rest of the DVD family, and therefore cannot be played in other DVD drives, unless they include special support for it. DVD-RAM discs come in several sizes and formats, both removable and stored in a separate caddy (refer to Figure 3.4). Panasonic Consumer Electronics (`www.panasonic.com/consumer_electronics/ dvd_recorder`) has been the most active supporter of the DVD-RAM format for both computer and consumer products. Panasonic introduced the first DVD recorder, the DMR-E10 at the end of 2000 for $3,999 (MSRP). In late 2001, Panasonic introduced its second-generation recorder, the DMR-E20, priced at $1,499 (MSRP), and available for under $999. This new recorder added DVD-R recording capability for making write-one recordings that are compatible with most DVD players. In June 2002, Panasonic announced the next generation DMR-E30 (see Figure 3.9), priced at around $899 (MSRP), with progressive scan display and long recording time.

FIGURE 3.9

Panasonic DMR-E30 DVD-RAM and DVD-R recorder.

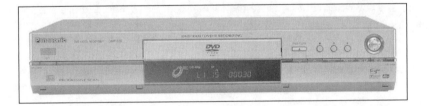

In June 2002, Panasonic also announced the DMR-HS2, a combination DVD recorder with hard disk recorder, at a target price of $1,199 (MSRP). The DMR-HS2 includes a 40GB hard disk drive, which holds up to 52 hours of recording. You can record shows or your own videos to the hard disk, create playlists, and then copy them to DVD to save and watch later. You also can copy from DVD to hard disk, edit the footage, and then record back to DVD.

DVD-RAM Recording

DVD-RAM discs can be used to record up to 12 hours on a double-side DVD-RAM disc (in EP mode, on both sides), or up to six hours on a DVD-R disc. On DVD-RAM media, you can record up to one hour in high-quality XP mode, two hours in standard SP mode, four hours in long-time LP mode, or six hours in the extended-time EP mode. The recorder also offers a Flexible Recording mode, which selects the best picture quality possible for the recording time and available space on the disc.

With DVD-RAM media, the recorder also can offer one-touch recording. You do not need to worry about cueing up the disc, or finding an empty segment to record to. Instead, the recorder will automatically find available space on the disc and start recording.

The DVD-RAM recorder offers video-editing functions to create multiple custom playlists of favorite scenes. You can select and rearrange the order of scenes, skip unwanted scenes, and copy selections. You can even trim the length of a clip by setting in and out points.

But the most impressive feature of the DMR-E30 recorders is the time-slip function, controlled by a roller on the front of the player. The disc access rate of the DVD-RAM disc is fast enough that you can record and play back material from the disc simultaneously. This is not just recording one program while watching another. This means you can pause a show you are watching, or watch a scene over again, and then continue with the rest of the show. Or you can come in late to a program that has already begun recording, and you can start watching it from the beginning, even while the rest of the show is still being recorded. You can even scan through the recorded section in a small onscreen window.

DVD-R Recording

The DMR-E20 includes support for recording on write-once DVD-R discs. You can record separate clips onto a disc; and perform editing functions, such as giving titles to discs and programs, and erasing programs (although this does not free up space).

After it finishes recording a clip, the recorder takes about 30 seconds to complete recording management information. The recorder optimizes the disc for each recording when you start recording after inserting the disc or turning the unit on. You can no longer record to a disc after it has been optimized about 50 times.

Compatibility Issues

DVD-R discs must be finalized before they can be played on regular DVD players. Finalizing takes up to 15 minutes. You cannot record to or edit a DVD-R disc if it was recorded with another unit, whether it is finalized or not.

After it is finalized, DVD-R discs should be playable on most DVD players, set-top and computer.

Some DVD-RAM discs are unformatted, or you can choose to format a disc to erase its contents. Formatting takes up to 70 minutes. You cannot erase data written to DVD-RAM with a computer.

DVD-RAM discs are playable only on set-top DVD players and computer drives that explicitly support DVD-RAM format. The DVD Forum has adopted a DVD-Multi logo to identify players that support all Forum formats, including DVD-R/RW and DVD-RAM.

DVD Camcorders

The DVD-RAM format also has found a home in digital camcorders, using the half-size disc format that also can be played on set-top DVD-RAM units.

The Panasonic VDR-M10 DVD-RAM camcorder offers up to an hour of MPEG-2 video recording for $2,499 (MSRP). In June 2002, Panasonic announced the new VDM-20 DVD-RAM and DVD-R camcorder (see Figure 3.10), planned for fall introduction at around $999 (MSRP).

FIGURE 3.10

Panasonic VDR-M20 DVD-RAM and DVD-R camcorder.

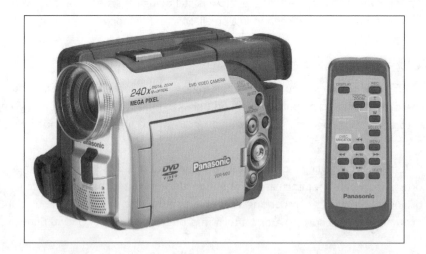

With the random-access disc, you can start recording immediately to an available space on the disc, instead of having to fast-forward or rewind to position a video-tape. You also can directly access the recorded clips for playback using thumbnail images, and even perform editing functions in the camera. Best of all, you can remove the disc from the camera and play it back immediately on a compatible DVD-RAM player (or even on a PC with a DVD-RAM drive).

The VDR-M10 offers two recording modes: 30 minutes at Fine quality (approxi-mately 6Mbps) or one hour at Standard quality (3Mbps). Panasonic warns that blocky noise can appear in recordings of difficult material in Standard quality, such as with complicated background patterns (trees) fast motion of the subject, or panning the camera. You also can record up to 999 still images to the disc in MPEG-2 format for TV display, at 704×480 resolution; or JPEG format for use on a computer, at 1280×960.

After recording clips on the camera, you can scan through your recordings or skip directly from one clip to the next. In disc-navigation mode, you can display thumb-nails of all recorded clips, delete unwanted clips, and edit clips into a playlist. You can add titles to clips; trim or split clips into two parts, or combine multiple clips; and add special effects, such as a fade or wipe. As you edit playlists, you can add or skip clips, rearrange the playback order of the clips, and add different titles and effects.

The smaller DVD-RAM discs are 8cm, compared to the standard 12cm size, and hold 1.4GB per side or 2.8GB for both sides. There are two kinds of 8cm discs, designed for use in video cameras (AV) or for personal computers. Some DVD-RAM discs for camcorders can be removed from their cartridges, so they can be inserted in the disc trays of set-top DVD players and computer drives.

The VDR-M10 includes analog video inputs and outputs, so it can record your VHS tapes and other videos to DVD, and display recordings directly on a televi-sion. It also includes a USB port to connect to a computer to download still images, or you can access the images directly from the disc on a computer with a DVD-RAM drive.

Hitachi also has been a leader in DVD camcorders (www.hitachi.com/dvdcam).

Summary

Although DVD recorders would seem to be a natural set-top accessory for recording and saving video, the market is unfortunately confused by all these different formats—and even modes within formats. But even so, there are some clear trends emerging.

If you want to record off-air material and watch it later (such as a disk-based video recorder), then use rewritable media. The DVD-RAM format provides the most flexibility for this use.

If you want to make permanent recordings from your old videotapes, then you should record direct to write-once media. DVD-R recorders are certainly highly compatible, and the newer DVD+R format that began shipping in the first half of 2002 promises to be the same.

It's the in-between uses that cause the confusion: recording material and then editing it, saving some clips and deleting others, or deciding after recording that you want to save the disc. In these cases, no matter the format, you will need to pay more attention to the recording mode. DVD-RW is more and more compatible with newer players, but you need to trade off editing capability and compatibility with the VR and Video modes. DVD-RAM is the most flexible, but requires players explicitly supporting that format. And the newer DVD+RW format promises both: clip-based editing features and at least reasonable compatibility.

If you want to create your own videos on DVD to save and share, these DVD recorders are great for converting your old tapes to DVDs, complete with chapters and a main menu. They also can be used to record a collection of shorter clips and then organize them with a playlist, but this kind of use stresses the capabilities of write-once DVD-R or can require compatibility compromises from using a rewritable format.

Beyond set-top DVD recorders are computers with DVD burners and authoring software. Part III describes computer-based authoring tools that can be used to transfer tapes to DVD and provide more control over organizing a collection of clips into a DVD production.

chapter 4

Digital Media and DVD on the Macintosh

APPLE REFOCUSED ITS PRODUCT LINE ON DIGITAL MEDIA in early 2001 with the introduction of the Power Mac G4 systems, along with the new Mac OS X operating system. Just as Apple established the graphical personal computer with the Macintosh and then helped create the desktop publishing revolution, now it is positioning the Macintosh as the "hub" of the digital media experience.

The Macintosh platform now includes all the necessary hardware components and software applications for convenient desktop video production—and even DVD authoring. Mac OS X provides a powerful platform for enhancing and optimizing digital media applications. The Macintosh system also includes a full set of built-in digital media applications with image, audio, and video tools.

This chapter explores the Macintosh digital media platform, including the Macintosh system hardware with USB and FireWire/IEEE 1394 ports and CD and DVD drives, and the Mac OS X operating system software and built-in applications for accessing digital media devices and playing digital media files. Chapter 6, "Playing DVDs on Macintosh OS X," will describe the Apple applications for playing audio CD and DVD movie titles.

These are the tools you can use to explore existing DVDs to understand how they are designed, and use to capture and edit material to use in creating your own DVD productions.

Macintosh systems and Mac OS X come loaded with a full complement of digital media tools built in for accessing digital media discs and devices to view and edit photos, music, and video (see Table 4.1).

TABLE 4.1   Mac OS X Digital Media Applications

Logo	Product Summary	Detailed Description
Maine 2 Clips	Burn to CD/DVD	You can access files on attached CD and DVD drives, and burn data files to recordable CD and DVD drives.
iPhoto	Import from USB digital cameras and organize photo albums using iPhoto	You can import images from digital cameras over a USB connection using the iPhoto application; and then organize, edit, and export your images in a variety of formats.
iTunes	Play and rip from CD with iTunes	You can use the iTunes application to play and import music from audio CDs, and also to burn your own mixes to CD to save them to a portable player.

Logo	Product Summary	Detailed Description
QuickTime Player	View Media with Quicktime Player	You can use the QuickTime Player application to view a tremendous variety of media formats—including images, audio, and movies—and also to play media over the Internet.
iMovie	Capture from DV and edit movies with iMovie	You can capture video and audio clips from DV camcorders over a FireWire/IEEE 1394 connection, and use the iMovie video editor to create your own movies.
DVD Player	Play movies on DVD with DVD Player	You can watch movies on DVD with the DVD Player application, full-screen with your computer sound system, or on a laptop during a long trip.
iDVD	Create DVD productions with iDVD	You can use the iDVD authoring tool to create your own DVD productions, and record them to DVD discs.

Mac OS X

The new Macintosh operating system, Mac OS X, also was introduced in 2001. Mac OS X combines the power of a UNIX core operating system with the traditional simplicity and elegance of the Macintosh interface.

Mac OS X starts up with the new Aqua interface. Aqua has a new look with larger and expressive icons, bright colors, and fluid motion. Background windows turn translucent, and objects have drop shadows.

OS X also includes a new Finder with a customizable toolbar for navigating folders; and the Dock area, which is designed to help you navigate and organize your system, and gives you instant access to your most frequently used applications, folders, and minimized windows (see Figure 4.1).

FIGURE 4.1

Mac OS X desktop with the Dock bar at the bottom and the Finder windows showing the built-in Applications folder and user folders.

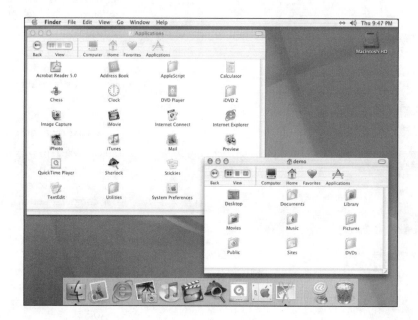

Mac OS X is intended to combine the simplicity and elegance of the Macintosh with the power and stability of a new underlying foundation: the UNIX operating system. The UNIX-based core operating system, called Darwin, provides Mac OS X with powerful advanced features, such as protected memory, pre-emptive multi-tasking, advanced memory management, and symmetric multiprocessing. This design can provide better performance for applications; for example, allowing iDVD 2 to compress your video clips in the background while you continue to work on authoring your DVD menus and navigation.

The graphics and media capabilities of OS X are built on three graphics technologies: the Apple Quartz 2D graphics engine with built-in PDF and PostScript support, the OpenGL standard for 3D graphics drawing and effects, and Apple QuickTime 5 for image and digital media playback.

As Apple made the transition from the Mac OS 9 to the next-generation Mac OS X in 2001, it shipped systems with both operating systems installed. This allowed customers to continue working with their existing applications in the familiar OS 9 environment; then to migrate to OS X to use newer applications designed to take advantage of the new operating system features, and to work with the new interface. The Macintosh can quickly switch between operating systems by using the Startup Disk control panel to select the appropriate System Folder for OS 9 or OS X, and then restarting.

Macintosh Systems and the CD/DVD SuperDrive

Apple helped kick-start DVD on the desktop when it introduced the Power Mac G4 systems in early 2001 and then upgraded the line in July 2001. These systems included all the components and interfaces required for end-to-end digital media processing, from capturing and editing DV video with iMovie to creating and burning DVD productions with iDVD.

These Power Mac systems introduced DVD burning to personal computers by including the SuperDrive, a combination CD-RW/DVD-R drive that reads and records both CD-R/RW and DVD-R discs. With this hardware, Apple also introduced its two DVD authoring tools, iDVD and DVD Studio Pro, and the new DVD-R format, aggressively priced at introduction around $10.

For plug-and-play convenience when interfacing to external devices, such as digital cameras and DV camcorders, the Power Mac G4 systems include both USB and FireWire (IEEE 1394) ports.

For interfacing to DV camcorders and other peripherals, such as digital cameras, the Power Mac G4 systems included 400Mbits/sec FireWire (IEEE 1394) port and 12Mbits/secUSB ports. For communications, they provided 10/100/1000BASE-T Ethernet networking, and a built-in 56K V.90 modem. For future expansion, the systems also included 33MHz PCI slots, a 4X AGP slot for a NVIDIA GeForce2 graphics card, and disk expansion bays for hard drives and CD and DVD drives.

Burning Data to CD and DVD

With the introduction of DVD recording drives, such as the SuperDrive, you can use DVD discs just like CDs on the Macintosh to archive and share your data files. In addition, you can use the iTunes CD jukebox application to burn your own audio CDs, and the iDVD authoring tool to create your own productions and burn them to DVD (see Chapter 10, "Personal DVD Authoring with Apple iDVD"). But you can also use the DVD for removable computer data storage. Instead of archiving and sharing your files by burning them to 650MB CDs, you can now burn 4.7GB of data to a DVD disc. With 7 times more capacity, DVDs are especially useful for storing your large digital media files.

This section steps you through the process of burning data files and folders to a recordable CD or DVD disc. With Mac OS X, you can do all this directly in the Finder.

Formatting a Recordable Disc

Mac OS X has built-in support for burning data files to DVD. The process is actually the same for both CD and DVD: You insert and initialize the disc, drag and drop the files that you want to burn to it, and then start the burn. Compared to CD/DVD recording applications for Windows, you do not get many options for burning, but it cannot get much simpler than this: Just insert, drag, and eject.

When you first insert a blank recordable disc (CD-R/RW or DVD-R), the Mac recognizes the disc format, and displays a dialog box that offers to initialize it to prepare it for burning (see Figure 4.2). Click on the Prepare button, and the Finder mounts the disc on the desktop—empty and ready to receive files.

After you record to a rewritable CD-RW disk, you need to erase its contents before you can record to it again. Use the Erase option in the Disk Utility control panel to erase the information on the disc so that it will appear as a blank disc again (see Figure 4.3).

Copying the Files to Burn

To record data to a blank disk, drag and drop the files and folders that you want to record to the empty disc volume on the desktop. This actually does not burn the files; instead, you are accumulating the list of files that are to be recorded to the disc. You can display the disc contents in a Finder window, and add and remove files. Pull down the File menu, and choose Show Info to check the size of the accumulated files and the available size on the disc (see Figure 4.4).

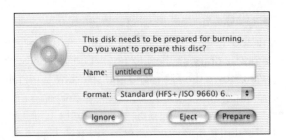

FIGURE 4.2

Before you can use a blank CD or DVD disc for recording you must first prepare (initialize) it.

FIGURE 4.3

Use the Disk Utility control panel to erase a previously recorded CD-RW rewritable disc.

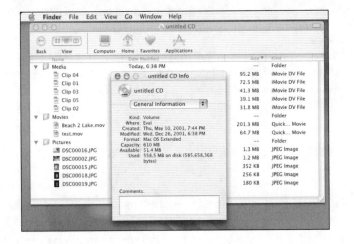

FIGURE 4.4

Drag and drop files that you want to burn to the disc's folder. Use Show Info to display the available space.

Burning the Disc

When you are done adding files to the disc, it is time to actually burn them. You can start a burn simply by dragging the CD or DVD disc icon to the Trash icon in the Dock, or by pulling down the File menu and selecting Burn Disc. If you drag a previously recorded disc to the Trash, it changes to an Eject icon, and the result is the disc is ejected. But when you drag a blank disc to the Trash, it changes to a Burn icon because the disc is ready to be recorded (see Figure 4.5).

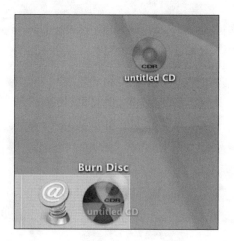

The Mac displays a confirmation dialog box, and starts burning the disc. When the burn is complete, the files and folders that you selected have been recorded to the disc.

To eject the disc, you can drag it to the Trash/Eject icon in the Dock, press the Eject key on the keyboard, or pull down the File menu and choose Eject. The data discs that you create can then be read on any Macintosh or Windows PC.

Accessing USB Digital Cameras with iPhoto

Mac OS X provides built-in support for connecting to digital cameras through the USB (Universal Serial Bus) interface. Macintosh systems also can use USB to connect the keyboard and mouse because the USB specification was explicitly designed for sharing multiple devices. USB also provides a very convenient "plug-and-play" connection: You can plug in and remove devices while the system is running, and it even provides power, so small devices do not need a separate power supply.

With a data rate of 12Mbits/sec (1.5MBytes/sec), USB can be used to connect to other devices, such as printers and scanners. A new version, USB 2.0, is starting to enter the market, with data rates up to 480Mbits/sec. USB also has become popular for interfacing to external disk drives, especially with removable media, such as CD burners.

Because an IEEE 1394/FireWire connection is significantly faster than the original USB specification, FireWire is used for interfacing to the current generation of DV camcorders and other fast devices, such as large hard disks and DVD recorders.

This section shows you how to use the iPhoto application under Mac OS X to download images from a USB digital camera; and organize, edit, export, and share your images. It demonstrates how USB devices, such as mountable disk drives, are handled under Mac OS X.

About iPhoto

The iPhoto application is included with Mac OS X to help you download images from a digital camera to your hard disc. iPhoto is designed to work with digital cameras that provide a computer interface through a USB connection. It launches automatically when you connect your camera to a USB port.

With iPhoto, you can import photos from your digital camera or from local folders, organize them into albums, edit and save them, and organize them into photo books to print and share.

Before Apple released iPhoto, Mac OS X included two other applications for accessing and viewing digital photos. The Image Capture application was designed to help download images from a digital camera to hard disc. It can be set up to automate the process of downloading the images, opening them in an application, and even creating a web page from them. Image Capture can also access video and audio clips from these cameras. The Preview application was designed for viewing images and PDF (Portable Document Format) files. It also can be used to rotate images and convert them to different file formats.

Connecting to the Camera

To start iPhoto, simply connect your digital camera to the Macintosh by using the USB interface cable supplied with your camera. Then, turn your camera on and set it to the appropriate mode to interface to a computer (typically the Play setting for PC mode or Transfer mode).

iPhoto then launches automatically when the Macintosh recognizes the camera (see Figure 4.6). See the online documentation if your camera does not work with iPhoto.

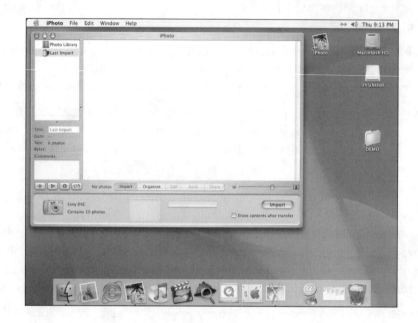

The digital camera also appears on the desktop as a new Untitled disk, just as if it were a new external disk drive or removable disk. Independently from the IPhoto application, you can use the Finder to browse the contents of the camera memory as if it were an external disk drive, and access the individual image files stored in it (see Figure 4.7).

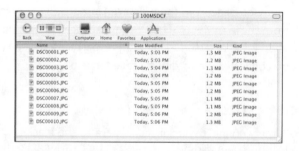

Importing Photos from a USB Camera

When iPhoto launches automatically after you connect a USB camera, it starts up in Import mode (indicated by the Import mode button in the button bar below the main screen). iPhoto also displays information about your camera in the bottom-left corner of the screen, including the number of photos stored on it.

To import your photos, click on the Import button on the bottom right of the window. You can also enable the check box to erase the photos after they are transferred. iPhoto then transfers the photos to files on your hard disk (see Figure 4.8).

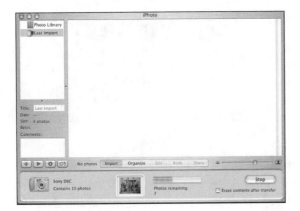

FIGURE 4.8

iPhoto imports the photos from your USB camera into the Photo Library.

iPhoto displays all the images that you import in your Photo Library. The default album is listed at the top left of the window. After the import is complete, it displays just the more recently transferred photos under the Last Import album with a thumbnail for each image file (see Figure 4.9).

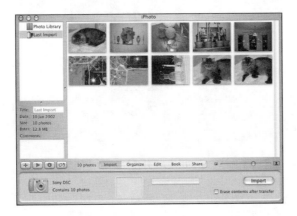

FIGURE 4.9

Click on the Last Import album to view the collection of photos that you most recently imported into iPhoto.

Disconnecting Your Camera

Before turning off or disconnecting your camera, drag the disk icon for the camera to the Trash icon in the Dock (which turns into an Eject icon; see Figure 4.10).

You can then disconnect the camera. The iPhoto window then changes to indicate that no camera is attached.

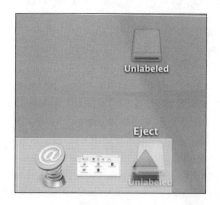

Importing Photos from Local Disk

iPhoto can also import photos from local disks, CDs, or other storage devices. To import local image files, pull down the File menu, and choose Import. Use the Import Photos dialog box to select one or more image files, or an entire folder.

iPhoto then imports the images, and displays them as the Last Import (see Figure 4.11).

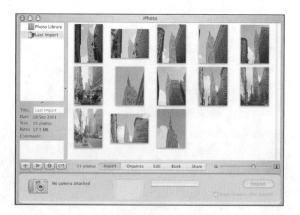

Organizing Your Photos

To view all your photos, click on the Organize mode button below the photos. You can then browse your photos and organize them into albums.

To have iPhoto arrange your photos automatically, pull down the Edit menu and choose by Film Roll or by Date, or choose Manually.

To change the display size of the photos, drag the Size Control slider at the bottom right of the window. iPhoto then dynamically adjusts the album display as you shrink or enlarge the photos. To zoom in on a specific photo, click to select it, and adjust the slider (see Figure 4.12).

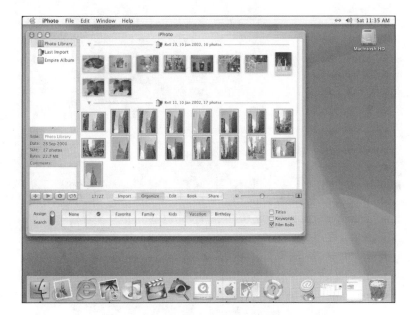

FIGURE 4.12

Use Organize mode to view and organize your photos. Use the Size Control slide to change the size of the photos.

You can also use the area at the bottom of the window to Assign keywords to photos, and then Search for photos matching specific keywords. Use the check boxes to display Titles and Keywords with the photos, and show Film Roll dividers.

Pull down the File menu, and choose New Album to create a new photo album for grouping your photos (or click on the New Album + button below the album list). You can then drag your photos into albums to help organize them by topic or theme. The albums are just for organizing; the full photo collection always remains in the main Photo Library, and you can include the same photo in several libraries.

Editing Your Photos

To view and edit an individual photo, click on the Edit mode button below the photos.

You can then use the controls at the bottom of the window to rotate the photos; and select a rectangular region of the photo to Crop, remove Red Eye, and convert to Black and White (see Figure 4.13).

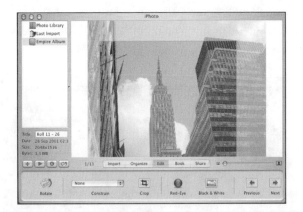

You can also double-click on a photo to open it in a separate window. Then, click the button in the top-right corner of the window to display the Edit toolbar to access and customize the editing tools (see Figure 4.14).

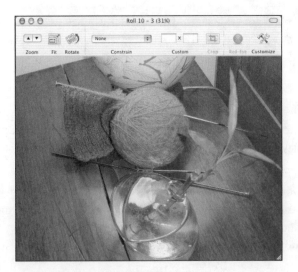

Before you make changes to a photo, you may want to pull down the File menu and choose Duplicate to make a copy of it. You also can use Undo to undo a series of changes. In addition, iPhoto saves the original version of any photo you edit, so you can always pull down the File menu and choose Revert to Original to remove any changes and restore the original photo.

Creating Books from Your Photos

iPhoto also helps you create photo books of your images, which you can print out; or you can have them professionally printed and bound. Click on the Book mode button below the photos.

You can then choose a Theme for the graphical design of your book, change the overall Page Design, lay out your photos, and add titles and text (see Figure 4.15). When you are done, you can print the book on your printer, save it in Acrobat (PDF) format, or order a professionally printed copy through an Internet connection.

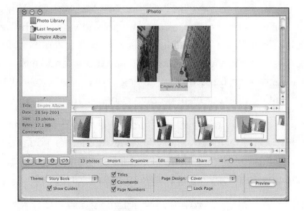

FIGURE 4.15

Use Book mode to create a photo book design.

Exporting Your Photos

To share and export your photos, click on the Share mode button below the photos (or pull down the File menu and choose Export).

Use the buttons at the bottom of the window to Print selected photos; create a Slide Show with musical accompaniment; Order Prints or a Book over the Internet; publish to a HomePage; or Export to image files, a web page, or to a QuickTime file (see Figure 4.16).

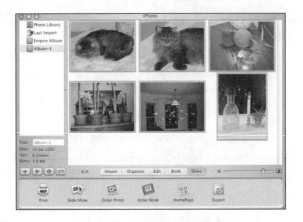

FIGURE 4.16

Use Export mode to save and share your photos.

Displaying Video Files with QuickTime Player

Just as you can use iPhoto to view and edit image files, Mac OS X also provides built-in support for viewing movie files with audio and video with the QuickTime Player. The QuickTime Player actually can display a wide variety of different digital media formats, including video, audio, animations, and stills. And with the QuickTime Pro upgrade, it becomes an editing tool as well, so you also can perform simple editing operations and convert media formats.

Apple has worked diligently to develop QuickTime as a cross-platform digital media system, for both Macintosh and Windows. Whether you are on the Mac or Windows, QuickTime Pro is an inexpensive and convenient tool for both simple cut-and-paste editing and converting between media formats.

On the Macintosh, Apple also provides the iMovie video editor for capturing clips from a DV camcorder and editing video and audio, complete with transitions, titles, and effects. You can then save and share your video productions as digital files, or share them on your personal web page with iTools. You also can use iDVD to author video productions to DVD.

About QuickTime Player

The QuickTime Player can display and play a wide range of more than 200 media file formats, including still images, motion video, and audio. It can also play streaming media files and broadcasts over the Internet.

Apple also offers the QuickTime Pro upgrade for $29.99 to add the capability to edit and export multimedia files in a variety of formats.

Playing Movie Files

Double-click on a QuickTime movie file in a Finder window to open it (or pull down the File menu and choose Open). The QuickTime Player application opens a window to play the movie (see Figure 4.17).

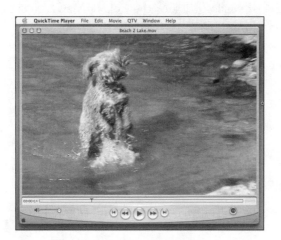

FIGURE 4.17

Use the QuickTime Player application to view movies.

Use the play controls on the bottom of the window to play through the movie, or drag the slider at the bottom of the window to move to a specific point. Use the Movie menu to Loop playback; and to resize the display to Half, Normal, Double Size, or Full Screen.

Viewing Information on Movie Files

To view more detail on the movie file, pull down the Movie menu and choose Get Movie Properties. QuickTime displays a Properties window (see Figure 4.18).

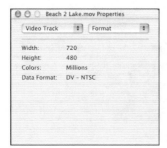
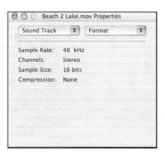

FIGURE 4.18

Use the Properties window to display information about the movie and its tracks.

Use the left drop-down menu to view information about the overall Movie, Video Track, or Sound Track. Then use the right drop-down menu to view details of the Format, Annotations, or other properties for the movie or the selected track.

You can also preview digital video files and find out information about them from the Finder. In a Finder window, click on the Column View icon in the top-left corner of the Finder window to display the full hierarchy of folders. Click a movie file to see the details about that movie, including its format, size, resolution, and duration (see Figure 4.19).

FIGURE 4.19

Use the Column View in the Finder window to display information about movie files.

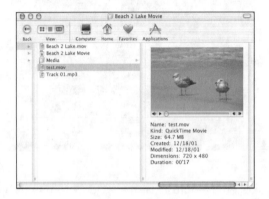

You can also select the media file in the Finder, pull down the File menu, and choose Show Info. The Finder displays an Info window; choose Preview from the drop-down menu to see information about the file and to play a preview of it (see Figure 4.20).

FIGURE 4.20

You can also display a preview of the file in an Info window.

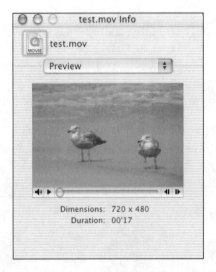

Playing Sound Files

You can also use the QuickTime Player to play other multimedia formats, including sound files. Some media file formats (that is, MP3) are associated with other applications, so they will open in that application (that is, iTunes) when you double-click on them in the Finder. However, you still can play these files with the QuickTime Player by dragging them to the QuickTime Player icon in the dock or on the desktop. You also can open media files from within the QuickTime Player by pulling down the File menu and choosing Open Movie in New Player.

When you open a sound file, the QuickTime Player application opens another window to play it (see Figure 4.21).

Use the same play controls on the bottom of the window to play through the clip. To adjust the sound, pull down the Movie menu and choose Show Sound Controls (or click on the meter display to the right of the slider). You can then adjust the audio Balance, Bass, and Treble.

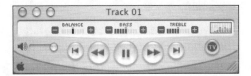

FIGURE 4.21

You can also play sound files with QuickTime Player, with audio controls.

Viewing Information On Sound Files

Again, pull down the Movie menu and choose Get Movie Properties to display information about the sound file in a Properties window (see Figure 4.22).

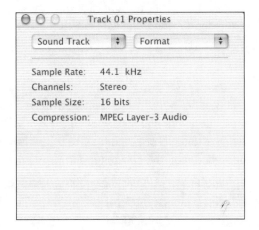

FIGURE 4.22

Use the Properties window to display information about the audio format.

Editing and Converting Media Files with QuickTime Pro

QuickTime Player is more than just a viewer for digital media file formats. With the QuickTime Pro upgrade, you can use the QuickTime Player to edit and convert digital media formats. The Pro upgrade adds the capability to cut and paste portions of clips; add, extract, and delete tracks; and export and save in a wide variety of formats.

You also can enhance movies and still pictures with filters and effects. In particular, QuickTime Pro can resize movies, create slide shows with a music track, prepare and compress streaming content for viewing on the web, and work with the full-quality DV camcorder format.

You can edit clips by simply selecting segments on the slider and then trimming and combining them by using cut and paste (see Figure 4.23).

FIGURE 4.23

Use the QuickTime Pro upgrade to edit tracks by cutting and pasting segments.

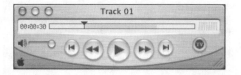

DV Video Editing with iMovie

Apple popularized the FireWire interface on the Macintosh system for interfacing to DV (digital video) camcorders. (Although Apple calls the interface FireWire, it is also known as IEEE 1394 as it was standardized, and Sony also calls it i.Link.) Because FireWire provides a much faster interface than the original USB specification at 400Mbits/sec (versus 12Mbits/sec for USB 1.0), it has been adopted for use with digital camcorders and external disk drives.

Like USB, FireWire provides a plug-and-play interface, and you can connect and disconnect multiple devices as the system is running. But DV camcorders are not treated like an external disk (as were USB cameras). Instead, interfacing to a DV device requires an application with knowledge of both how to control the camcorder (play, pause, rewind, and so on), and how to transfer video and audio over the FireWire connection between the computer and the camcorder.

This section shows you how to use the iMovie application under Mac OS X to capture video and audio clips from a DV camcorder over a FireWire connection, and then perform some simple video editing.

About iMovie

Apple provides the iMovie application to work with DV camcorders to quickly and easily capture, edit, enhance, and share desktop movies. You can use iMovie to quickly capture clips from a DV camcorder, arrange them in a storyboard, and export the final movie back out to DV tape. Or you can import a variety of clips, and use the Timeline display to edit them together and add transitions, titles, effects, and audio. Then, you can export to QuickTime files or directly to iDVD format.

Version 2 of iMovie, introduced in late 2001, added significant new video and audio editing tools and effects, but without damaging the simplicity of the user interface.

Capturing from DV

To start working with iMovie, first launch the iMovie application. Unlike using USB digital cameras, the application is not launched automatically when you connect a camcorder to a FireWire cable.

When iMovie starts up, it prompts you to start a new project or reopen an existing project. Click New Project (see Figure 4.24).

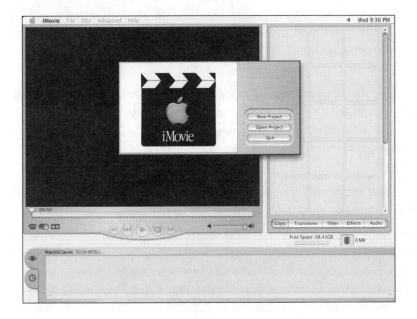

FIGURE 4.24

When you first launch iMovie, choose to start a new project or open an existing project, you will get this display.

iMovie displays the Create New Project dialog box (see Figure 4.25). Navigate to the folder in which you want to save your project, and type a name for the project. Click on the down arrow icon at the bottom right of the dialog box to display a column view to help you browse through the hierarchy of folders.

FIGURE 4.25

Use the Create New Project dialog box to specify where your new project will be saved.

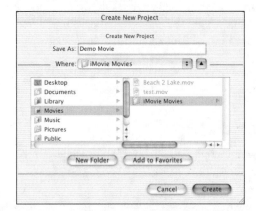

iMovie then displays an empty new project with the Monitor window on the left, the Clip Viewer along the bottom, and the Clip storage shelf along the right side of the display. The Camera Mode/Edit Mode toggle at the bottom left of the Monitor window is set to DV Camera mode, and the display shows Camera Disconnected.

Plug in your DV camcorder using a FireWire cable, turn it on, and set it to the playback or VCR mode. iMovie automatically recognizes that the camera is attached, and the Monitor window now shows Camera Connected, and displays the current timecode on the tape (see Figure 4.26).

You can watch the tape in the Monitor window while using the play controls under the window to play and scan through the tape. When you have positioned the tape and are ready to start capturing, click on the Import button.

iMovie immediately starts importing the video and audio in full-resolution DV format to clips on your hard disk. As it captures, iMovie detects scene changes in the video and adds individual clips to the Clips storage shelf on the right side of the display, each marked with their name and duration (see Figure 4.27). You can click on the Import button to start and stop capturing each clip, or iMovie can automatically start a new clip each time there is a scene change in the input videotape.

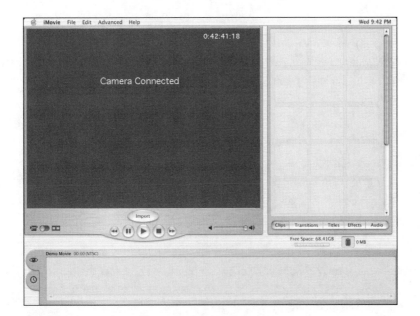

FIGURE 4.26

iMovie recognizes that a camera is connected, and displays the current timecode.

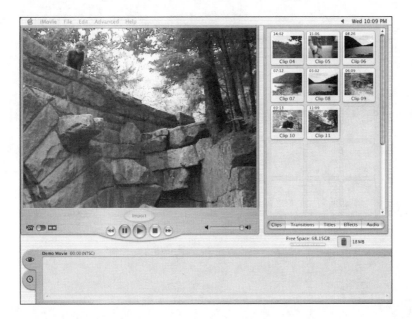

FIGURE 4.27

While capturing video, iMove automatically detects scene changes and adds individual clips to the storage shelf.

You can also import clip files from hard disk, in DV stream format (as captured from DV tape), or in a variety of still image formats. iMovie does not import QuickTime video files in any arbitrary compression format or resolution. However, you can use the QuickTime Player Pro to convert full-resolution, full-rate video files into streaming DV format.

Editing Your Movie

After you have finished capturing the clips, click on the Camera Mode/Edit Mode toggle at the bottom left of the Monitor window to switch into editing mode, or just click on a clip thumbnail.

When you click on a clip, it is displayed in the Monitor window, and you can use the play controls to play through the individual clip.

To make a quick movie from your clips, simply drag and drop them into the Clip Viewer storyboard at the bottom of the display, and arrange them in the order that you like (see Figure 4.28).

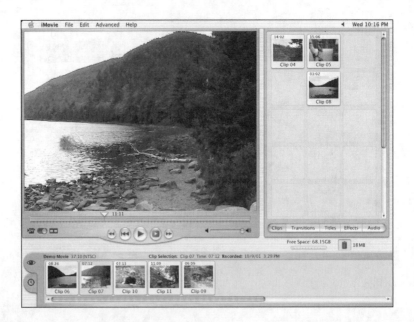

FIGURE 4.28

Switch to Edit mode, and drag and drop clips into the Clip Viewer to arrange them into a movie.

iMovie also provides editing operations on the video and audio tracks of your clips. You can trim individual clips in the Monitor window by clicking and dragging trim markers below the scrubber bar. Use the Edit menu to split video clips and to create a still clip. Use the Advanced menu to reverse the clip direction, extract audio, and lock audio.

To enhance your movie with more sophisticated effects, click through the design panel tabs to the right of the Monitor window to select Transitions, Titles, Effects, and additional Audio tracks or effects. You can control the direction of transitions and the speed of effects.

For more advanced control over the video and audio tracks, click on the Timeline Viewer tab below the Monitor window to switch to a timeline view (see Figure 4.29). You can then position and view your clips with multiple audio tracks, and with transitions and effects.

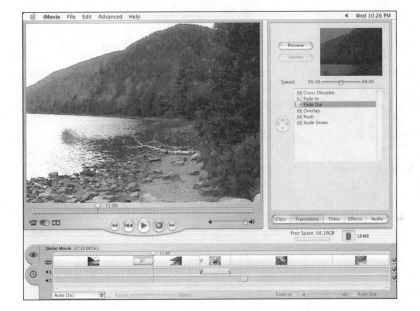

FIGURE 4.29

Add elements from the Transitions, Titles, and Effects design panels, and use the Timeline Viewer for more sophisticated productions.

Exporting Your Movie

When you finish editing, you can export your movie to a QuickTime format or in iDVD-ready (DV) format. For exporting to a QuickTime file, iMovie provides presets for small web formats, medium-size CD-ROM formats, and full-quality DV format; or you can select any supported QuickTime video and audio formats. iMovie can also export a movie back to your DV camcorder to record it to a DV tape.

Summary

This chapter provided a walkthrough of how the Apple Macintosh platform is evolving toward a digital media hub, powered by the Mac OS X operating system and a complete set of built-in applications. On these systems, you can import digital media with built-in interfaces to digital cameras over USB and DV camcorders over FireWire. You can save and share digital files by burning to CD and now DVD discs. And you can view, edit, and convert digital media files with the preloaded Apple applications.

For working with images, you can capture from USB digital cameras with iPhoto, and organize and share your photos in albums.

For working with a wide variety of digital media formats and movies, you can use the QuickTime Player to view files and the QuickTime Pro upgrade to edit and convert them.

For working with movies on DV camcorders, you can use iMovie to capture, edit, and enhance video productions. You can then save and share your video productions as QuickTime movie files, export to iDVD, transfer back to DV camcorders, or share them on your personal web page with iTools.

These applications are provided with all Macintosh systems (with the associated hardware), based on capabilities that are built in to Mac OS X. With these tools, you can import and prepare the multimedia materials that you can then use to author DVD productions.

If you want to work with a more advanced video-editing tool, you can step up from iMovie to Apple's Final Cut Pro professional video-editing software, which provides sophisticated editing, compositing, and special effects.

For the next step in working with prerecorded music and movie titles on CD and DVD, see Chapter 6, which describes the iTunes application for playing audio CDs and DVD Player for playing DVD movies. Chapter 10 then describes how to create your own DVD productions with the iDVD application.

chapter 5

Digital Media and DVD on Windows

As DESCRIBED IN THE PRECEDING CHAPTER, Apple has refocused its Macintosh product line to provide built-in support for digital media right out of the box, including the necessary hardware ports and disc drives, and associated software-editing tools. As you will see in this chapter, Microsoft is moving in a similar direction with Windows XP, but the picture for the PC and Windows world is more complicated. There are wide variations in the hardware capabilities of different computer systems, differences in the digital media support built into various versions of the Windows operating system, and more use of third-party tools that also differ between systems.

This chapter discusses digital media under Windows XP, which has become a complete environment for acquiring, viewing, and editing digital media. You can transfer photos from a digital camera through a USB port, and capture digital video and audio from a DV camcorder through a FireWire/IEEE 1394 connection.

Of course, you also can import media from other sources, such as scanners and analog capture devices, as well as download and transfer materials over the Internet. Many of the issues in this discussion (and certainly the general concepts) also apply to earlier versions of Windows—especially Windows 2000 and Windows ME for the home.

Even as most PCs were shipping in 2002 with Windows XP, however, it is still possible to purchase a Windows computer with limited digital media capability, such as only a CD-ROM reader, and therefore with no capability to read DVDs or write CDs or DVDs. When you buy a Windows computer for digital media, make sure you get the appropriate digital media hardware and software components, as shown in Table 5.1. If you purchase a Windows XP computer with these components pre-installed, the vendor also should install all the associated drivers and utility software.

TABLE 5.1   Suggested Hardware for Digital Media Under Windows XP

USB/USB-2 port	Universal Serial Bus that is standard on most current Windows computers. A standard interface for connecting to peripherals at moderate speeds (12Mbits/sec). Used for transferring digital photos from a digital camera. Also used to reduce wires, to replace the serial and parallel ports by chaining together the keyboard and mouse, and for devices, such as printers and scanners. The new USB-2 port that started appearing in mid-2002 offers higher-speed connections for external devices, including hard disk drives and DVD drives.
FireWire/IEEE-1394 port	Added cost option for most Windows computers. A standard interface for connecting to peripherals that require higher speed (400Mbits/sec). Used for transferring digital video from a DV camcorder. Also used for connecting to external drives, such as DVD recorders and hard disks.
CD-R/RW drive	Read/write CD drive (Recordable and ReWritable). Still an added cost option on many Windows computers, but becoming standard.
DVD-ROM drive	Read-only DVD drive. Reads data and video DVDs, and typically also CDs. Still an added cost option on many Windows computers, but becoming standard.
DVD-R or DVD-RW drive	Read/write DVD drive (Recordable/ReWritable). There are multiple competing and incompatible standards for recordable DVD drives. Reads data and video DVDs, and sometimes also records CDs. Added cost option that is becoming more available on Windows computers.

This chapter explores Windows XP as a platform for digital media, including burning data to recordable CD and DVD drives, acquiring and organizing digital photos in the My Pictures folder, and importing motion video and editing movies with Windows Movie Maker. Chapter 7, "Playing DVDs in Windows XP," describes how to use Windows Media Player to organize and play music and videos, especially audio CDs and movies on DVD.

Using these tools, you can acquire and prepare the materials that you then can import into the DVD authoring tools described in the following parts of the book. These materials include video clips, additional audio tracks, still image backgrounds for menus, and even photo slide shows.

Burning Data to CD and DVD

Although we think of CD and DVD discs in terms of music and movies, a computer sees these discs as just another digital data storage device. The disc contents may be audio or video, but it is all just data to the computer. A computer with a recordable CD or DVD drive can write any type of data to the CD or DVD—not just music or video. Hence, you can use recordable CDs and DVDs to back up, archive, or share files. A CD holds 650 to 700MB of data, and a DVD holds about 4.7GB.

T I P

Originally, the CD data recording applications described worked only with CDs, not with DVDs, so writing DVDs required different tools. More recently, the built-in support in Windows XP and in these applications has been expanded to supporting both CDs and DVDs. However, many of the application dialog boxes and explanatory language still refer only to CD, not to DVD. This chapter generally refers to both, with some differences between the way recordable and rewritable drives work.

Windows XP Desktop CD and DVD Recording

Windows XP now includes the capability to burn data to a CD or DVD directly from the desktop by copying files to the CD or DVD drive in Windows Explorer. Windows actually builds a temporary disc image file with the files that you have copied. When you have accumulated all the files you want to record, you then start the process of burning the data to disc. This works much like desktop CD burning on the Macintosh, as described in Chapter 4, "Digital Media and DVD on the Macintosh."

In addition, many Windows systems also ship with third-party CD burning tools, such as Roxio (formerly Adaptec) Easy CD Creator and Direct CD (www.roxio.com). Easy CD Creator allows you to create Audio CDs, and to organize data files and folders to be burned to a data CD and then burn the entire set in one operation. DirectCD adds itself to the Windows file system to allow you to drag and drop files to a CD as if it were a hard disc, so it writes out small packets of data continuously as you add items to the disc.

However, using both the Windows XP desktop CD recording feature and DirectCD at the same time can be confusing. Instead, you can disable the Windows recording feature, or you might find that it is already disabled on some systems when DirectCD is installed. To check your system, open My Computer to see your disk drives, click to select the recordable CD (or DVD) drive icon, and right-click and choose Properties from the pop-up dialog box.

In the CD Properties dialog box, click on the Recording tab (see Figure 5.1). To disable Windows desktop CD recording, uncheck Enable CD Recording on This Drive. (If DirectCD has been installed, the Recording tab might be removed, and new Settings and DirectCD Options tabs are added instead.)

FIGURE 5.1

Use the Recording tab in the CD Properties dialog box to control Windows desktop CD recording.

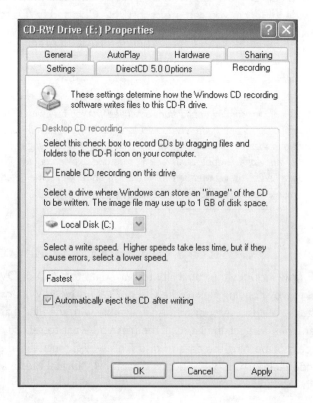

Choosing Recordable Disc Formats

Before you burn data to a CD, it must be formatted or prepared for adding directories and files. Blank discs that you buy in the store are unformatted. For CD-R (Recordable) write-once discs, you format them once and then can burn one or more groups of data until the disc is full. For CD-RW (ReWritable) discs, you can format and write to them like a CD-R, and reformat them to erase their contents before using them again.

CDs can be formatted to several different standards, depending on the intended use and the need to be compatible with older platforms and players. These include the following:

- CD-Audio
- UDF 1.5, the new universal disc format
- High Sierra ISO 9660, the Windows standard for CD-ROM
- Macintosh HFS

These standards define the file system used to organize data files on the disc, including whether the files can have long names or must comply to the 8.3 (eight-letter filename and three-letter file type) convention of the original DOS. For the most part, you can ignore these details and accept the appropriate format used by the disc-burning tools. Just be aware that after a disc is formatted for a particular purpose to an audio or data format, you cannot combine a different format on the same disc.

After you burn data to a CD disc, you can leave the disc in one of two states: open or closed. If you expect to add more data to the disc, you can leave it open for further writing. If you are done writing data and want to read the disc on another drive, then you should close or finalize the disc to mark it as complete. Many audio CD players can only read discs that have been closed.

Formatting Recordable Discs

Although you must format a recordable (R) disc before you write data to it, this formatting process is often combined with the burning operation. Therefore, you typically do not need to perform a separate formatting operation when a blank disc is inserted in the computer.

ReWritable (RW) discs can be reformatted to erase data stored on them and prepare them to be reused. You can do this by right-clicking on the disc icon in Explorer and selecting Format, or by using Easy CD Creator to pull down the CD menu and choose Erase (see Figure 5.2). Use the DirectCD Format dialog box to prepare a disc for use with DirectCD (see the section, "Writing Flles with DirectCD," later in this chapter for more information). Use Quick Erase to prepare the disc to be reused, or Full Erase to actually erase the entire contents of the disc.

FIGURE 5.2

Use Easy CD Creator to reformat a CD-RW or DVD-RW ReWritable disc.

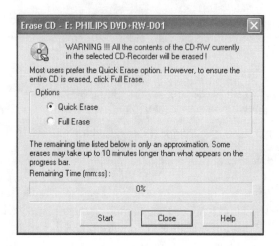

Burning Data Discs with Windows Desktop Recording

To burn data to recordable CDs or DVDs on the Windows desktop, first copy the files to the CD disc icon and then start the burning process.

You can copy files by dragging and dropping them to the disc icon, or by using Copy from the menus. You also can select the files in an Explorer window and then click on Copy on the Explorer task pane. Windows displays the Copy Items dialog box, so you can choose the destination recordable disc device.

Windows then builds a temporary image file of the data to be written to CD. Open the CD drive in Windows Explorer to view the files and folders that are ready to burn (see Figure 5.3).

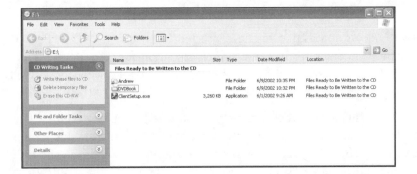

FIGURE 5.3

Use Windows Explorer to assemble the files to copy to a CD or DVD.

Finally, click on Write These Files to CD in the Explorer task pane. Windows then displays the CD Writing Wizard to step through the process of burning the data to CD (see Figure 5.4).

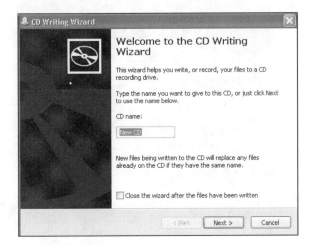

FIGURE 5.4

Then, use the CD Writing Wizard to write the files to CD.

T I P

In Windows Explorer, click on the Folders button to alternate the left Explorer Bar panel between a hierarchical list of folders and a context-sensitive Taskbar. The Taskbar displays appropriate actions for files and folders, depending on their type. Use the View menu (or Views icon drop-down menu) to choose different views for the list of files in the right pane.

Setting the Disc AutoPlay Option

When Windows notices that you have inserted a new disc in a CD or DVD drive, it examines the contents of the disc. It then can automatically perform a specified AutoPlay function based on the type of data, such as launching Windows Media Player to play an audio CD.

To set the default action when a blank disc is inserted, right-click on the CD or DVD disc icon in Windows Explorer, and choose Properties from the pop-up menu. In the Properties dialog box, select the AutoPlay tab and then choose Blank CD from the drop-down list (see Figure 5.5).

You can than select an AutoPlay option, such as automatically launching Roxio Easy CD Creator to create a new data CD. You can choose to have Windows prompt for an action each time you insert a blank disc, or choose Take No Action so that you can launch the desired application directly.

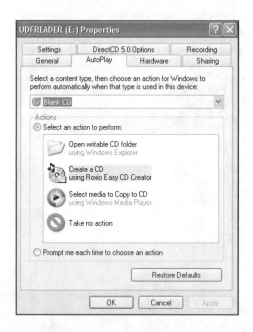

FIGURE 5.5

Use the AutoPlay options in the CD Properties dialog box to set the action to be performed when a blank disc is inserted in your system.

The AutoPlay option actually launches the Easy CD Creator Project Selector when you insert a blank disc (see Figure 5.6). Use the Project Selector to choose the operation to perform with this disc: creating an audio or MP3 CD, creating a data CD or DVD with Easy CD Creator or DirectCD, creating a photo or video CD, or copying an existing disc.

The basic version of Easy CD Creator that is bundled with many new systems does not have all the options for music and photos. You can upgrade to the Platinum version to enable all the functionality.

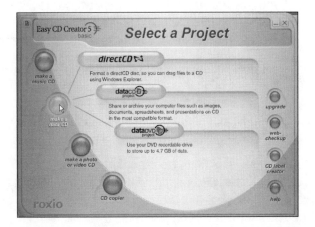

FIGURE 5.6

Use the Easy CD Creator Project Selector to begin a project with a blank disc.

Burning Data Discs with Easy CD Creator

To create a data CD or DVD, choose Data Project from the Project Selector, or launch Easy CD Creator directly (see Figure 5.7). Use the bottom pane of the Easy CD Creator window to organize the data that you want to burn to disc. You can drag and drop folders and files from the top pane, and create new folders and reorganize the folder hierarchy in the bottom pane. Watch the Project Size bar at the bottom of the window to ensure that the files that you have selected will fit on the disc.

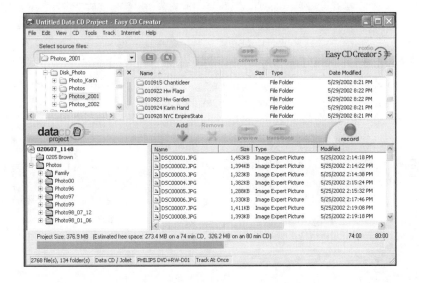

FIGURE 5.7

Use Roxio Easy CD Creator to organize files and folders to burn to a data CD or DVD.

Finally, click on the Record button to start recording the data to disc. Easy CD Creator displays the Record CD Setup dialog box. Select the target Drive and the Number of Copies to record. Set the Write Speed based on the speed of your drive, the rating of your disc media, and your experience with recording. You may want to experiment with using lower speeds for greater reliability and compatibility, especially if you are using unbranded media or need the discs to be readable on a wide array of possible players.

You can check Copy to hard drive first to create a disk image file before writing, but this is typically not required on current machines. Make sure Buffer underrun protection is checked; most PCs and CD drives should then be fast enough to record your disc without the glitches that used to plague the recording process.

Click on the Options button to set the Record Options. It is a good idea to use Test and Record CD to check the burning process the first few times you use it. Use the Record Method to specify when you finish recording. Use Disk-at-Once to record the entire disc in one operation, and close it so that it can be read on other platforms. Use Track-at-Once to record data in multiple operations and to finalize each recording session. When the disc is full, you can finalize and close the CD.

Writing Files with DirectCD

Besides using Windows desktop recording or Easy CD Creator to write entire collections of data in one recording session, Roxio DirectCD offers an alternate approach that makes the CD act like a normal disk drive, so you can drag and drop individual files to write them to disc. DirectCD implements a packet-writing technique that enables you to write files to the disc and then come back later to add additional files. It does this at the cost of compatibility with other format standards, however. After you finish writing to a disk using DirectCD, you then can modify the disc to be compatible with either the UDF or the ISO 9660 format.

Depending on your system configuration, the version of DirectCD installed on your system, and the DirectCD options settings, it can automatically launch when you insert a blank disc and offer to close a disc when you eject it.

To use a recordable CD or DVD disc with DirectCD, you need to first format it for DirectCD access. Use the DirectCD Format Utility to format a blank CD for drag-and-drop recording (see Figure 5.8). Click on the Format CD button to begin the format, which can be completed in less than a minute for a blank CD-R. A full format of a CD-RW with a check of the format can take 15 to 60 minutes, depending on the speed of your drive.

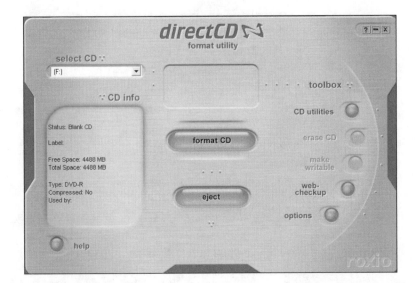

FIGURE 5.8

Use the DirectCD Format Utility to format a blank, recordable CD or DVD for drag-and-drop access.

When the format is complete, the disc appears in Windows Explorer, just like any other disc. You can drag files onto it, delete files, and use it in Save File dialog boxes within your applications. You also can rename, move, and delete files. The only differences are that access to the disc is slower than a hard disk; and when you delete a file on a CD-R, the file goes away, but the space that it occupied is not freed for use by other files.

Ejecting a DirectCD Disc

When you eject a recordable disc formatted for use with DirectCD, it displays the Eject Options dialog box (see Figure 5.9). You can either choose Leave as Is to keep the disk in the DirectCD state so that it can continue being used for DirectCD access, or choose Close to Read on Any Computer to reformat it to be accessible on standard CD-ROM or DVD-ROM drives.

If you are using CD-RW media, when ejected it can be read by CD-RW and most current CD-ROM drives. When reinserted, you can still continue to use it with DirectCD drag-and-drop access.

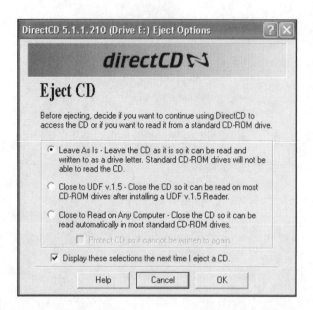

Importing and Browsing Pictures in Windows XP

Windows XP has built-in support for connecting to most USB digital cameras. Importing photos is as easy as connecting the camera like a removable disk, browsing the stored pictures on it in Windows Explorer, and then copying the photo files to your hard disk.

Windows XP provides the My Pictures folder for storing and organizing your photos. Windows Explorer also includes enhanced support for browsing folders of pictures, with options in the Taskbar that include viewing the folder as a slide show.

You can then use the Windows Paint accessory or other third-party tools to edit your images.

Connecting and Disconnecting Your USB Camera

Windows XP has built-in support for connecting to most USB digital cameras.

First, connect your camera to the USB port on your computer and then turn the camera on in playback mode. Windows automatically recognizes the device and mounts it as a new external disk drive on your system. You can then browse the photo files stored in your camera's memory as if they were stored on a disk drive attached to your computer.

The first time you connect your camera, Windows XP displays a Found New Hardware notification in the Taskbar at the bottom right of the display.

When the camera is connected, Windows adds a Safely Remove Hardware icon to the Taskbar. Before you disconnect or power off your camera, you should use this to dismount the camera and associated disk from your system. This prevents the danger of breaking the electrical connection while the computer and the camera are in the middle of an operation.

To prepare to disconnect the camera, click on the Safely Remove Hardware icon and select Safely Remove Hardware. Windows dismounts the disk and then displays a Safe to Remove Hardware notification (see Figure 5.10). You then can disconnect your camera safely. Windows uses this same process when mounting and disconnecting other devices, such as external drives—both USB and FireWire.

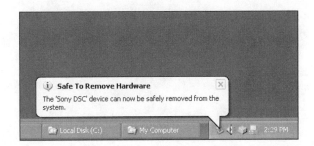

FIGURE 5.10

Use the Safely Remove Hardware icon to dismount the camera from your system before disconnecting it.

Accessing Your USB Camera

When your digital camera is connected and mounted on your system as a disk, you can access its contents like any other disk drive. Open a Windows Explorer window from My Computer and then browse the contents of the camera disk. Windows recognizes its contents as a collection of pictures, and displays the files as photo thumbnails (see Figure 5.11).

Explorer provides a viewer interface with buttons to step through the photos; it also provides options under Picture Tasks, including viewing the photos as a slide show.

The photos are still stored on the digital camera, however, and accessed through the relatively slow USB connection. You should copy the files to your hard drive to save and edit—typically into the My Pictures folder. You then can delete the pictures stored in the camera.

FIGURE 5.11

Use Windows Explorer to browse the photos stored on your digital camera.

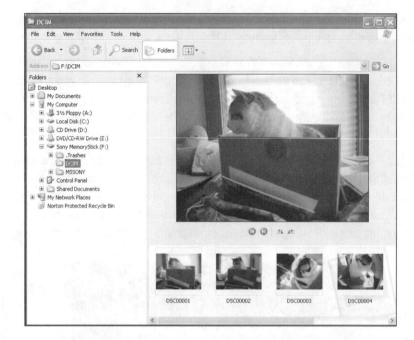

Similarly, you can import photos from other cameras using USB readers for their removable media. You can acquire images yourself from a scanner, or have film processed and digitized and then returned on a CD or posted on the web for you to download.

Organizing Your Photos and the My Pictures Folder

Windows provides standard folders that you can use to organize your files—including the My Documents folder for various word processing, spreadsheet, and other kinds of documents. Windows XP extends this support by providing a My Pictures folder within My Documents that can be used to organize pictures. Under Windows XP, each user login has its own copy of the My Documents folder.

When you use Windows Explorer to view the My Pictures folder (or actually any folder with image files), Explorer enhances the window for viewing pictures. This is shown by the faint photo watermark at the bottom-right corner of the Explorer window. Of course, because your pictures are simply files, all the normal file-browsing features and actions also are available.

Use the View menu to select the viewing mode for your files. Choose Filmstrip to display a viewer to step through your files (refer to Figure 5.11). Choose Thumbnails to view thumbnails of each picture and folders with small thumbnails of some of the images inside them embossed on their covers (see Figure 5.12).

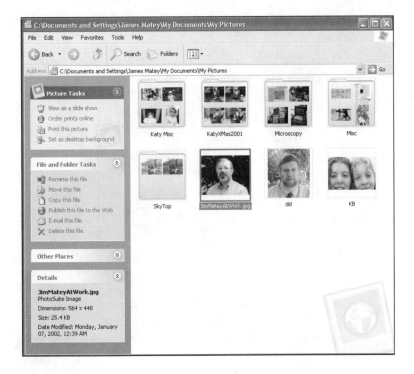

FIGURE 5.12

Use the Windows Explorer View options to browse the My Pictures folder.

Click on the Folders button to alternate the left Explorer Bar panel between a hierarchical list of folders and the context-sensitive Taskbar. The Taskbar includes specific Picture Tasks for photo files, general File and Folder Tasks for all files, Other Places, and Details of the currently selected file.

Under Picture Tasks, you can view the contents of any folder as a slide show, and even order prints of your photos online.

You also can right-click on a file to see a pop-up menu with both general Explorer actions and picture-specific actions. Choose Properties to examine the image file characteristics. Select the Summary tab, and click on the Advanced button to display the information that the camera stored with each photo, including lens type and exposure time (see Figure 5.13).

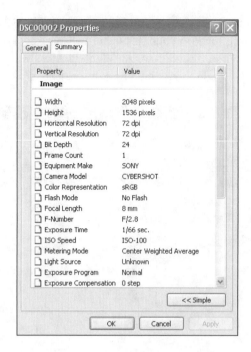

You can organize your pictures using folders and shortcuts. For example, you might keep all your vacation photos in a Vacation folder, with subfolders for each year. If you decide that you want to create a highlights slide show, you could select and Copy photos of interest, move to a Highlights folder, and then use Paste Shortcut to create shortcuts to the originals in the Highlights folder. Your originals remain in place, and the shortcuts take up little space.

If you choose to store photo files in other folders besides My Pictures, Windows Explorer can provide the same kinds of View options as Filmstrip or Thumbnails. You also can customize a folder as a Photo Album by using the Customize tab in its Properties dialog box.

DV Video Editing with Windows Movie Maker

As with digital photos and the My Pictures folder, Windows XP provides built-in support for browsing and viewing video files in the My Videos folder.

Windows also includes the Windows Movie Maker application to capture, edit, and export video from DV digital cameras over a FireWire/IEEE 1394 port. You can edit and save movies, download them to a portable device, and share them over the web.

Browsing Video in the My Video Folder

Just as the My Pictures folder is enhanced with built-in photo-viewing capabilities, Windows XP also includes a My Video folder enhanced for browsing video clips (see Figure 5.14). As with pictures, Windows Explorer automatically provides these enhancements for any folder containing video files, as shown by the filmstrip watermark at the bottom-right corner of the Explorer window.

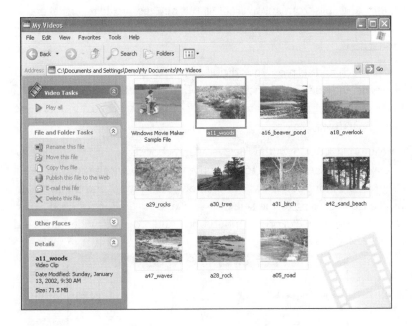

FIGURE 5.14

Windows Explorer provides enhanced capabilities for viewing the My Videos folder.

The My Video folder works much like the My Pictures folder, with a thumbnail for each file displaying a single frame of the video sequence. You can organize your videos using the same methods you use for your pictures—including renaming, moving, copying, publishing to the web, emailing, and deleting. You can select and play back single videos or all the videos in a folder.

About Windows Movie Maker

Windows Movie Maker is the basic video-editing tool built into recent versions of Windows. It is normally found under Accessories in the Start menu. With Movie Maker for Windows XP, you can import media files, capture video from DV camcorders or record from other devices, and import and edit clips into projects; you can then export your movie to a video file, copy it to a portable device, or post it to a web site.

Capturing from DV with Windows Movie Maker

A Movie Maker project is built around a collection of media material. You can import video, audio, and still images in a variety of formats. You also can capture video, audio, and stills from any available input devices, including digital and analog sources. Movie Maker can record to files from digital camcorders with FireWire or USB connections.

When you attach and turn on your digital camcorder, Windows recognizes the type of device and adds it as an icon to the Taskbar. Note that unlike with digital cameras, a camcorder is not treated like a disk device, so you cannot browse its contents in Windows Explorer.

To start capturing, pull down the File menu and choose Record to display the Record dialog box (see Figure 5.15). Use the Change Device button to select between multiple input devices as available on your system, and the available options change according to the selected device. Use the Record drop-down menu to select between recording Video only, Audio only, or Video and Audio.

FIGURE 5.15

Use the Record dialog box in Windows Movie Maker to capture input material from a DV camcorder.

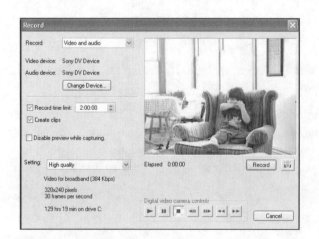

You also can set a Record time limit and use the Create Clips check box to have Movie Maker split the input recording into individual clips based on recognizing scene transitions.

Movie Maker always records files in Windows Media format. Also use the Setting drop-down menu to choose the compression type: Low, Medium, or High Quality; or choose Other to select specific target data rates for dial-up to broadband web streaming, or for PDA devices.

For digital camcorders connected by a FireWire interface, you can use the play controls to play the tape and position it to the start of the material that you want to control.

Finally, click on Record to start recording to disk. Press Stop to finish recording the clip.

In the Timeline view, you also can record audio clips by pulling down the File menu and choosing Record Narration. The audio source can be any source on your computer, including microphone or line input, an audio CD, or the output of your sound mixer.

If you already have audio or video clips from another source in your system, you can use the Import menu item to add them to your collection to use in the movie.

Editing Your Movie

When you have imported and recorded your clip collection, you then assemble your movie into the Storyboard area at the bottom of the window. You also can use the View menu to switch to a Timeline view to precisely control the overlap of the different streams (see Figure 5.16).

As you work with clips, you can edit their order by dragging them on the Storyboard or Timeline. Use the Clip menu to Trim, Split, and Combine adjacent clips. Select Set Start Trim Point, and a set of movable sliders appears at each end of the clip. Move the sliders to set the trim points, and the video display changes to display the frame at the current trim point.

To create a transition between adjacent clips, drag the second clip so that it overlaps the first. Movie Maker automatically creates a dissolve transition from the first clip to the second for the duration of the overlap. Use the Zoom buttons on the left of the Timeline to zoom in and out for more control.

FIGURE 5.16

Use the Timeline display for more precise control while editing your movie.

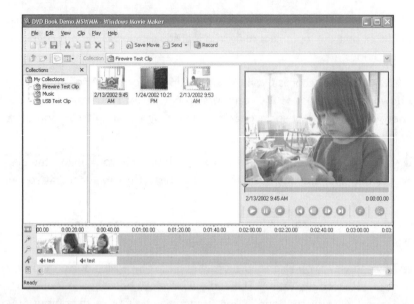

As you edit, you can use the play controls under the video window to preview the entire duration of the assembled clips, or drag the slider to move to a specific section of the movie. You also can use the Play menu options to work your way through the movie scene by scene or even frame by frame.

Exporting Your Movie

After previewing your movie, you can export it to disk, and play and share it by writing it to CD or copying it to a portable device, such as a PocketPC handheld. You also can save a movie directly to a web site, or send it by email.

Pull down the File menu, and choose Save Movie to use the Save Movie dialog box to select the output video file format (see Figure 5.17). You can export to a Windows Media file and choose the compression format and target data rate, or save the movie as a DV-AVI file in DV NTSC or PAL format. You also can supply properties information that can be displayed in the browser window for the My Videos folder. After the video clip has been saved, you can use Windows Media Player to play back the movie.

You can also use the Send Movie to menu option to send the movie to a web server or via email. Especially for email, make sure you compress it to a reasonably small size.

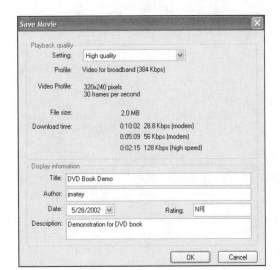

FIGURE 5.17

Use the Save Movie dialog box to export your movie in Windows Media or DV-AVI format.

Summary

This chapter provided a walkthrough for using Windows XP on a PC to import, organize, edit, and export digital media. On a system with the appropriate USB and FireWire ports and recordable disc burners, you can record data files to CD and DVD; import and browse digital photos; and import, edit, and save video and audio movies.

Windows XP provides built-in support for accessing digital cameras via the USB port and digital camcorders via the FireWire (and USB ports), as well as capturing from other analog video and audio devices using compatible hardware. Windows Explorer also provides enhancements for browsing and viewing folders of still image files and motion video clips.

You also can use Windows Movie Maker to perform basic video editing to prepare clips for importing into DVD authoring tools.

Now that you have explored how to connect to digital media hardware devices and access them on the Macintosh and under Windows, you can move on to Part II, "Exploring DVDs on Your Computer" to play movies on DVD and explore how they were designed.

You can then use these capabilities to import and prepare your own video, audio, and still image media content, and use the tools described in Part III, "Automated DVD Authoring" to quickly create your own DVD production, complete with navigational menus and slide shows.

Part II

Exploring DVDs on Your Computer

Now that you have seen DVD in action in Part I, it's time to play and explore DVDs on your computer. By playing through movies on DVD and exploring their structure, you can better understand how different DVD authoring tools organize and automate all the various capabilities of the DVD-Video format.

Playing the content of commercial pre-recorded CDs and DVDs on a computer requires both that the computer has both a disc drive with the capability to read the physical disc, and the appropriate software applications that understand the data files stored on the disc and can decode and play their contents.

However, although the CD-Audio format is quite straightforward, with plain files of uncompressed audio tracks, the DVD-Video format is much more sophisticated, with multiple tracks of video and audio, compressed in different formats, and linked with menus and navigation.

This Part shows you how to use the Mac and Windows player tools, not only to play discs, but also to explore and understand their contents and structure.

Chapter 6, "Playing DVDs on Macintosh OS X," shows you how to use the built-in OS X iTunes and DVD Player applications to access and play music CDs and DVD movies. It also explores the actual data contents of the discs using the Finder.

Chapter 7, "Playing DVDs on Windows XP," shows you how to use Windows Media Player similarly on the PC platform. It then uses the CyberLink PowerDVD and InterVideo WinDVD players to go beyond simple playback to explore the navigational and track structure of the DVD content. It also demonstrates another aspect of DVDs, the capability to include additional computer-readable information and data, along with the movie content. Using tools like the InterActual/PC Friendly Player, these enhanced DVDs can include computer applications to provide access to additional information stored on the disc, online material and events accessed over the web, and even games and activities linked to the movie.

Playing DVDs on Macintosh OS X

CHAPTER 4, "DIGITAL MEDIA AND DVD ON THE MACINTOSH," described how Apple has developed the Macintosh platform and the Mac OS X operating system as a digital media "hub" for capturing, editing, and recording digital video and audio. It also showed how to use recordable CD and DVD drives to write data files to discs. This chapter then explores the built-in Macintosh applications for playing premastered music CDs and DVD movies.

Macintosh systems can serve as digital media players for commercial audio CDs and movies on DVD, just like a set-top player—and more. All that is required to play discs on a computer is a hardware drive that can read the disc, and the appropriate software application that can understand and play the audio and video data prerecorded on the disc. Apple provides two built-in applications on the Macintosh for this purpose: iTunes to play, rip, and burn audio CDs; and DVD Player to play movies on DVD (see Figure 6.1).

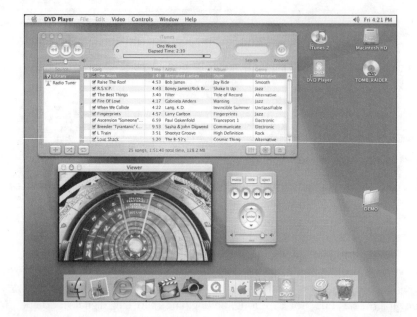

FIGURE 6.1

Mac OS X desktop with player applications: iTunes for music CDs and DVD Player for movies on DVD.

DVD Content ©Paramount Home Entertainment

Playing back commercial CD and DVD discs does not require a recordable drive. You can play music CDs on any CD drive, from a CD-ROM player to a CD-R/RW recordable drive. And similarly, you can play movies on DVD on any DVD drive, from a DVD-ROM player to a DVD-R/RW recordable. These days, combination drives are becoming more common. DVD-ROM drives can read CDs, CD-R/RW recordable drives are being combined with DVD-ROM readers; and drives, such as the SuperDrive, can do it all—reading and recording both CD and DVD.

This chapter explores the CD-Audio and DVD-Video formats using the player applications, and also explores using the Finder to view the data on the discs. With this understanding of the formats, you can then move on to Chapter 10, "Personal DVD Authoring with Apple iDVD," to create your own DVD productions with the iDVD application.

Playing Audio CDs with iTunes

The CD-Audio format was originally designed as a relatively simple format for use in consumer audio systems, but the disc file format was also readable by computers. The CD-Audio disc format simply contains one file per song on the disc, with each file containing uncompressed audio data. There is no other information on the disc, even to identify its contents.

At first, it was amazing just to be able to play these audio CDs on a computer. However, times have changed with the continued dramatic growth in the power of home computers, the availability of gigabytes of disk storage, improvements in audio compression technology, and access to Internet resources. It is now not only feasible, but common to "rip" copies of an entire CD collection into MP3 format on a hard disk, organize the collection and create custom playlists, and then burn your own mixes to a CD or download them to a portable player.

This section provides a hands-on tour of the Apple iTunes application, which combines all these functions into a common interface. The focus is on playing and exploring the CD-Audio format, but it also provides an overview of how to use each major function in iTunes.

About iTunes

iTunes is the Macintosh audio jukebox application for playing, importing, organizing, and saving music. You can import and convert music CDs to MP3 files, create playlists, and burn your own mixes as music CDs.

A new version, iTunes 2, was released in late 2001 as a free download for both Mac OS 9 and Mac OS X. It includes a 10-band equalizer, sound enhancer, crossfader, burner of MP3 CDs, and automatic synchronization with the Apple iPod portable music player.

Exploring iTunes

When you first launch iTunes, it displays the Library window with an eclectic sampler of preloaded music across a variety of genres (see Figure 6.2). The Library shows a list of all your songs, with information on the song title, duration, artist, album, and genre. Click on the column headings to sort the list by each category.

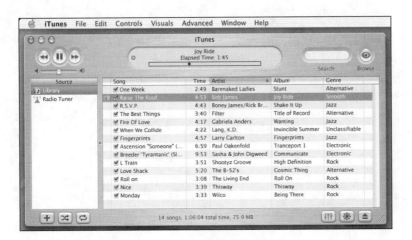

FIGURE 6.2

iTunes window with sampler Library of preloaded music.

To start playing a file, just double-click on its entry in the list. The speaker icon on the left of the list shows the currently playing song. Use the play controls in the top left of the window to adjust the volume, play or pause, and skip between songs.

Playing and Exploring Audio CDs

You can also use iTunes to play music directly from an audio CD. Insert a music CD in your Macintosh. OS X will recognize the disc format as an audio CD, and show an Audio CD icon on the desktop. It will also launch iTunes if it is not already running. The new audio CD will also appear as a new Source in the left column of the iTunes window (see Figure 6.3).

FIGURE 6.3

When you load an audio CD the disc appears on the desktop, and then iTunes launches and is ready to play it.

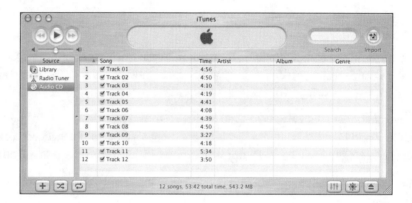

To play directly from the CD, just double-click on the track in the iTunes listing.

Unlike DVDs, the CD-Audio format was not designed to include computer-readable information about the contents of the disc, such as the album name, artist, or song titles. As a result, if your computer is not connected to the Internet, iTunes can display only generic names for each track.

If your computer is connected to the Internet, iTunes can search the CD Database (CDDB) to retrieve this information for the CD to save in your library (see Figure 6.4). See the GraceNote web site for more information on the CDDB (www.gracenote.com).

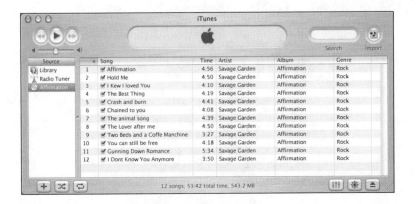

FIGURE 6.4

When connected to the Internet, iTunes can retrieve album information from the Internet CD Database.

Courtesy of Sony Records

Next, double-click on the Audio CD icon to open a Finder window to display its contents. Click on the List View icon to see the file sizes (see Figure 6.5).

Name	Date Modified	Size	Kind
Track 01.cdda	Today, 8:39 PM	49.9 MB	CD Audio Track
Track 02.cdda	Today, 8:39 PM	48.9 MB	CD Audio Track
Track 03.cdda	Today, 8:39 PM	42.1 MB	CD Audio Track
Track 04.cdda	Today, 8:39 PM	43.6 MB	CD Audio Track
Track 05.cdda	Today, 8:39 PM	47.4 MB	CD Audio Track
Track 06.cdda	Today, 8:39 PM	41.8 MB	CD Audio Track
Track 07.cdda	Today, 8:39 PM	46.9 MB	CD Audio Track
Track 08.cdda	Today, 8:39 PM	48.8 MB	CD Audio Track
Track 09.cdda	Today, 8:39 PM	34.9 MB	CD Audio Track
Track 10.cdda	Today, 8:39 PM	43.5 MB	CD Audio Track
Track 11.cdda	Today, 8:39 PM	56.2 MB	CD Audio Track
Track 12.cdda	Today, 8:39 PM	38.7 MB	CD Audio Track

FIGURE 6.5

Open the audio CD in a Finder window to view the tracks as files.

Again unlike DVDs, the CD-Audio disc format is extremely straightforward, with each individual track stored in a separate file. The files contain uncompressed music data, requiring approximately 10MB per minute of stereo music. You can therefore store more than 74 minutes of music on a 650MB CD disc, or around 80 minutes on a 700MB CD.

Click on the Audio CD disc icon on the desktop to select it, and then pull down the File menu and choose Show Info. The Finder displays an Audio CD Info window (see Figure 6.6).

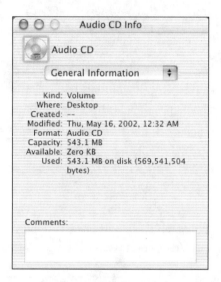

FIGURE 6.6

The Info window shows that the Macintosh recognizes the CD-Audio disc format.

The disk was created in CD-Audio format, and it is readable across different platforms: Macintosh, Windows, and UNIX. As a result, the folder names and filenames are limited to eight characters, with three-character file type extensions. The disk capacity values show how much of the 650MB available on a CD are used for this album.

T I P

Technically, CD-Audio is sampled at a 44.1KHz sampling rate (44,100 samples per second), with two 16-bit stereo samples, which works out to 10.09MB/min.

Recordable CD disc capacity was originally 650MB, also described as 74 minutes; and newer CDs are now available with 700MB, or 80 minutes.

Importing Music from CD

Although you can use your Mac simply as a CD player to spin your discs, iTunes can do much more. By using today's larger hard disk drives and by compressing the audio files, it becomes quite feasible to import and organize your CDs as files on your hard disk. You can then access and play any song instantly without needing to find and load the CD, and you can even create your own custom playlists that span many different albums.

To import the song tracks from the current audio CD, click on the Import button on the top right of the iTunes window. iTunes then compresses each track into the MP3 audio format, and adds them to the Library. Click on Library in the Source column to view the new songs (see Figure 6.7).

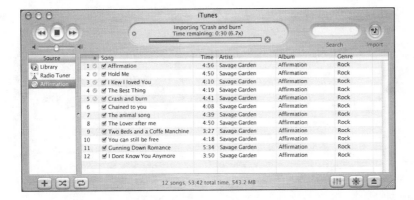

FIGURE 6.7

Use iTunes to import song tracks from an audio CD to files on your hard disk.

Courtesy of Sony Records

To see how much the song files have been compressed, click to select a song, pull down the File menu, and choose Show Song File. iTunes opens a Finder window. Click the List View icon to see the file sizes (see Figure 6.8).

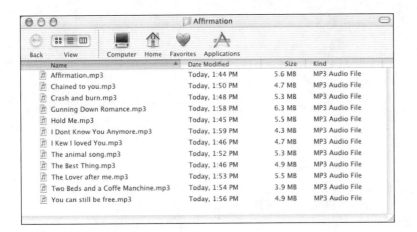

FIGURE 6.8

Use Show Song File to open a Finder window to view the song files compressed in MP3 format.

Courtesy of Sony Records

The MP3 files are significantly smaller than CD-Audio (almost 10 times smaller), typically compressed at 128Kb per second to around 1MB per minute of music, compared to 10MB for the uncompressed CD-Audio format. As a result, an entire album in compressed MP3 format can use only about 60MB of hard disk space, compared to 650MB for the original album on an audio CD. (The size of MP3 files can vary because audio files in the MP3 format can be compressed at different rates.)

M P 3   A U D I O   C O M P R E S S I O N

The audio compression format popularly called MP3 is actually MPEG-1, Layer 3 audio com-pression, which is brought to you by the same Motion Picture Experts Group (MPEG) standards group that defined the MPEG-1 and MPEG-2 video compression used for DVD-Video.

*MP3 is a **lossy** compression technique: Some of the audio signal is removed or lost during the compression process to significantly reduce the amount of data. However, this loss is typically not noticeable for casual listening because MP3 uses a **perceptual** compression technique, which attempts to remove only those portions of the original sound signal that are not noticeable to most listeners.*

The MP3 format also provides a great deal of flexibility and control over parameters, including the sample rate and compression data rate, so that you can select different amounts of com-pression to trade off the file size and sound quality.

Setting MP3 Compression Options

To change MP3 compression options, pull down the iTunes menu and choose Preferences to display the iTunes Preferences dialog box. Under the Importing tab, you can choose to import audio in MP3, Macintosh AIFF, or Windows WAVE formats (see Figure 6.9).

For the MP3 format, you can select a standard Configuration of Good, Better, or High Quality—corresponding to a 128, 160, or 192Kbits-per-second data rate. The 128Kbps rate is used quite commonly, and corresponds to around 1MB per minute.

Pull down the Configuration drop-down menu, and choose Custom to display the MP3 Encoder dialog box (see Figure 6.10). iTunes provides MP3 compression options to adjust Mono or full Stereo, change the CD Sample Rate, choose a custom Bit Rate, and enable additional Smart Encoding and other techniques to improve the sound quality and lower the data size.

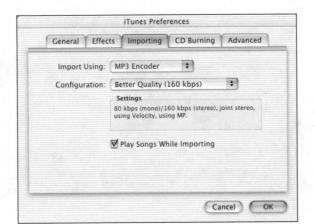

FIGURE 6.9

Use the iTunes Preferences dialog box to control how music is compressed when importing.

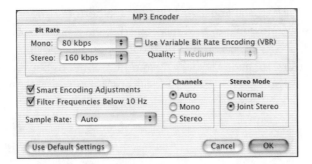

FIGURE 6.10

The iTunes MP3 Encoder dialog box provides control over compression parameters.

Organizing and Sharing Music with iTunes

As a music jukebox, iTunes can do much more than just play and import audio CDs; you can use it to organize your music library for customized playlists, and to burn your collections to CD or download them to a portable player, such as the Apple iPod. Click on the Playlist button at the bottom-left of the iTunes window to create a new playlist.

If you are connected to the Internet, you can also click on Radio Tuner in the Source column to access Internet radio stations around the world.

iTunes provides several methods to work with a large collection as you add more music. Click on the Browse button at the top right of the window to view your collection by artist and album, or use the Search box to display only matching entries for the first few letters of a song, album title, or artist name.

To entertain your eyes, click on the Visual Effects button at the bottom right of the window (or use the Visuals menu) to display onscreen graphics that pulse to the beat of your music (see Figure 6.11).

FIGURE 6.11

iTunes displays visual effects choreographed to your music.

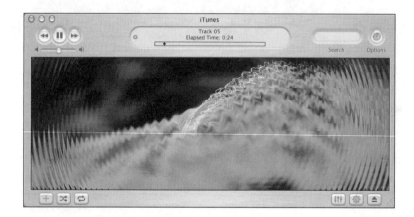

For your ears, click on the Equalizer button at the bottom right of the window (or select it in the Window menu) to display the 10-band Equalizer control with built-in EQ presets (see Figure 6.12). Also, in the Preferences dialog box, click on the Effects tab to use Crossfade Playback to smooth transitions between songs on your playlists and Sound Enhancer to add life and richness to your music.

FIGURE 6.12

Use the Equalizer presets to adjust the audio frequencies for your type of music and listening environment.

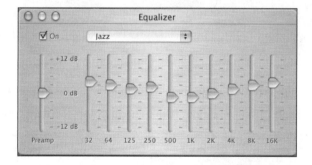

Playing Movies on DVD with DVD Player

Like CDs in CD-Audio format, OS X can recognize DVD discs in DVD-Video format, and automatically launch the associated DVD Player application so that you can play the contents of the disc. You can play DVD movies on Macs equipped with a DVD drive, whether it is a DVD-ROM drive for reading DVDs or the SuperDrive for DVD recording.

This section provides a hands-on tour of the Apple DVD Player application, which provides a simple interface for navigating DVD menus and controlling playback. It uses DVD Player to explore how movies on DVD are authored: organized onto different title sets, segmented into chapters, and accessed through navigational menus.

About DVD Player

DVD Player is the Macintosh application for playing movies on DVD. It provides a clean and simple interface, like those you are used to, for controlling DVD playback on the Mac with a graphical remote control for a set-top DVD player.

You can configure DVD Player to automatically launch when you insert a DVD disc and then start playing your movie full-screen on your display. All you have to add is the soda and popcorn.

Starting DVD Playback

When you install a DVD-Video movie disc in the DVD drive, the Mac recognizes its format, and automatically launches the DVD Player so that you can watch the movie. (You can set DVD Player to automatically start playing, and even to display full-screen, using the Preferences dialog box.)

The main DVD Player screen is a Viewer window used to watch the video (see Figure 6.13). You can position and size the Viewer window to fit your needs and mood. Choose a desired size from the View menu: Half Size to shrink the window in a corner of the screen as you are working, Normal Size to fit the size of the video on the DVD, or Maximum Size to enlarge it to the full width of the display.

Choose Enter Full Screen to hide the Mac desktop and display the movie full-screen as you lean back and enjoy your popcorn. You can also use the Preferences dialog box under the Player tab to specify how the movie and controller are displayed in this mode. Double-click to restore the desktop, or move the cursor to the top of the screen to display the menu bar.

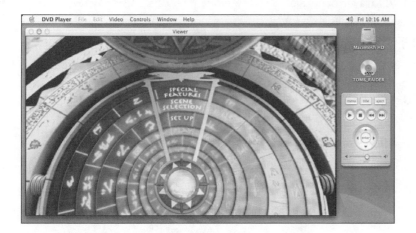

FIGURE 6.13

When you insert a DVD disc, the DVD disc icon appears on the Mac desktop, and the DVD Player application can launch automatically.

©Paramount Home Entertainment

The DVD Player also provides a Controller window to act like a DVD remote control. If necessary, pull down the Window menu and choose Show Controller to display the Controller window. You can control the DVD playback by clicking on buttons on the controller or by selecting the equivalent entries in the Controls menu. You also can use the Controller Type entry to switch the controller between a Horizontal layout (for positioning under the Viewer window) or a Vertical design (for positioning next to the window).

Click on the Play button on the left of the controller to start DVD playback. DVD Player automatically resizes the Viewer window, if needed to match the widescreen format of the movie.

Movies on DVD typically have a main Title menu that is the first thing displayed when you start playing the DVD (sometimes after an introductory clip). Besides letting you just play the movie, Title menus typically also provide access to additional material and features. This is part of the fun of watching movies on DVD (besides the ability to easily jump around and watch favorite scenes.)

Click on the Up and Down arrows on the navigation pad in the center of the controller to step through the menu entries. You then can click on the center Enter button to select the current option. But you can do even better. After all, you are playing the DVD on a computer with a mouse, so you can just point the cursor at a DVD menu entry to select it, and click to activate it.

Click on Play in the Title menu to begin playing the movie.

Controlling DVD Playback

The DVD Player controller has very simple controls, especially for playback. The play controls combine a lot of capability into four buttons: Play/Pause, Stop, Reverse, and Forward.

Click on Play to begin playing the movie. It then turns into a Pause button. Click on Pause to temporarily pause the playback with the current frame frozen on the display.

Click on Stop to stop playing the movie. Clicking on Stop and then Play restarts playback at the beginning of the disk.

Click on Reverse and Forward to skip to the next or previous chapter point, as defined when the DVD was originally authored.

In addition, you can click and hold down the same Reverse and Forward buttons to scan quickly through the movie. Pull down the Controls menu and choose a Scan Rate for 2x, 4x, or 8x fast scanning speed.

As you click on the play controls, DVD Player displays an onscreen display to confirm your actions. Next, pull down the Window menu and choose Show Info to display the Info window. It gives you status information about the chapter and titles that you are currently watching (see Figure 6.14).

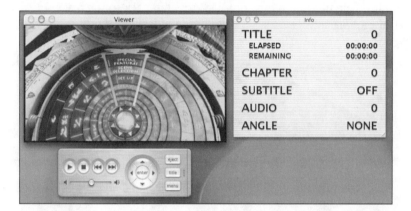

To examine the movie in more detail, click on the right side or bottom of the controller (depending on its orientation) to display the additional controls (see Figure 6.15).

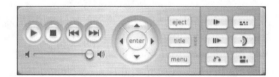

Click on the top-left Slow button to play the movie in slow motion. Click on the Slow button again to cycle though 1/2x, 1/4x, and 1/8x speeds.

Click on the next Step button to step through the movie frame by frame.

DVD Navigation

Besides the full-length movie, the DVD also contains other materials, which are accessed from the main menu. One form of navigating the DVD is to skip between chapters, but this moves you only through the movie portion of the DVD, which is typically contained by itself in one title set in the DVD-Video format. All the other segments of the disc can then be accessed through the navigational structure designed into the menus.

Click on the Title button on the controller to jump back to the main Title menu (see Figure 6.16).

FIGURE 6.16

Click on the Title button to display the main Title menu.

©Paramount Home Entertainment

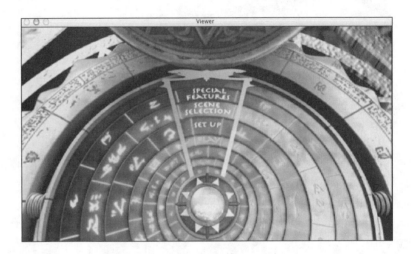

Besides offering a Play option so that you can just play the movie, movie title menus typically include a Set Up option to provide access to additional DVD features, a Scene Selection option with a visual index of the movie to jump to your favorite part, and a Special Features option that links to additional material, such as trailers and outtakes.

Click on Scene Selection to see a visual index of the movie (see Figure 6.17).

Many movies include scene or chapter indexes of each major section of the movie, with thumbnails of the scenes so that you can jump directly to that scene. The scene index is typically spread across several linked menus, so you can page through each set of scenes and get a visual summary of the entire movie.

You can click on a specific scene to jump into the movie portion of the disc, or click on the navigational elements on the scene index menu to look at the different scenes. The menus also need to include an entry to return back to the Main menu.

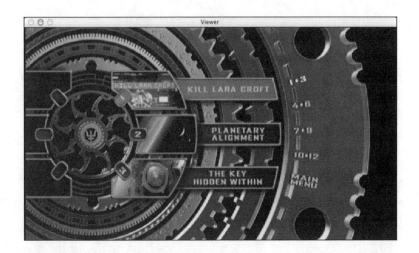

FIGURE 6.17

The scene index menus provide a thumbnail index of the movie contents.

©*Paramount Home Entertainment*

In addition, the DVD-Video format includes several direct navigational controls for moving within a hierarchy of nested and linked menus.

As you have seen, the Title button is designed to jump directly to the main or top Title menu.

The Menu button (next to Title) is intended to be used to jump to whatever menu is appropriate for your current location on the disc, typically the main menu for the current title set.

The Return button (on the additional controls) is intended to be used to jump up a level in the menu hierarchy, something like a Back button in a web browser.

Unfortunately, although the use of these controls is defined as a convention for the DVD-Video format, the way they actually work on an individual DVD is determined by the DVD developer when the disc contents are authored. As a result, their use on different movies is inconsistent.

DVD Features

Click on the Title button to jump back to the main Title menu. Select the Special Features option, and play some of the additional material stored on the disc, such as trailers, documentaries, or deleted scenes.

As you play through the additional material, watch the title and chapter information in the Info window display (see Figure 6.18). You will see that the additional material is stored in title sets that are different from the main movie. Each type of material—trailers or deleted scenes—is often placed in its own separate title set and then can also be separated into chapters.

FIGURE 6.18

Watch the Info window display as you explore the additional contents of the DVD to see how it was authored into different title sets and chapters.

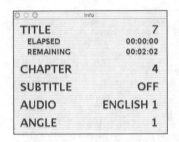

But the DVD-Video format not only supports multiple groups of material in different title sets, but it also supports multiple alternate tracks of video, audio, and subtitles. Like the navigational structure, these can be accessed through the menu structure of the disc or directly from the remote control. Again, the available tracks for a specific movie depend on how the DVD for that movie was designed and authored.

Click on the Title button to jump back to the main Title menu. Select the Set Up option to display the Set Up menu (see Figure 6.19).

FIGURE 6.19

Use the Set Up menu to choose between the available alternate tracks for audio and subtitles.

©Paramount Home Entertainment

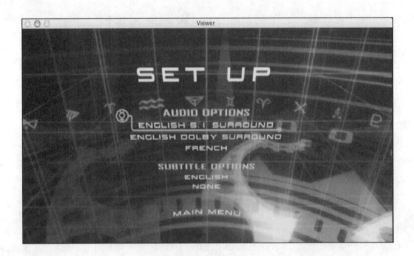

The Set Up menu authored on the disc allows you to set the current option for which audio track and subtitle text is displayed as the movie is played. They are often used for selecting multiple languages, director's commentary, and different surround-sound formats. But because of the flexibility and even limited programmability of the DVD-Video format, you may find other interesting uses on various movies.

Support for multiple languages is actually built into the DVD-Video specification, so that you can specify a desired language for the DVD player, and it can automatically display that language when it plays any DVD, since the tracks can be tagged as specific languages when the DVD is authored.

In DVD Player, use the Disc tab in the Preferences dialog box to set the default language settings for the audio, subtitles, and DVD menu, or to use the default for each individual disc.

Select different audio and subtitle options, and watch the Info window display to see the associated track number. Then go back to the main Title menu and start playing the movie. The Info window display changes to show the associated language for the selected tracks (see Figure 6.20).

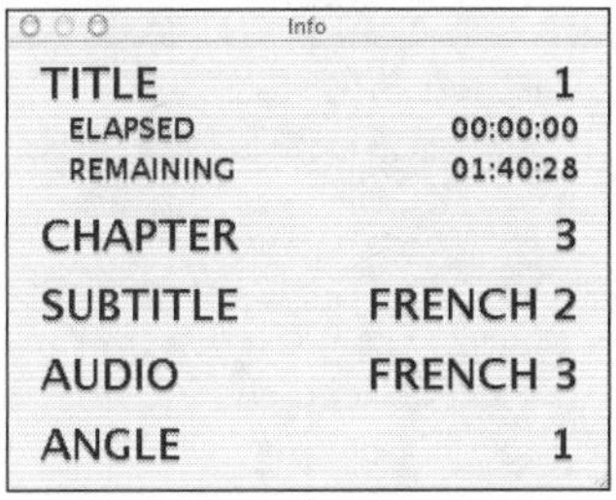

Info	
TITLE	**1**
ELAPSED	00:00:00
REMAINING	01:40:28
CHAPTER	**3**
SUBTITLE	**FRENCH 2**
AUDIO	**FRENCH 3**
ANGLE	**1**

FIGURE 6.20

The Info window displays the current subtitle and audio track numbers plus the associated language name.

Again, the design of the Set Up menu can be quite varied on different DVDs. Some list all possible options so that you can select different languages for the audio and subtitles, whereas others group the selections.

Similarly, many movies on DVD now include a director's commentary, which is actually an alternate audio track with the director discussing the movie over the background soundtrack. Some DVDs are designed with this option in the Set Up menu, whereas others provide the same option under Special Features. In both cases, you are simply selecting the same alternate audio track.

As with DVD menu navigation, DVD remote controls typically include dedicated buttons for selecting between the alternate tracks. The DVD Player controller provides these buttons on the slide-out additional controls. Click on Subtitle to cycle through the available text subtitles, and click on Audio to cycle through the audio tracks.

If the DVD provides alternate video tracks, perhaps for a concert filmed from different video angles, for example, you also can use the Angle button to switch viewing angles.

Exploring DVD Data

You can use DVD Player to explore the structure of the DVD disc, as it was designed when the disk was authored: divided into multiple title sets, marked with chapter points, and linked together with the menu navigational structure. However, the DVD disc also has another structure: as a computer-readable storage medium with a directory structure and data files.

Click on the DVD disc icon on the desktop to select it, and pull down the File menu and choose Show Info (see Figure 6.21).

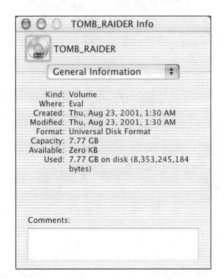

FIGURE 6.21

The Info window for the DVD disc shows that the Macintosh recognizes the DVD-Video disc format.

©Paramount Home Entertainment

The disc was created in Universal Disc Format (UDF), a standard interchange format for DVD discs. Like audio CDs, the DVD disc format is readable across different platforms: Macintosh, Windows, and UNIX. As a result, the folder names and filenames are limited to eight characters, with three-character file type extensions.

For some movies, the disc capacity number may be larger then the 4.7GB DVD disc size that you are used to seeing. The larger size indicates that the movie was mastered to a double-layer disc, in order to fit the entire movie and all the additional material on a single side of the disc.

Double-click on the DVD disc icon on the desktop to open a Finder window to display the files on the disc (see Figure 6.22).

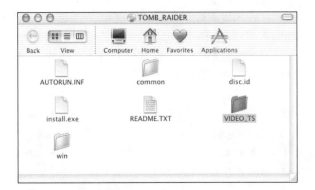

FIGURE 6.22

Open a Finder window to display the data contents of the DVD disc.

Depending on the movie that you are viewing, you may see only a single VIDEO_TS folder, or you also may see other files, as discussed in the following section. But to play on set-top DVD players and on computers with DVD player software applications, the DVD-Video format requires only the VIDEO_TS folder. All the rest of the folders and files are ignored for normal DVD playback.

The VIDEO_TS folder contains the title sets for the DVD-Video content. (Similarly, DVD-Audio discs contain an AUDIO_TS folder.)

Double-click on the VIDEO_TS folder to open it, and choose the List view (see Figure 6.23).

```
000                    VIDEO_TS
  ◄►   [ 88 ≡ □ ]    💻    🏠    ♥    A
  Back      View     Computer Home Favorites Applications
  Name                Date Modified         Size    Kind
  VIDEO_TS.BUP        8/23/01, 1:30 AM      22 KB   Document
  VIDEO_TS.IFO        8/23/01, 1:30 AM      22 KB   Document
  VIDEO_TS.VOB        8/23/01, 1:30 AM     760 KB   Document
  VTS_01_0.BUP        8/23/01, 1:30 AM      18 KB   Document
  VTS_01_0.IFO        8/23/01, 1:30 AM      18 KB   Document
  VTS_01_0.VOB        8/23/01, 1:30 AM     226 KB   Document
  VTS_01_1.VOB        8/23/01, 1:30 AM      10 KB   Document
  VTS_02_0.BUP        8/23/01, 1:30 AM      18 KB   Document
  VTS_02_0.IFO        8/23/01, 1:30 AM      18 KB   Document
  VTS_02_0.VOB        8/23/01, 1:30 AM     226 KB   Document
  VTS_02_1.VOB        8/23/01, 1:30 AM     86.8 MB  Document
  VTS_03_0.BUP        8/23/01, 1:30 AM      82 KB   Document
  VTS_03_0.IFO        8/23/01, 1:30 AM      82 KB   Document
  VTS_03_0.VOB        8/23/01, 1:30 AM    249.6 MB  Document
  VTS_03_1.VOB        8/23/01, 1:30 AM   1,023.9 MB Document
  VTS_03_2.VOB        8/23/01, 1:30 AM   1,023.9 MB Document
  VTS_03_3.VOB        8/23/01, 1:30 AM   1,023.9 MB Document
  VTS_03_4.VOB        8/23/01, 1:30 AM     840 MB   Document
  VTS_04_0.BUP        8/23/01, 1:30 AM      32 KB   Document
```

FIGURE 6.23

The VIDEO_TS folder lists the information and data files that contain the movie content.

The VIDEO_TS folder contains all the content displayed when you play the movie, including the menus; navigational structure; and video, audio, and subtitle tracks. Unlike the CD-Audio format, there are a lot of different kinds of data, and they are all combined together, instead of breaking out each chapter or track into a separate file.

The Information files (.IFO) contain menus and control information for accessing the video and audio, and the Video Object files (.VOB) contain the actual compressed video and audio data, with additional navigation information. The Backup (.BUP) files contain a copy of the data in the IFO files.

The first VIDEO_TS files contain the root information needed to start playing the disc. THE VTS_xx_x files then contain the data for different video title sets. To avoid possible file size limitations on some platforms, the .VOB files are limited to a maximum of 1GB, and the data for that title set is continued in additional files with sequential numbers.

You can see why you need a special DVD player application to read through and understand the DVD disc format and files to decode and play the DVD content.

Exploring Enhanced DVD Data

As shown in Figure 6.22, movies on DVD can contain more than just the DVD-Video material. They also can contain computer-readable files to provide an enhanced experience for viewing on a computer. These Enhanced DVD features can include both computer applications, such as games that run on your machine and web pages and links to online resources.

These additional files are often described as "DVD-ROM" features because the disc contains both the DVD-Video files and computer data read on computer DVD-ROM drives. Many such DVDs use the InterActual "A" or "PC Friendly" logos on the back of disc cases to identify discs that use the InterActual Player interface (see the following chapter for more information).

In exploring these DVD discs, you may find installation programs for the applications, copies of web pages, and even entire sites to explore locally. You also could find combined material, such as web pages with Flash animation and applications that can run in the web browser.

Even better, Enhanced DVDs can combine the best of both worlds: viewing your local copy of a DVD movie while simultaneously accessing associated information over the web. This is the promise of WebDVD, combining the full quality of the stored DVD with updated and interactive material on the web.

Unfortunately, many Enhanced DVD applications are supported only under Windows. On the Mac, you still can access stored web pages and run web applications developed using tools such as Macromedia Flash.

Apple also has implemented its "DVD@CCESS" feature in the Mac DVD Player application to permit DVD-Video content to link to web pages (see Chapter 12, "Professional DVD Authoring with Apple DVD Studio Pro"). This feature is also supported under Windows with some DVD player applications.

Summary

The Macintosh provides a comfortable platform for playing and exploring audio CDs and DVD movies, with the bundled iTunes and DVD Player applications under Mac OS X.

This chapter has used these applications to explore audio CDs and movies on DVD to understand the CD-Audio and DVD-Video formats, and to see examples of how to use the capabilities of the DVD format.

Chapter 10 describes how to create your own DVD productions with the iDVD application. As you work with iDVD, you will see how DVD authoring applications are designed to hide some of the more complex DVD features, either by automatically generating features—such as the up/down navigation between entries on a DVD menu, or by not supporting advanced features, such as multiple audio and video tracks. This degree of both automation and simplification is what separates personal DVD authoring tools, such as iDVD, from more professional tools, such as DVD Studio Pro (see Chapter 12).

The next chapter provides a similar look at playing CDs and DVDs on Windows (Chapter 7, "Playing DVDs in Windows XP").

Playing DVDs in Windows XP

Personal computers are becoming the preferred way to experience and manage digital music and video. As movies on DVD have become such a success for set-top viewing, it is also fun—and useful—to also be able to watch DVDs on your PC.

Of course, you can watch movies on stand-alone consumer electronics products, such as set-top DVD players, as described in Chapter 2, "Consumer DVD Players: DVD Video and Audio." But you can do more on your computer, and you have more control over customizing the playback. In particular, if you are interested in authoring your own DVDs, you can use the software DVD player applications to explore and understand how movies on DVD were designed.

This chapter describes how to play CDs and DVDs using your Windows computer. It continues the discussion that began in Chapter 6, "Playing DVDs on Macintosh OS X," to show you how to use the applications included with Windows XP to first explore and play audio on CD, and then play and analyze movies on DVD.

This chapter begins with Windows Media Player, Microsoft's all-in-one tool for organizing and playing both audio and video material. It then presents other third-party DVD tools from CyberLink and InterVideo that provide even more capabilities for exploring the navigational structure of a disc. Exploring DVDs on your computer can be helpful, both for understanding how commercial discs were designed and for testing your own discs. Finally, the chapter explains the Enhanced DVD features found on many commercial DVDs. These DVD-ROM features, including games and web links, can be viewed only on a computer, and commonly use the InterActual Player (previously PC Friendly).

After you have seen how commercial movies are organized on DVD discs, you can then move on to Part III, "Automated DVD Authoring," to begin to create your own DVDs.

Playing Digital Media on Windows XP

Viewing DVDs on your computer requires both hardware and software: a DVD-ROM drive to physically read the disc and DVD player software to decode and display the data on the disc. Just as CD-ROM drives have become standard equipment on today's PCs, DVD-ROM drives are also becoming a common option, and are even standard on some models.

For playing digital media, Windows XP includes a new version of the Microsoft Windows Media Player, an audio and video player that also organizes and manages digital media on your hard disc between removable discs, the web, and even portable devices. Microsoft further upgraded the Windows Media Player in September 2002 with the release of Windows Media version 9 (www.microsoft.com/windows/windowsmedia).

PC Hardware for Digital Media Playback

The first step in accessing and playing CDs and DVDs on a Windows PC is to ensure that your system has the necessary disc drives. As described in Chapter 6, the newer Macintosh systems come equipped with both DVD drive hardware and iTunes and DVD Player software. Because the Macintosh systems and software are all designed and integrated by Apple, you can be sure that they will play CDs and DVDs out of the box.

This is not necessarily the case with PC systems. The drive hardware on your system depends on how the system was originally configured, or how it may have been upgraded since then. These days, essentially all PC systems come equipped with at least a CD-ROM drive because most software is now distributed on CD. And CDs are not just for reading anymore—most CD drives now include the capability to record in both CD-R/RW Recordable and ReWritable formats. DVD capability is often an added cost option, however.

As prices for these drives have continued to drop, it makes sense to have both kinds of drives in your system: a DVD-ROM drive for reading DVDs (and CDs) and a CD-R/RW writable drive. DVD-ROM drives also can read compatible recordable DVD formats, especially DVD-R.

Another option that is becoming more popular is a single combination drive, with both DVD-ROM reading and CD-R/RW writing capability (although it still is often handy to have two drives available at the same time). In addition, recordable DVD drives in a variety of formats are starting to become available as standard equipment, even on consumer PCs (as discussed in Chapter 1, "Making Sense of DVD" and Appendix A, "DVD Technical Summary").

In addition to the DVD drive, you need PC system hardware components to play sound and video. For audio playback, most standard audio cards can provide great sound quality to amplified speakers or headphones. You also may want to add a subwoofer for low bass effects or even step up to a surround-sound audio system.

For video playback, again most PC video cards now use the AGP bus instead of the PCI bus for faster graphics performance, and provide a separate hardware overlay plane for displaying video in an onscreen window. Many video cards also provide hardware acceleration for display and even video decoding under the Windows DirectX interface, which also can offload your processor when playing a DVD. The video card and monitor should have at least the resolution of the base DVD frame size: 720×480 (NTSC) or 720×576 (PAL). You probably want more resolution, however (1024×768 or better), so that you can devote part of the screen to software menus and controls, and other applications.

Finally, you need enough system horsepower and capacity in the processor, memory, backplane, and hard disk drive to keep up with the demands of processing a continuous compressed audio/video data stream. Depending on your system hardware, a 400MHz machine with at least 32MB of system memory should be capable of playing DVDs without glitches. This would include new complete PC systems, available under $900, as well as a wide range of older machines. It is also possible to upgrade an existing machine to play DVDs by adding a DVD-ROM drive.

PC Software for Digital Media Playback

If your PC has the necessary hardware to read DVDs and CDs, then playing them should be as easy as inserting a disc. Windows XP can recognize the disc format and launch the Windows Media Player to play the content. Media Player is an all-in-one media organizer and manager. It can rip songs from CDs, download associated CD album and DVD movie information from an online database, find and download audio and video material from the Internet, organize it all into a media library, download playlists and videos to portable devices, and burn custom collections to CD discs.

However, Media Player depends on third-party add-ins for DVD decoding and MP3 compression capabilities, so most new PCs with DVD drives also ship with alternative software DVD players, which also enable playback in Media Player. As described as follows, products such as CyberLink PowerDVD and InterVideo WinDVD provide a wide range of features to enhance DVD playback, including multiple subtitle display, single-step to fast-forward playback, video adjustments and zooming, and enhanced sound clarity. These applications are especially useful for exploring movies on DVD to understand their navigational structure and design.

In addition, many movies on DVD also include Enhanced DVD (also called DVD-ROM) features, with additional features and web access when played on a computer. Most of these DVDs use the InterActual Player (previously called PC Friendly) for playing the DVD and accessing these enhanced features.

SETTING AUTOPLAY FOR CDs AND DVDs

One result of all these options for DVD playback is that these software products are competing to be your preferred application. As a result, when you start one up, it offers to register itself as the default application for a wide range of uses, including playing various multimedia file types when you double-click to open them and playing a new disc when it is inserted in the system. As a result, you may find your system behaving differently after you run different multimedia applications.

You can set the default action for when you install different types of media (such as audio CDs or DVD movies) using the AutoPlay tab in the Properties dialog box (see Figure 7.1) for the DVD or CD drive (click the drive icon in Windows Explorer to select it; then right-click and choose Properties).

Under the AutoPlay tab, select the media type from the drop-down menu (Music CD or DVD movie); then select the action you want Windows XP to perform when you insert a disk (that is, play using Windows Media Player).

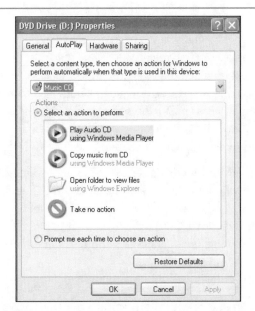

FIGURE 7.1

*Set the AutoPlay
options in the
Properties dialog
box for the DVD
or CD drive.*

In addition, you can set the default player for different types of media files, such as for files of
type .WMA for Windows Media Audio. To set file associations, pull down the Tools menu in
Windows Explorer, and choose Folder Options. Use the File Types tab in the Folder Options
dialog box to select the file type extension, and use the Opens With dialog box to choose the
program to use to open files with that extension (see Figure 7.2). Windows displays the recommended programs that are associated with that file type, or you can restore the default settings.

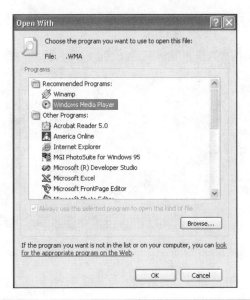

FIGURE 7.2

*Set the associated
application for a file
type in the Opens
With dialog box.*

Exploring Windows Media Player

Since the introduction of Windows 98, Microsoft has developed Windows Media Player as an all-in-one application for playing digital media, accessing media over the Internet, and organizing and managing the Media Library. With audio CDs, Media Player can rip songs from CD, download album information from online databases, and write playlists to CD and portable devices—from music players to Pocket PCs. With video, Media Player can download information from online databases, play local and streaming web video, and transfer video clips to Pocket PCs.

Windows Media Player for Windows XP extends the new interface design that was introduced with Windows Media Player 7 in 2000: CD audio access, Internet media guide and radio, and portable device access. New features in the Windows XP Media Player include direct CD access from the My Music folder, MP3 encoding (using plug-ins), support for multiple CD and DVD drives, and DVD playback (using plug-ins).

The default Media Player interface includes the main display window, playback controls at the bottom, fields with information about the current selection, and a Taskbar down the left side that provides one-click access to the main features (see Figure 7.3). This full display mode can be collapsed to save screen space and to hide the Taskbar and menu bar, minimized with various skin graphics to just show the playback window and controls, or expanded to full-screen over the desktop with floating playback controls.

FIGURE 7.3

Use Windows Media Player to organize and manage your Media Library.

Courtesy of Sony Records

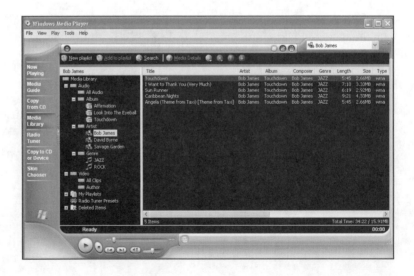

The Taskbar tabs are as follows:

- **Now Playing**. A control panel for the current playlist. You can change playlists; select a particular track from a playlist; control the playback; adjust volume and equalization; and look at information about the album, title, author, and artist.

- **Media Guide**. A built-in Internet browser to access the Microsoft WindowsMedia.com web site. You can access music, radio, video clips, movies, and other entertainment content to play over the Internet or download to your local machine.

- **Copy from CD**. A tool that enables you to copy (rip) the tracks from a CD onto your hard disk.

- **Media Library**. A browser to view and organize your audio and video tracks and clips. Even better, Media Player can download information about CD albums and DVD movies (for example, titles, album art, artist, and author information), and incorporate it into the Media Library.

- **Radio Tuner**. A browser for Internet radio sites.

- **Copy to CD or Device**. A tool that enables you to copy audio tracks and playlists from your hard disk onto CDs or portable devices, including portable music players and Pocket PC handhelds. You also can transfer video clips to Pocket PC devices.

- **Skin Chooser**. A browser for the graphical skins loaded on your computer to personalize the Media Player interface.

Playing Audio CDs with Windows Media Player

Windows Media Player is designed as an end-to-end tool for importing, organizing, playing, and exporting music. Music tracks can be imported into albums, organized into playlists, and burned to CD or downloaded to portable devices.

This section provides an overview of using Media Player to access and manage audio CDs under Windows XP before moving on to DVDs in the following section.

Playing and Exploring Audio CDs

Playing audio CDs under Windows XP should be as easy as inserting the disc into a CD or DVD drive—Windows automatically loads Media Player, switches to the Now Playing tab, and begins playing the first track on the disk. However, this feature may be disabled on your machine, or another program may be installed as the default player (see the sidebar at the beginning of this chapter, "Setting AutoPlay for CDs and DVDs," for more details).

In addition, the graphical look of Media Player can be very different. Media Player can switch between full and more minimized displays, match your Windows XP desktop theme, and it also can be customized with add-on skins, or graphical looks (see Figure 7.4).

FIGURE 7.4

Play your CDs with Media Player, using a minimized skin style and the graphic equalizer.

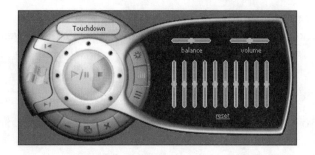

The skins typically provide the common buttons for a CD player, including Play/Pause, Stop, Skip Reverse/Forward, and Volume control. Most skins also provide buttons to display a graphical visualization of the music, a graphic equalizer, or the current playlist. The graphic equalizer lets you adjust volume, balance, and equalization; the playlist lets you select a track to play.

If your computer is connected to the Internet, Media Player can download information about the current CD, including artist information, song titles, and even album art. If your computer is not online, however, none of this information is available. Unlike the DVD-Video format, the CD-Audio format was not designed with these kinds of uses in mind.

Open Windows Explorer to browse through the contents of the CD-Audio disc in your CD drive. Audio CDs contain only the data files of raw uncompressed music, with no text or graphics identifying them (see Figure 7.5).

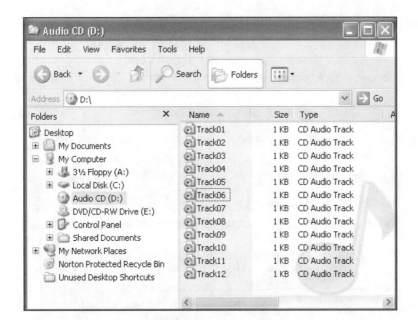

FIGURE 7.5

Use Windows Explorer to view the track files on a CD-Audio disc in your CD drive.

T I P

When Media Player downloads album information from the Internet, the server that it accesses can collect information about your usage patterns and the albums that you are listening to. The server makes use of cookies that personalize your media experience, and each copy of Media Player has a globally unique ID that can be transmitted by Media Player to any server that it contacts. You can disable the unique ID for your copy of Media Player under the Player tab in the Options dialog box.

Importing Music from CD

Besides playing discs in your CD drive, you also can use Media Player to copy entire CDs or selected tracks onto your hard disk to organize and play as part of your Media Library.

Click the Copy from CD tab to prepare to rip the CD to your hard drive. Use the check boxes to select individual tracks to be copied. Click the Get Names button to look up the CD information online, and click the Copy Music button to start copying the tracks to the Media Library (see Figure 7.6).

Media Player also compresses the audio as it is being copied so it takes much less space on your hard disk. Today's computers can copy and compress tracks from CD much faster than real-time playback, so you can rip an entire CD in minutes. Media Player also keeps track of the album and song information in your Media Library.

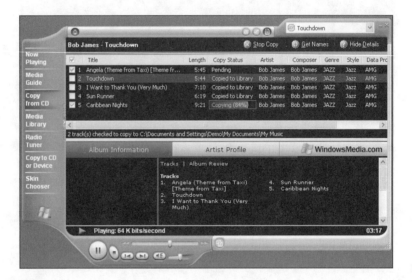

Exploring the My Music Folder

For convenient storage and browsing of different kinds of multimedia files, Windows XP provides built-in folders—including My Pictures for still images and My Videos for working with video clips in Windows Movie Maker (see Chapter 5, "Digital Media and DVD on Windows"). Windows XP also includes a new My Music folder that provides convenient access to your music, separate from Media Player.

Media Player stores the music files in the My Music folder on your hard disk. By default, Media Player organizes your music in folders by artist and album, and names the file for each track with the track number and song title.

You also can use the My Music folder to view your albums by using the cover art (if available). You can use the Music Tracks panel to rearrange your music folders, play selections, and even create audio CDs from selected albums or tracks (see Figure 7.7).

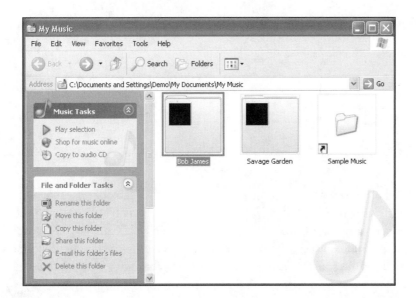

FIGURE 7.7

You also can organize, play, and create CDs from the My Music folder.

Courtesy of Sony Records

Setting WMA and MP3 Compression Options

The music data on CD-Audio discs is not compressed, so the files require approximately 10MB per minute of stereo music. You can therefore store about 74 minutes of music on a 650MB-CD disc or about 80 minutes on a 700MB-CD.

Modern compression algorithms can significantly reduce the size of a music file—by a factor of 10 or 20—without significantly affecting the playback quality. Although these are lossy compression algorithms that do remove some of the audio data, they use perceptual compression techniques that attempt to remove only those portions of the original sound signal that are not noticeable to most listeners.

By default, Media Player compresses music to disk using Microsoft's Windows Media Audio compression format. It can compress to "near-CD" quality at rates as low as 48Kbps, or at custom rates up to 192Kbps for high quality. View the file details in the My Music folder to see the compressed file sizes (see Figure 7.8).

FIGURE 7.8

Use Windows Explorer to view the copied tracks, which are stored in the My Music folder in compressed format.

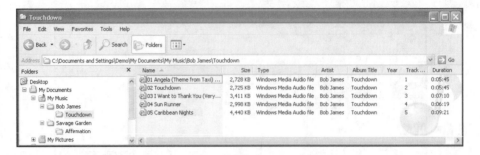

Media Player also supports third-party add-in packs for encoding in MP3 audio format (actually MPEG-1, Layer 3 audio compression). The MP3 standard is used widely for sharing audio files, storing more songs on a CD, and for downloading audio to portable devices. Microsoft states that Windows Media Audio now can provide the same sound quality as MP3 in half the file size.

Use the Copy Music tab in the Media Player Options dialog box to select the compression format and data rate to use when copying files into your Media Library (see Figure 7.9).

FIGURE 7.9

Use the Copy Music tab in the Options dialog box to set the compression format.

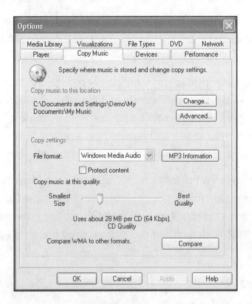

Organizing the Media Library

When you have imported music into Media Player, you can browse and select albums and tracks, and organize them into custom playlists.

Click the Media Library tab to browse and sort your content (refer to Figure 7.3). The left pane shows a hierarchical view of your stored media, with Audio organized by Album, Artist, and Genre. The right pane shows information about each track. You can then sort or search your content—to see all the music within a specific genre, for example.

Click the New Playlist button to create a new entry in the My Playlists folder. You then can drag items into your personal playlist to create a new custom mix with tracks from a variety of albums.

Sharing Music on CD

After you have organized your music into custom playlists, you can then burn them to CD or download them to portable devices.

To burn a CD, click the Copy to CD or Device tab (see Figure 7.10). Select the playlist or tracks in the left pane, choose the output CD burner from the list of available devices in the right pane, and then click on Copy to CD to start recording the CD. You also can burn CDs directly from the My Music folder by clicking Copy to Audio CD from the Music Tasks area on the left side of the folder (refer to Figure 7.7).

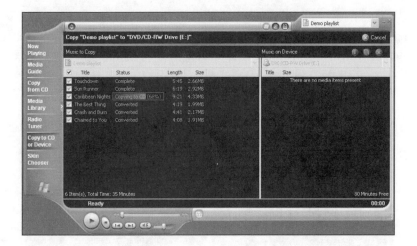

FIGURE 7.10

Use the Copy to CD or Device tab to burn your audio to CD.

Besides creating standard audio CDs that can play in any CD player, you also can pack more music on a CD by burning files in compressed Windows Media Audio or MP3 format. You can play these CDs in other PCs, of course, but some newer CD and DVD players also now can play WMA and MP3 files on CD.

You also can transfer your music to portable devices, including portable music players and Pocket PC handhelds.

Playing Movies on DVD with Windows Media Player

Windows Media Player is much more than an audio player; it also can be used to access and organize video files (see Chapter 5). Plus, it also can be used as a DVD player, including retrieving information about the movie from the Internet. You can even download entire movies (over a broadband connection), and rent and buy movies for a long trip.

However, Media Player does require a third-party DVD decoder to play movies on DVD. These are available as add-in packs from companies such as CyberLink and InterVideo (see the following sections). Even better, if you purchase a complete Windows PC with a DVD drive, you typically will find that a DVD decoder has already been pre-installed on the system.

Playing DVDs with Windows Media Player

As with CD-Audio discs, Media Player should launch automatically when you insert a DVD-Video disc in your system. (If your system is configured differently, you can change the behavior using the AutoPlay tab in the Properties dialog box for the DVD drive. See the previous discussion of CDs.)

In full mode, Media Player plays the DVD video in a window, along with information about the movie and the list of DVD chapters as a playlist for quick access (see Figure 7.11). As with CDs, you can use the controls under the window to Play/Pause, Stop, Skip Reverse/Forward, and adjust the Volume.

FIGURE 7.11

Media Player also can play DVDs, and display movie information and chapter names.

©*Paramount Home Entertainment*

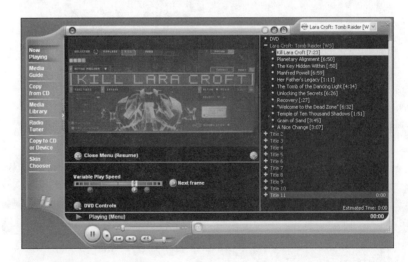

It is also possible to view a DVD in a small window using a minimized skin mode, as shown previously. Alternatively, you can view the DVD in full-screen mode, with playback controls that appear when you move the mouse, and then hide again so you can watch the full screen. Pull down the View menu, and choose Update DVD Information to download online information about the movie. The Media Player playback and navigation controls are similar to what you would find on the front panel of a DVD player. You can also use the mouse cursor to directly select DVD menu items.

Pull down the View menu, and choose Now Playing Tools to display additional controls—including DVD Controls, Video Settings, Graphic Equalizer, and Media Information.

Pull down the View menu, or right-click and choose DVD Features to DVD navigation playback options. Select Top Menu to return to the main menu for the disc, or Title Menu to jump to the menu for the currently playing section within the disc. You also can choose an alternate Audio, Subtitle, and Camera Angle track.

As described in Chapter 6, movies on DVD typically have a main or top menu for the disc that provides access to playing the movie. There are also added capabilities, such as a Scene Selection menu with thumbnail images of scenes, a Set Up menu that provides access to additional DVD features (especially for audio), and a Special Features menu that links to additional material, such as trailers and documentaries. However, this menu navigation structure is only a convention, not a standard. Like the graphical design of the menus, it is completely determined by the designer of the disc.

The following sections describe how to use several different DVD software players to explore the navigational structure of DVDs to understand how they were designed, and to find material on the disc that may not be easily accessible from the built-in menu structure.

Exploring DVD Movies with CyberLink PowerDVD and InterVideo WinDVD

Windows Media Player is built in to Windows XP to provide playback for both audio and video, CD and DVD; and enhanced with media information downloaded from Internet databases. Although Media Player requires a third-party decoder to play DVDs, new computers with DVD drives typically ship with a DVD decoder preinstalled. Otherwise, especially when upgrading a system, you can purchase DVD decoder add-in packs from several vendors, including CyberLink and InterVideo.

These companies also sell stand-alone DVD player applications as alternatives to Media Player. You may prefer a particular player for the quality of the video playback; for the overall look and feel of the interface; or for particular features, such as video adjustments and zooming, enhanced audio quality, fast playback with audio, and the capability to take screen shots of the DVD video.

In mid-2002, Sonic also released the Sonic CinePlayer DVD player application to complement its DVD authoring tools (see Chapter 9, "Automated DVD Authoring with Sonic MyDVD").

About DVD Players

CyberLink PowerDVD and InterVideo WinDVD are both popular DVD player applications. Each of these companies also has a broader product line of video and audio capture, editing, and playback applications, including video-editing applications with DVD authoring capabilities (see Chapter 8, "Integrated Video Editing and DVD"). You often will find these applications bundled with new PC systems, DVD add-in drives, and even DVD authoring software. Note that these players are available in several versions with different feature sets, and the bundled versions may not include all the features described here.

If you are interested in how DVDs for movies are designed, these players provide enhanced interfaces for viewing and exploring the navigational structure of a DVD, including hierarchical menus to access each title and chapter; the capability to browse through alternative video, audio, and subtitle tracks (and to display multiple subtitles simultaneously); and visual displays of chapter points.

For DVD authors, these tools provide the ability to test out a DVD design by playing the DVD volume files from hard disc, even before burning to a DVD disc. You not only can click through each menu and play each clip, but you also can use these tools to explore and verify the overall navigational structure and chapter points.

Use the Menu button on the control panels to access a specific menu defined by the DVD designer, including the Title menu (main or top), Root menu (for the current section), Subtitle and Audio set-up menus, and Chapter menu (scene). These players also can remember your location in the DVD so that you can easily resume from where you left off.

You can use the Configuration dialog boxes to display information about the video player, audio and video playback modes, and computer system.

However, be aware when you edit and author video clips for use on DVD, the video on DVD is designed for set-top playback on interlaced television displays, whereas computer displays are progressive. DVD video is stored in NTSC or PAL television format, with alternating lines from two consecutive fields captured at slightly different points in time. To display interlaced video on computer monitors, these DVD player applications deinterlace the video to remove the alternating lines, but you will see the interlacing if you view the video in a video editor. Therefore, you should burn your production to DVD, play it on a set-top player, and view it on a consumer television to completely verify that it works properly and looks good on the kind of systems in which you intend to show it.

T I P

As discussed in Chapter 1, one of the copy-protection features designed into the DVD-Video format is region management, an anti-piracy mechanism that marks a disc with a region code so that it is playable only on players in specific geographical regions of the world. Unlike set-top players, DVD drives for PCs typically are not manufactured with a hard-coded region code. Instead, they are designed to allow the player software to set a region code so that a disc with the corresponding code can be played on the drive. However, the region code can be changed only a small number of times before it is permanently fixed. As a result, if you alternate between playing discs from different regions in the same DVD drive, you will cause it to be locked to a specific code.

About CyberLink PowerDVD

CyberLink PowerDVD (www.gocyberlink.com) provides powerful tools for playing and exploring DVDs. It supports a wide range of video hardware acceleration, including dual-view monitors. It also supports surround-sound decoding, virtual surround sound, and audio enhancement. PowerDVD 4.0 XP, released in November 2001, supports a wide range of disc and multimedia file formats, provides built-in surround-sound decoding, and provides preset video profiles for enhancing the video contrast and brightness. PowerDVD 4.0 XP is available in a Standard version for around $49 and in a Deluxe version with DTS digital Surround and SRS TruSurround XT audio enhancement for around $69.

For video playback, PowerDVD offers preset and adjustable contrast and color-viewing controls, dual-view monitor support, digital zoom, and full-screen video playback. For audio playback, PowerDVD offers dynamic range control, bass enhancement, and virtual surround sound through two speakers or using Dolby Headphone.

PowerDVD is compatible with a wide variety of DVD formats, including DVD-Video, Video CD (VCD 2.0), Super Video CD (SVCD), and the VR (Video Recording) format used on set-top DVD players. PowerDVD also is a general media player, and plays a wide variety of video and audio files from hard disk, including AVI, QuickTime MOV, Windows Media, MPEG, and MP3.

Exploring with PowerDVD

PowerDVD provides a customizable user interface through the use of skins to design the controls and button layouts (see Figure 7.12). During playback, the controls can be minimized to the Windows Taskbar, or can be switched to a minimized skin design with only the basic navigation functions. You also can use a pop-up Tool Bar Navigator for easy access to controls without using the controller interface.

FIGURE 7.12

Use the PowerDVD pop-up menus to explore the title and chapter structure of the DVD.

©Paramount Home Entertainment

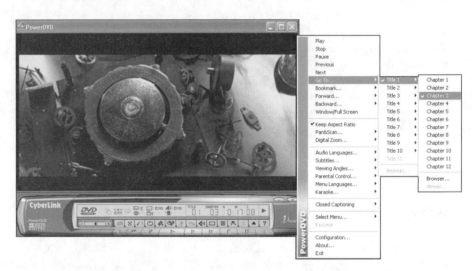

Depending on the current skin design, the controls include the basic navigation buttons: Play, Pause, and Stop; and Step, Scan, and Chapter Backward/Forward. You also can rotate the Shuttle control to scan quickly forward or backward up to 32X. The additional buttons provide access to other DVD and control functions, including the menus and alternate streams.

The display area includes the current Title, Chapter, and Time; plus indicators for the current disc Location and Type, Audio mode, alternate streams (video Angle, Audio, and Subtitles), and even Region and Parental Control.

PowerDVD provides a hierarchical menu for exploring the entire navigational structure of your disk. Right-click in the video window to display the pop-up menu and then choose Go To. The menu then shows a list of all the title areas in the disc and the chapter points defined in each title. Typically, the first title set contains the entire movie, with the chapter points corresponding to the scene index menu. The remaining title sets then contain the auxiliary material, such as trailers, documentaries, and deleted scenes (refer to the discussion of the Special Features menu in Chapter 6).

Even better, PowerDVD provides a DVD Browser window to display a tree view of each title on the disc and the chapters within each title (see Figure 7.13). You also can define a Bookmark to remember a specific point on the disc, and it also will appear in the Browser.

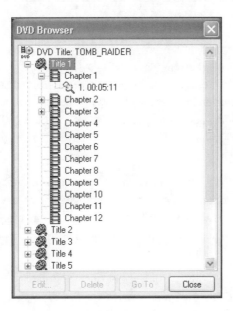

FIGURE 7.13

The PowerDVD DVD Browser displays the full title and chapter structure of the disc.

In addition, PowerDVD provides a graphical Viewer to display thumbnail images of each chapter point defined in a title (see Figure 7.14). This is particularly useful for checking chapter points that you have set in your own DVDs.

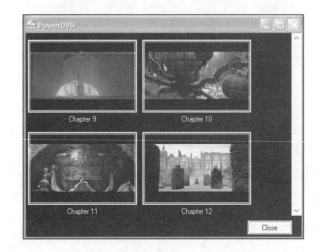

About InterVideo WinDVD

InterVideo WinDVD (www.intervideo.com) provides a flexible interface for playing and exploring DVD content. It includes extensive support for enhanced audio playback, and a time-stretching feature to play back faster or slower while still preserving normal-sounding audio. Version 4, released in May 2002, is available for around $49 or in a Plus version for around $79 (with features including enhanced surround sound).

For video playback, WinDVD offers contrast and color controls, multiple monitor and TV out support, zoom and pan, and video playback as the desktop background. For audio playback, WinDVD offers dynamic range enhancement, dialog enhancement, audio equalization and effects, and virtual surround sound through two speakers or using Dolby Headphone.

WinDVD is compatible with a wide variety of DVD formats, including DVD-Video, Video CD (VCD 2.0), Super Video CD (SVCD), Audio CD, and the VR (Video Recording) format used on set-top DVD players. WinDVD also plays DVD, MPEG, MP3, and other video and audio files from hard disk.

Exploring with WinDVD

The WinDVD controls include a large Transport control on the left side that surrounds a large Play button; and includes buttons to Pause, Stop, and Step Forward or Backward by individual frames (see Figure 7.15). Click and drag the Jog Dial on the left side of the circle for smooth variable-speed playback up to 20X for zipping through a movie. The WinDVD time-stretching feature can play at speeds from $1/2$

to 2X, but still with normal sounding audio. Click the Time-Stretch Clock button to choose to play a movie in a fixed amount of time: Specify a time to Finish By or Play In, and WinDVD will adjust the playback speed accordingly.

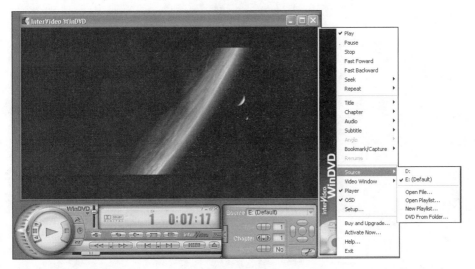

FIGURE 7.15

Open the WinDVD subpanel to access additional controls, or use the pop-up menus to directly jump to a specific chapter.

©Paramount Home Entertainment

Use the buttons along the bottom of the control to navigate through the DVD: Scan Fast Reverse or Forward (or set a specific rate from the pop-up menu), or jump to the Previous or Next Chapter (or select a specific chapter from the pop-up menu). You also can drag the slider underneath to move rapidly to any point in the current clip.

The Display Panel at the top of the controls shows the current chapter or track and elapsed time. Click the subpanel hinge to the right of the controls to access additional controls. Use the Navigation and Language subpanels to access and view the DVD structure and alternate streams, and the Display and Audio subpanels to set video and audio features.

WinDVD provides several different mechanisms to explore the DVD structure. Select the Navigation subpanel to view and change the current chapter, and use the right-click pop-up menu to jump directly to a specific chapter.

Open the Bookmark Browser, and click Include Chapters to have WinDVD automatically create thumbnail images for each chapter point (see Figure 7.16). You also can click the Bookmark button to add your own bookmark points to the browser. WinDVD provides a second Capture browser to review screen shots that you have captured from the DVD.

FIGURE 7.16

Use the WinDVD Bookmark Browser to view thumbnails of each chapter point.

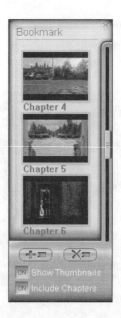

DISPLAYING VIDEO IN GRAPHICAL WINDOWS

Video playback under Windows (and on the Macintosh) is accelerated by video display cards. In particular, the motion video frames are actually drawn in a separate region of memory, and then are mixed with the user interface graphics by the video card. As a result, when you drag around a video window, you may see its video contents jumping to follow the enclosing window. The graphics display actually draws a black rectangle inside the window, which shows through to the background video plane.

Another result of this design is that when you capture a screen shot of a video widow, you get an image of the surrounding graphics, but with only black where you see the video on your monitor. Even odder, if you display the captured screen shot in a window that overlaps the video background, you actually can see the video showing though the screen shot.

As a result, DVD player applications, such as PowerDVD and WinDVD, include a screen-capture function to capture the background video from the DVD.

Exploring DVD Discs and Files

To a computer, a DVD disc is simply yet another storage medium with directories and files. To play in a set-top DVD player, however, a DVD disc must conform to the DVD-Video format, with specific information placed in specified locations and order on the disc. But because the discs use a standard file system, we can examine their content to see how the directories and files are laid out for DVD-Video, DVD-Audio, and other disc formats.

Exploring DVD-Video Discs

To explore a DVD disc, insert the disc in your computer and then view it with Windows Explorer (see Figure 7.17). The root directory of the disc contains two required directories: VIDEO_TS for DVD-Video data and AUDIO_TS for DVD-Audio data (the TS stands for title set, the mechanism for including multiple independent groups of material on a disc).

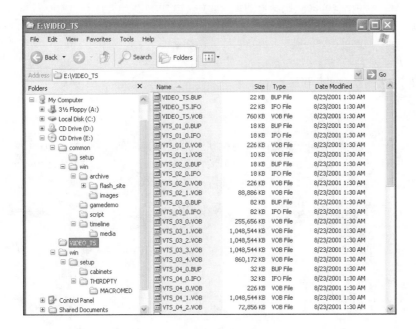

FIGURE 7.17

Use Windows Explorer to view the VIDEO_TS directory on a DVD-Video disc.

Expand the VIDEO_TS folder to view the files that contain all the content displayed when you play the movie, including the menus; navigational structure; and video, audio, and subtitle tracks.

Unlike the simple CD-Audio format, there are a lot of different kinds of data in a DVD, and they are all combined together instead of breaking out each chapter or track into a separate file. You can see why you need a special DVD player application to read through and understand the DVD disc format and all these files to decode and play the DVD content.

The first VIDEO_TS files contain the root information needed to start playing the disc. The numbered VTS_01_0 and similar files then contain the data for different title sets. To avoid possible file-size limitations on some platforms, the VOB files are limited to a maximum of 1GB, and the data for that title set is continued in additional files with sequential numbers.

The Information files (.IFO) contain menus and control information for accessing the video and audio, and the Video Object files (.VOB) contain the actual compressed video and audio data with additional navigation information. The Backup (.BUP) files contain a copy of the data in the IFO files.

Besides these DVD-Video directories and files, a DVD-Video disc also can contain additional files that are accessible only when the disc is read on a computer. Such a disc is sometimes called a hybrid disc, with both the DVD-Video portion and a DVD-ROM computer data. Many movies on DVD contain these DVD-ROM features, including games and activities, additional information about the movie, and web links to associated content (see the following section called "Enhanced DVD with the InterActual Player").

Exploring DVD-Audio Discs

Not surprisingly, the format of DVD-Audio discs is very similar to that of DVD-Video discs, except that the files are clustered under the AUDIO_TS folder, and the files are named Audio instead of Video (see Figure 7.18).

FIGURE 7.18

Use Windows Explorer to view the AUDIO_TS directory on a DVD-Audio disc.

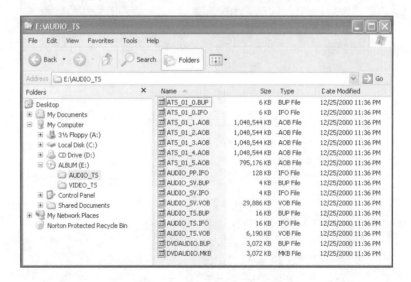

In addition, because DVD-Audio is a newer format designed for audiophiles, some DVD-Audio discs also contain a DVD-Video portion with copies of the same music mixed for DVD-Video audio format (including 5.1 surround sound). In this way, the same disc can be played in set-top DVD players and with computer DVD player applications that do not support the DVD-Audio format. DVD-Video players see the files under the VIDEO_TS folder and play them instead.

Exploring Video CD Discs

The Video CD (VCD) format, by comparison, is totally different from the DVD-Video and DVD-Audio formats. The Video CD format supports a simple menu that links to clips compressed in MPEG-1 video format.

The VCD disc contains several folders with files of control information about the disc, and the MPEG clips are stored in the MPEGAV folder (see Figure 7.19). Each of the DAT files is actually just a MPEG file with video and video for a clip, so you can play it with a DVD or MPEG player (although you may have to rename the file to .MPG).

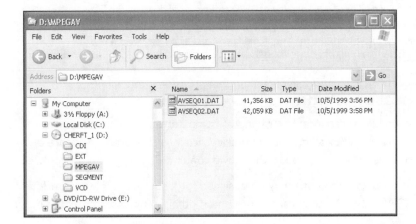

FIGURE 7.19

Use Windows Explorer to view the MPEGAV directory on a Video CD disc.

Enhanced DVD with the InterActual Player

Many commercial movies on DVD include two kinds of additional material: special video features such as movie trailers and "making of" documentaries that can be accessed from the DVD menus, and DVD-ROM material that can be accessed only by a personal computer. As described earlier, the movie and all its special features are stored in DVD-Video format under the VIDEO_TS folder on the disc.

Set-top DVD players simply play the DVD-Video portion, and ignore any other files stored elsewhere on the disc. However, computers can read the entire contents of these hybrid discs—both the DVD-Video portion, plus any additional data stored on the discs, which is accessed as regular files as stored on a DVD-ROM data disc.

The enhanced features included on commercial DVDs can include computer applications, web pages, links to additional online resources, and dynamic links between the DVD playback and online web content.

T I P

You may hear several different names used to refer to these kinds of dual-use DVDs. Most generally, these are described as Enhanced DVD, as in DVD-Video plus additional computer content.

WebDVD is a specific form of Enhanced DVD, with web links between the DVD content and associated web information. The packages on commercial movies often describe these discs as having two types of special features: DVD features (included with the DVD-Video content) and DVD-ROM features (for computers). DVD packaging also includes the InterActual (or PC Friendly) logo to indicate the use of the InterActual player for this content.

Accessing Enhanced DVD Content

Enhanced DVDs can include any kind of computer-readable files, including data such as web pages and executable computer applications. The applications are often entertainment that is related to the movie content, such as games and puzzles.

However, the applications may be designed for a specific computer platform such as PC/Windows, so they cannot be run on other platforms such as the Macintosh.

Another platform-independent way of distributing applications is to use a player, such as Macromedia Flash, that runs across platforms and even from a web browser.

In addition to video playback or stand-alone applications, DVD playback on a computer can offer the best of both worlds: real-time video playback from your local DVD disc combined with online access to additional information, including new updates and even interactive activities. The InterActual Player provides an environment to combine DVD video with computer content in this way.

Apple has designed a different approach to WebDVD, with its DVD@CCESS feature. This feature in the Mac DVD Player application permits DVD-Video content to automatically open a web browser and link to web pages (see Chapter 12, "Professional DVD Authoring with Apple DVD Studio Pro"). This feature also is supported on Windows when using some DVD player applications.

About the InterActual Player

InterActual Technologies (www.interactual.com) is the leading provider of software and services for Enhanced DVD content with commercial movies. More than 80% of the top 25 U.S. major studio box office movies for 2001 used InterActual technology. InterActual reports that its player software was installed on more than 7.4 million PCs by the end of 2001. DVDs that are enhanced with InterActual technology are identified by the InterActual logo on the case ("i" in "A"), or by the PC Friendly logo used in earlier releases.

The InterActual Player 2.0 replaced the previous PC Friendly player in the summer of 2000. It is fully backward-compatible with all PC Friendly enabled titles, and offers support for the Macintosh, as well as Internet-connected set-top DVD players. It supports both DVD-Video and CD-Audio, and is DVD-Audio-ready. It also provides a customizable look through skins. Unfortunately, the InterActual technology is not supported on Macintosh OS X, due to the inability to synchronize DVD-Video and DVD-ROM content.

Use Windows Explorer to examine an enhanced DVD that uses the InterActual technology. Besides the VIDEO_TS folder, the disc also includes directories with the Player installation files and the enhanced disc content (see Figure 7.20). The root directory of the disc contains the installer for the InterActual Player, which even runs automatically, depending on how your system is set up (see the sidebar at the beginning of this chapter, "Setting AutoPlay for CDs and DVDs," for more details).

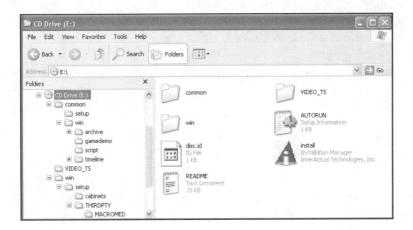

FIGURE 7.20

Use Windows Explorer to view the installation files on an InterActual Enhanced DVD.

TIP

The InterActual Player (or PC Friendly) is included with the movie on each Enhanced DVD. You can install the player from the first such disc that you play on your computer, and then when you play other enhanced discs you then need to install only the disc-specific content for that movie.

However, the InterActual Player does not include a built-in MPEG decoder. It requires that you have some other DVD player application or MPEG decoder installed to decompress and display the DVD data. If you can play your DVD with Media Player or with another DVD player application, you should be all set.

Playing Movies with the InterActual Player

The InterActual Player provides a single environment to play your DVD and to access the interactive computer features.

When you run the Player, it displays a main menu screen to access all this content. One selection is to just play the movie; others may include background information on the movie, games or other entertainment applications; a local archive of the movie web site; and an online experience, combining the movie with updated online content.

Use the View Content button (disc icon) in the top left of the window to switch between the two main viewing modes: the DVD-ROM InterActual Content and watching the DVD-Video movie.

When watching the movie, the InterActual Player displays a Controller bar below the main window, and provides a Web Link frame with links to related content. You also can right-click to use the pop-up menu to choose specific audio and subtitle streams (see Figure 7.21). You can resize the movie in a window or play it full-screen.

Viewing Enhanced Content with the InterActual Player

Use the View Content button to switch back to the DVD-ROM InterActual Content. From the main menu, you can play games and browse through web content on the DVD. Click the Browser Controls button (vertical arrow) on top of the window to display the web browser toolbar at the top of the window as you explore the information.

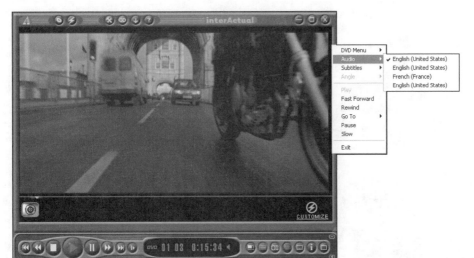

FIGURE 7.21

When playing a movie with the InterActual Player, use the Controller bar or pop-up menu to select DVD-Video features.

©*Paramount Home Entertainment*

In addition to viewing the information stored on the DVD, you can go online to access additional material (even beyond what could fit on a DVD) and updated after the movie was shot. With some movies, your DVD disc serves as a key to unlock bonus material that cannot be accessed directly on the web without a disc.

Even better, you can realize the potential of WebDVD by choosing special features that combine DVD-Video playback with web content. For example, you could review a discussion of the filmmaking process while simultaneously viewing the associated movie scenes, or play a trivia game based on viewing portions of the movie (see Figure 7.22).

Summary

This chapter has shown how to use the Microsoft Windows Media Player for Windows XP to provide an all-in-one environment for not only playing digital audio and video; but also enhancing, organizing, and sharing the experience.

When playing commercial CDs and DVDs, you can use Media Player to access online information, including album and track information for CDs, and movie and chapter information for DVDs. You also can use it to import material from CDs and the web, organize your Media Library, create personal playlists, and copy your own mixes to CD or portable devices to take with you.

FIGURE 7.22

Use the InterActual
Player to view the
movie video while
participating in
an interactive
web activity.

©Paramount Home
Entertainment

One-K for Paramount
Home Entertainment

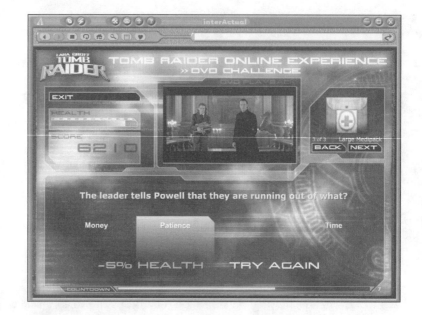

You can further enhance your movie-viewing experience with third-party tools, such as CyberLink PowerDVD and InterVideo WinDVD, and also explore the design and navigational structure of DVDs to help with authoring your own DVDs. And although fully integrated Enhanced DVD capability is not yet available for desktop authoring, you can create your own hybrid DVDs that play on a set-top box and include additional computer-readable data.

The following sections of the book then describe how to put this knowledge to use by authoring your own productions on DVD.

Automated DVD Authoring

Part III introduces several examples of quick-and-easy tools to create DVDs with a minimum of fuss. The idea behind these "automated" tools is to minimize the effort required to create a DVD—just capture some video or import some clips, choose a graphical style, and these tools will automatically create the menu layout and navigational structure. Even with this simplification, they also do provide some capability to customize your productions, such as entering title text or reorganizing the menu structure.

Chapter 8, "Integrated Video Editing and DVD," introduces CyberLink PowerDirector and InterVideo WinProducer as examples of video-editing tools that also include DVD authoring capabilities. These two applications take quite different approaches to providing simple interfaces for video editing and DVD authoring, and therefore are useful to demonstrate capabilities that you will also find in other applications.

Chapter 9, "Automated DVD Authoring with Sonic MyDVD," walks through Sonic MyDVD, an automated tool that can go direct from DV video in to DVD disc out with only a couple of clicks. But MyDVD also provides a wide range of additional features to customize a production, including nested menus, photo slide shows, customizable styles, and background audio. And MyDVD introduces the Sonic OpenDVD format, which permits you to import a DVD disc and re-edit it to add new material or even totally change the design.

chapter 8

Integrated Video Editing and DVD

ALTHOUGH DVD AUTHORING ONCE REQUIRED expensive and complex authoring tools, the new generation of "automated" tools introduced in 2001 has made creating productions on CD or DVD much more accessible by using step-by-step wizard interfaces with design templates and automated layouts.

This rapid development of DVD-authoring software also has blurred the lines between traditional video-editing tools and DVD authoring tools: Traditional video-editing tools are beginning to have the capability to export to DVD, and DVD authoring tools are adding more editing capabilities. Some of the most exciting developments are occurring with the lower-priced consumer tools because they are updated more rapidly, and therefore can adopt new technology more quickly than the more professional tools.

Another trend has been the growth of digital video entertainment software, such as the two popular Windows DVD Player applications, CyberLink PowerDVD and InterVideo WinDVD, described in Chapter 7, "Playing DVDs in Windows XP." Both CyberLink and InterVideo have expanded from DVD players to digital VCR applications for watching and recording TV on your computer, and now have added inexpensive video-editing tools that include basic DVD authoring.

This chapter describes these tools (CyberLink PowerDirector and InterVideo WinProducer), showing how they combine video editing and movie file creation with DVD authoring capabilities. For about $80, these products provide full-featured consumer video-editing capabilities, including DV capture, scene detection, effects, and overlays; and for about $120, they add integrated DVD and Video-CD authoring capability with menus, chapters, and slide shows.

CyberLink PowerDirector is a storyboard-based tool with which you apply edits and effects to individual clips and then arrange them on the storyboard (see Figure 8.1). InterVideo WinProducer provides a more sophisticated timeline-based interface, in which you can apply effects across multiple clips (see Figure 8.2).

You will find the basic editing concepts to be similar to the Apple iMovie and Microsoft Movie Maker consumer-editing tools that were introduced in Chapter 4, "Digital Media and DVD on the Macintosh," and Chapter 5, "Digital Media and DVD on Windows." You should also check out the ArcSoft ShowBiz video editor bundled with Sonic MyDVD, as described in Chapter 9, "Automated DVD Authoring with Sonic MyDVD." However, PowerDirector and WinProducer each take different approaches to providing a convenient interface for editing, and each provides different sets of technical capabilities for processing digital media.

FIGURE 8.1

The CyberLink PowerDirector video editor uses a storyboard interface to easily arrange individual video clips and apply effects to them.

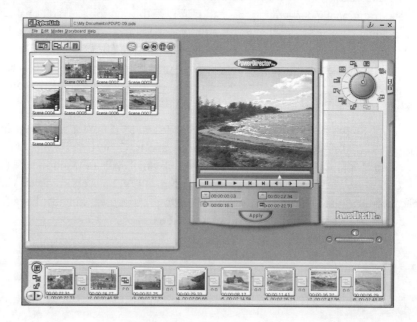

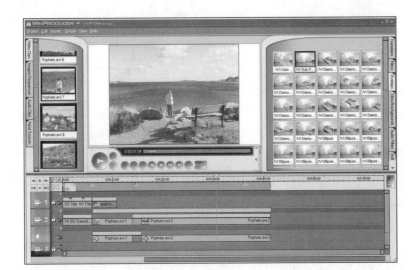

FIGURE 8.2

The InterVideo WinProducer video editor uses a timeline interface, in which you can overlay clips and apply effects across multiple clips.

Video Editing and DVD Authoring

Traditionally, video-editing tools involved importing and capturing video and audio clips, and organizing multiple tracks into a production on a storyboard or timeline. The sophistication of the editors came in the capability to control multiple tracks in a timeline; and in the variety and flexibility of the available tools to add interest and advance the story, including transitions between clips, overlays of multiple tracks and logos, video and audio effects, keyframed animations, and text titles.

Consumer video-editing tools have traditionally emphasized ease of use by constraining the user interface, simplifying the layout process (that is, using a storyboard instead of a timeline), restricting the number of parallel tracks, and providing a step-by-step process for adding effects.

At the same time, dueling new releases of consumer video editors were quick to adopt and support new technological developments by adding support for DV digital camcorders and FireWire/IEEE 1394 import and export; the capability to import and export MPEG-1 and MPEG-2 formats; and the capability to export streaming web media formats, including Apple QuickTime, Microsoft Windows Media, and RealNetworks RealVideo. Other more professional features that were often lacking in these products in the past have included batch capture, scene cut detection, real-time previews, and support for very large files under Windows.

Meanwhile, DVD authoring tools traditionally have been focused on designing the navigational menus to provide interactive access to the DVD content, and assumed that the content was already assembled and edited. For a compilation DVD, this involved importing a collection of clips and then laying out menus with thumbnails of each clip as buttons to jump to the associated clip. For a long production (such as movies on DVD), this involved marking chapter points in the production and then building menus to provide direct access to each chapter. But you still need some editing capability, even in a DVD authoring tool—at least to combine and split clips, and to trim the ends of clips. And it is so easy to add even more capabilities from traditional video editors, such as transitions between clips, titles, and overlays; audio soundtracks; and even video enhancement filters and effects.

With DVD tools, the consumer products have driven technology innovation, particularly by introducing real-time MPEG compression and DV to MPEG-2 transcoding. You can capture DV video live over a FireWire cable, convert it to MPEG-2, package it in DVD format, and burn the video to DVD. In addition, the capability to use the same tools to author productions to CD as Video CD (VCD) and Super Video CD (SVCD) meant that DVD authoring tools were useful to a much larger market, even when the cost of DVD burner drives was exorbitantly high.

Related Products

By the end of 2001, the leading consumer video-editing applications were adding DVD authoring capability to their new releases.

VideoWave 5 from MGI Software (www.mgisoft.com), which was released in September 2001 for $129, included scene detection, video mixing, text animation, transition and effects filters, time warp fast or slow motion, and built-in DVD authoring.

Similarly, VideoStudio 6 from Ulead Systems (www.ulead.com), which was released in February 2002 for $99, included batch capture, scene cut detection, real-time previews, DV and MPEG support, and template-driven DVD authoring (also available in a separate Ulead DVD MovieFactory application). See Appendix D, "DVD Authoring Software Gallery," for more information on the latest version of these and other related video-editing and DVD-authoring tools.

Editing and Authoring Process

CyberLink PowerDirector and InterVideo WinProducer include a broad range of video-editing functionality. They are designed for native editing in the MPEG-1, MPEG-2, and AVI/DV formats. They support real-time MPEG encoding, scene cut detection, and immediate previews without rendering.

The general editing process with these tools is quite traditional:

1. Create a new project to organize and save your work.

2. Organize the video, image, and audio content that is to be used in your production. You can import existing media files, and capture clips from analog or DV sources.

3. Split long clips into shorter contiguous scenes that can be edited separately.

4. Assemble the clips in a storyboard or timeline in the desired sequence.

5. Add special effects, including transitions between adjacent clips, video filters, video and image overlays, text titles, and additional audio tracks.

6. Preview the edited movie.

7. Export, or produce, your final movie production.

In addition, these tools include integrated DVD authoring for assembling your edited clips into a DVD presentation, organized into interactive menus:

1. Create a new project for a specified disc type (DVD, VCD, SVCD, DVD on CD).

2. Select the video clips to use in the project.

3. Split clips into chapter points.

4. Select still images and audio background for slide shows.

5. Select a graphical theme for menu backgrounds and title text.

6. Lay out the clips and chapters onto nested menus.

7. Edit the menus with background images, title text, and so on.

8. Preview the DVD presentation and navigation.

9. Burn the presentation to a DVD or CD disc, or save it to hard disk.

CyberLink and InterVideo

Meanwhile, both CyberLink (www.gocyberlink.com) and InterVideo (www.inter-video.com) have deep roots in DVD player software, with real-time decoding of MPEG video for DVD playback. From this background, CyberLink and InterVideo expanded into video encoding with digital VCR applications: CyberLink PowerVCR and InterVideo WinDVR. These applications turn your computer into a digital VCR by using TV tuner hardware—both to show live television, and to capture and record TV shows for later viewing.

With the system performance and disk speeds of today's computers, these digital VCR applications can capture live TV, compress to MPEG, and store hours of video and audio on hard disk—all without bringing your system to its knees. You can dial out to download the next week's schedules from an online program guide and then schedule shows to be taped in the future. You even can use these applications to time-shift live broadcasts, pausing for a while and then picking up where you left off, or even skipping forward through commercials.

From this background in DVD players, MPEG decoding and compression, and managing recorded video clips, CyberLink and InterVideo expanded their suites of digital media entertainment tools into video editing and DVD authoring with PowerDirector and WinProducer. These tools are designed to take you end to end, from captured video clips to polished movie productions to interactive presentations on CD and DVD.

CyberLink PowerDirector

CyberLink PowerDirector 2 Pro is a storyboard-based video editor with an integrated Disc Wizard for creating productions on CD or DVD. PowerDirector has a very interesting and visually simple interface design, without the profusion of windows and tabs of options that can make some editors appear cluttered and confusing.

PowerDirector 2.0 was released by CyberLink in January 2002 in two versions: the full PowerDirector 2.0 Pro (about $120) and PowerDirector 2.0 Standard without the DVD Wizard (about $80).

When you first launch PowerDirector, it runs a separate System Diagnostic application to verify that your IDE drives have fast DMA transfer mode enabled.

This section takes you on a tour of PowerDirector to see the different video-editing tools, and steps you through the DVD authoring process.

Using PowerDirector

The PowerDirector interface is centered around the main Preview window in the middle of the screen, in which you can view video clips during capture and editing (see Figure 8.3). The Library on the left side of the screen is where you import and organize your media files: video, audio, and images. The Storyboard runs along the bottom of the screen, with placeholders to lay out each clip in your production, and add transitions between them.

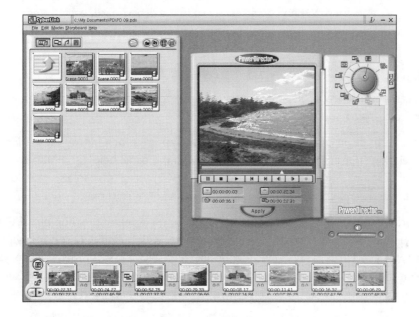

FIGURE 8.3

The PowerDirector interface includes the Library of clips, Preview window, Modes Wheel, and Storyboard.

All the components of the interface are in fixed positions in the PowerDirector window, which takes over your entire display screen.

The key interface feature is the Modes Wheel in the top-right corner of the screen. Instead of trying to offer all editing modes and alternatives at all times, PowerDirector enables you to turn the Modes Wheel to select each kind of editing and to reveal the associated interface elements for that mode. The panel under the Modes Wheel opens to reveal additional controls. In the Effects and Transitions modes, the Library area also is used to display thumbnails of the available effects.

The first two settings on the Modes Wheel are for capture and the default Preview mode for importing to the Library and reviewing clips.

Most of the Modes Wheel settings are used for applying different types of editing to clips as they are added to the Storyboard: Trim (split and resize), Speed adjustment (1/4X–8X), Titles, Video Effects, Picture-in-Picture (PiP) overlay, Audio mixing, and Transitions.

The last two Modes Wheel settings are used for saving your production: Produce Movie to a Disk File, and Disc Wizard to export to CD or DVD.

The Modes Wheel also provides a convenient visual summary of the editing that you have performed: When you select a clip in the Storyboard, each mode in which you have modified the clip is marked with a red line.

Capturing Video and Audio Clips

You can begin a new production in PowerDirector by capturing audio and video clips from analog sources and DV camcorders.

To set up to begin capturing, click on the first Capture mode button on the Modes Wheel. PowerDirector displays three buttons in the panel below the Modes Wheel: Capture Audio, Capture Video, and DV Capture. You can also pull down the File menu and choose one of these options under Capture.

PowerDirector can compress directly to MPEG during capture, either in real-time (if your system is fast enough) or in nonreal-time, with buffering (also for higher quality). CyberLink's Smart Video Rendering Technology (SVRT) then permits you to edit the MPEG video directly, without requiring the data to be recompressed during editing.

You can pull down the Edit menu and choose Preferences to display the Preferences dialog box to set options under the Capture tab. You can set the Capture directory, automatically add captured clips to the Library and the Storyboard, and save single-frame snapshots to the Clipboard as the wallpaper for the Windows display or to a disk file. Use the Performance option to display the captured video more efficiently with video overlay hardware.

For Video and DV capture, click on the Take Snapshot button at the bottom right of the panel under the Modes Wheel to grab a single frame of video.

DV Capture

PowerDirector can capture material from DV camcorders through a FireWire/1394 card, analog sources, or a digital camera. You also can batch-capture from a DV tape using timecodes, and take single snapshot images from the video source.

Click on the third DV Capture input source button under the Modes Wheel to
control and capture from a DV camcorder (see Figure 8.4). Use the play controls
under the Preview window to play through the tape, and use the shuttle control
under the controls to scan forward and backward at variable speeds.

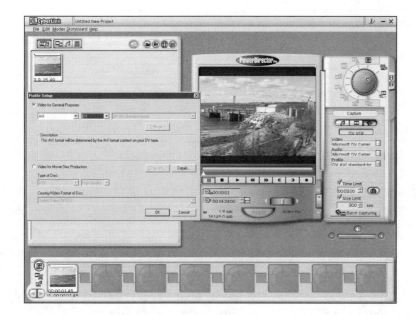

FIGURE 8.4

*Select Capture mode
to set up DV capture
and select the
capture format
profile.*

Click on the Profile output format button to display the Profile Setup dialog box.
Select Video for General Purposes to capture to MPEG-1, MPEG-2, or AVI format
for further editing. Choose a built-in compression format, or define a new custom
profile.

Select Video for Movie Disc Production to capture to a predefined MPEG format
compatible with VCD, SVCD, or DVD; optimized for high speed or high quality.

Click on Comments for system performance recommendations, and Details for a
summary of the compression parameters.

Before starting capture, use the Time Limit and Size Limit fields to specify a
maximum time and maximum file size for the captured clip.

You can then capture a single clip as done previously, or click on the Batch
Capturing button to enter a list of clips to be captured by specifying the start and
stop timecode for each clip using the Mark In and Mark Out buttons.

Click on the buttons on the bottom-right side of the Preview window to switch between Real-Time Capture and Non Real-Time Capture (button pressed in and lit on top). Use Non Real-Time Capture for higher-quality compression, but this will require waiting after the capture completes to encode the remaining buffered content.

Audio and Video Capture

Use the first two Capture Audio and Capture Video buttons to capture audio and video from analog devices, including TV tuner devices. You can capture and compress to AVI and MPEG format files, or compress directly to VCD- or DVD-compatible formats.

If you have capture hardware, click on the second Capture Video button to set up to capture video and its associated audio. PowerDirector displays the current video source below the buttons, with entries for the current video and audio input sources and the output capture format profile.

Click on the Video input source button to set the capture device (that is, TV tuner hardware), choose the capture source (that is, tuner or composite video input), and even to select the tuner channel for a TV tuner.

Click on the Audio input source button to set the audio device (that is, sound card or TV tuner) and audio input (that is, microphone or line in).

To start capturing, click on the Record button on the right end of the play controls under the Preview window. PowerDirector captures the clip in the specified format and then can add it to the Library and Storyboard, depending on the settings in the Preferences dialog box.

Importing Clip Files into the Library

Besides capturing new clips into the Library, PowerDirector also can import additional clips for your project from files on hard disk. PowerDirector can import a variety of common video, audio, and image file formats: AVI, MPEG-1, MPEG-2, and DAT (VCD) video; MP3, WAV, and Audio CD audio; and BMP, JPEG, and GIF images.

To import a file or folder of files, click on the Import Media or Import Folder buttons at the top right of the Library panel (or pull down the File menu and choose an option under Import, or right-click in the Library and chose an Import option from the pop-up menu). PowerDirector adds the selected media files to the appropriate section of the Library.

Click on the Show All Media button in the top left of the Library panel to display all the media files; or click on Show Video, Show Audio, or Show Images to display only those media types.

Click on the Large Icons and Details buttons in the top left of the Library panel to alternate between showing thumbnails of the clips and a detailed listing. Right-click in the Library window and choose Sort to rearrange the clip listing by name, date, or length.

Previewing and Splitting Clips

Click on the Preview mode setting on the Modes Wheel to preview the clips in the Library. Double-click on a clip thumbnail to display the clip in the Preview window. Then use the play controls to play through the clip.

Right-click in the Preview window to choose a display size from the pop-up menu. Some display sizes stretch the video frame to fill the Preview window area and therefore change the aspect ratio of the video.

If you capture long clips that contain multiple scenes, PowerDirector provides the capability to break a clip into separate parts so that you can edit them independently on the Storyboard.

PowerDirector also provides a flexible scene detection function that can find scene changes automatically.

Click on a clip in the Library to select it and then click on the Detect Scenes button on the top of the Library window (or right-click and select it from the pop-up menu). PowerDirector displays the Scene Detection dialog box (see Figure 8.5).

You can divide the clip into scenes manually by moving the slider to a split point and clicking on the Split button. PowerDirector then displays the individual scene cut points in the left pane of the dialog box.

PowerDirector also can detect scenes automatically. Click on the Advanced Settings button to display the Advanced Settings for Scene Detection dialog box. Select the Detection Method, either by analyzing changes in the actual video frames or based on the shot time from a DV tape. When analyzing the video content, you can ignore fade ins/outs and flashing lights (camera flashes), and adjust the sensitivity to how major a change is required to start a new scene.

Click on the Detect button to analyze the clip for scene cuts. Right-click on a scene cut thumbnail, and choose Remove Scene to remove that scene point and merge the adjacent scenes.

FIGURE 8.5

*Use the Scene
Detection dialog box
to split long clips by
using the DV time-
code or by analyzing
the scene content.*

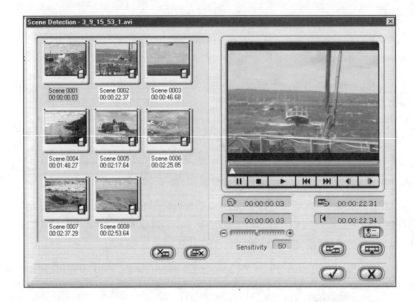

When you divide a clip into scenes, PowerDirector shows the original clip in the Library with a folder icon. Right-click on the thumbnail and choose View Scenes to access the individual scenes for that clip.

Editing in the Storyboard

To create a production in PowerDirector, you arrange a group of clips in order on the Storyboard by dragging or cutting and pasting. You can copy clips directly from the Library, or view and edit the clip in the Preview window and then add the clip to the Storyboard.

You can apply the editing functions on the Modes Wheel to a new clip from the Library or to a clip already in the Storyboard. First, select the clip so it displays in the Preview window, either by dragging a clip from the Library, or by double-clicking on a clip from the Library or from the Storyboard. Then, click on one of the editing operations on the Modes Wheel (or select an editing mode from the Modes menu).

PowerDirector then displays the options for that mode in the area under the Modes Wheel. You can then apply the editing operations and view the results on the clip in the Preview window.

When you finish adjusting the editing options, click on the Apply button at the bottom of the Preview window to apply the changes to the clip in the Storyboard.

Pull down the Edit menu and choose Preferences to choose how changes are applied to the Storyboard. Click on the General tab and then select an option in the Applying Clip Preferences section to specify whether changes are automatically applied after switching modes or making changes, and whether PowerDirector should prompt for confirmation before applying clips.

You also can use the Revert and Clear buttons at the bottom of the panel below the Modes Wheel to back out the most recent editing operations.

Trim Mode

Click on Trim mode on the Modes Wheel to set marker points and trim a clip (see Figure 8.6). You also can resize and crop video or images.

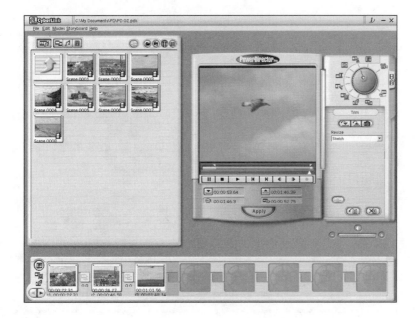

FIGURE 8.6

Use Trim mode to adjust the starting and end frames of a clip, and to resize or crop clips.

Specify a portion of the clip by setting the In and Out points for the trim operation. Use the play controls below the Preview window to position the Time Slider to the appropriate points, and click on the Mark In and Mark Out buttons under the play controls, or drag the sliders directly (above the Time Slider).

PowerDirector displays the In and Out times next to the buttons, with the current frame time (at the Time Slider) and total time of the trimmed region underneath.

You also can use the Resize drop-down menu to fit the clip to the display resolution, stretching it to fill the window, optionally maintaining the aspect ratio, and possibly cropping the sides.

When working with still images, use Trim mode to resize the images and set the time duration for the display.

Speed Mode

Click on Speed mode on the Modes Wheel to speed up or slow down the frame rate of a clip (see Figure 8.7).

FIGURE 8.7

Use Speed mode to adjust the frame rate of a clip from slow motion to fast playback.

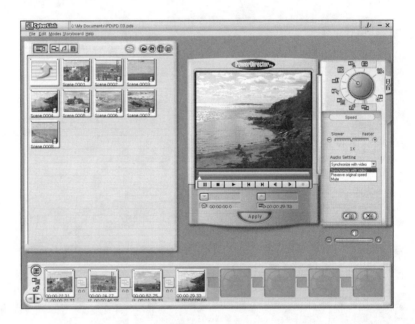

Adjust the slider from Slower to Faster, from 1/4X slow motion to 8X fast motion.

Use the Audio Setting drop-down menu to mute the audio, preserve the original speed, or synchronize the audio to the video speed (which then may be unintelligible).

Titles Mode

Click on Titles mode on the Modes Wheel to insert title text on a clip (see Figure 8.8).

Click on the + Add Title button to add a title entry to the list below the Modes Wheel. Type the title text in the list to have it appear in the Preview window. Then, drag the text to position it; click on the – Remove Title button to remove it; or click on the Set Font button to change the font, style, size, spacing, color, effects, and alignment.

Choose a motion effect and direction from the Titles Effects drop-down menu, and use the trim controls and Effect Length slider to control the timing of the motion effect.

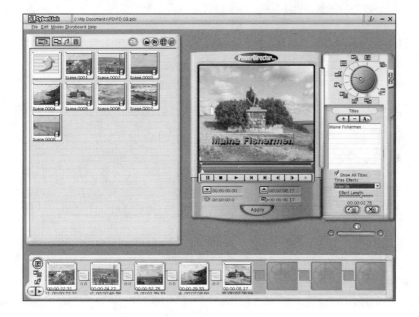

FIGURE 8.8

Use Titles mode to add text tiles to a clip and animate their movement.

Effects Mode

Click on Effects mode on the Modes Wheel to apply a variety of image and motion effects (see Figure 8.9).

PowerDirector displays the available effects in the Library panel. Hold the mouse cursor over each effect thumbnail to show an animation of the effect.

Click on an effect thumbnail to apply it to the current clip. For each effect, use the additional controls in the panel below the Modes Wheel to adjust the effect parameters.

Use the first Color effect to adjust the video appearance (Brightness, Contrast, Hue, Saturation, Sharpness). Or apply various image effects (for example, Emboss, Mosiac, Noise, Ripple) or motion effects (for example, Swing, TV Wall, Zoom), each with appearance and motion parameters.

FIGURE 8.9

Use the Effects mode to apply image and motion effects to a clip.

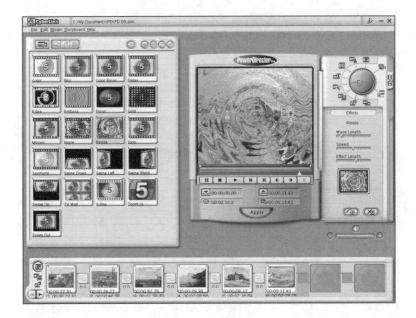

Picture-in-Picture (PiP) Mode and Master Watermark

Click on Picture-in-Picture (PiP) mode on the Modes Wheel to overlay an image or video clip on top of a video clip (see Figure 8.10).

Drag an image or video clip from the Library to the Preview window. Drag the overlay to position it, and use the handles to resize it. Use the Transparency slider to adjust how the overlay is blended with the background.

Use Apply Color Filter to select a background color in the overlay to be made transparent to show a non-rectangular shape.

Because these edit modes apply only to individual clips in the Storyboard, PowerDirector also supports a Master Watermark feature to provide an image overlay or logo over the entire movie. Click on the Master Watermark button to the left of the Storyboard, and select an overlay image (but not video) from the Library, with similar options. Note that this requires modifying every frame of the production, so the SVRT fast-rendering feature will be disabled.

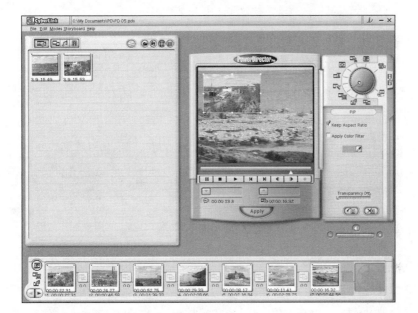

FIGURE 8.10

Use Picture-in-Picture (PiP) mode to overlay an image or video sequence on a clip.

Audio Mode and Master Audio

Click on Audio mode on the Modes Wheel to add up to three additional audio clips to a video clip—for a musical background or voice-over, for example (see Figure 8.11).

Click on the + Add Audio button to add an audio clip to the User-Defined list, or drag a clip from the Library. Click on the – Remove Title button to remove a clip from the list.

Select a clip, and click on the Trim Audio button to display a dialog box to trim that individual clip. Also, for each clip (including the audio from the original video clip), you can set the Fade In and Fade Out options, choose whether to repeat the clip, and set the Volume Mixing slider.

PowerDirector also supports a Master Audio feature to provide a background audio track for the entire production. Click on the Master Audio button to the left of the Storyboard, and choose a clip from the Library, with similar options.

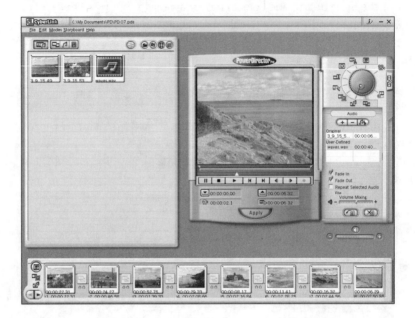

FIGURE 8.11

Use Audio mode to add additional background audio to a clip.

Transitions Mode

Click on Transitions mode on the Modes Wheel to apply transition effects between clips in the storyboard (see Figure 8.12), or click on the Transitions button between two clips.

PowerDirector displays the available transition in the Library panel. Hold the mouse cursor over each transition thumbnail to show an animation of the transition.

Click on a transition thumbnail to apply it to the current clip. Use the Transition Length slider to set the length of the transition, which is divided equally between the two adjacent video clips.

Previewing and Exporting the Production

As you edit your production on the Storyboard, you can preview the result at any time by playing back the entire Storyboard or from the current clip. When you finish your editing, you can then export your production by saving, or producing, it to hard disk, or by using the Disc Wizard to author it to CD or DVD disc.

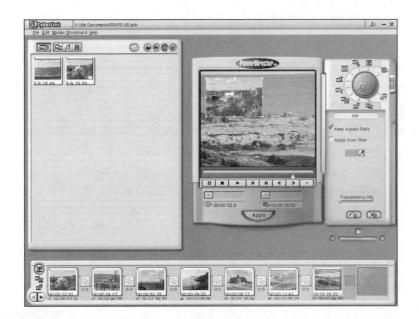

FIGURE 8.12

Use Transitions mode to add transition effects between two adjacent clips.

Play Movie

To preview your production from the Storyboard, click on the top Play Movie button to the left of the Storyboard. PowerDirector blanks the screen and plays the production in a small window on the screen.

Pull down the Edit menu and choose Preferences to select preview options, including the window size, whether to ignore effects or audio, and whether to play from the beginning of the Storyboard or from the selected clip.

Produce Movie

To save your production as a video movie file on disk, click on the final Produce Movie button on the Modes Wheel (or pull down the File menu and choose it under Export). PowerDirector can export to MPEG-1 and MPEG-2 formats, Windows AVI (including DV), and Windows Media formats. It also can export directly to VCD, SVCD, and DVD-compatible formats.

PowerDirector displays the Produce Movie Wizard dialog box to step through the production process.

First, choose whether you are exporting Video for General Purposes or Video for Movie Disc Production.

If exporting a general video file, use the drop-down menu to choose the video format (MPEG-1, MPEG-1, Windows Media, or AVI).

If exporting for CD or DVD disc production, then use the drop-down menus to choose the type of disc (VCD, SVCD, or DVD) and the Country/Video Format (NTSC or PAL, depending on the country).

Next, specify the details for the general file and compression format that you selected.

For the MPEG-1 and MPEG-2 profiles, choose a predefined profile based on video resolution and compressed bit rate, or create a custom profile. The profile also can include preprocessing options for improving the video quality, including Smoothing, Deinterlacing, and Noise Removal.

For the Windows Media profile, choose a predefined profile for single or multiple video and audio streams to match a specified distribution bandwidth, from modems to broadband and networks.

For the AVI profile, choose a Windows format to save in a standard Windows AVI file, or use the Settings button to specify the video and audio format and compression. Or choose a DV format to save in a DV AVI file, in Type I (new) or Type II format (with a separate duplicate audio track for compatibility with older applications). You also can use the Write to DV Tape option to write your entire production directly to your DV camcorder.

For the MPEG and AVI DV formats, choose to use the default Smart Video Rendering Technology (SVRT). This intelligently recompresses only the edited portions of your production, saving compression time and preserving quality by not recompressing.

Finally, select the output filename and directory and export the production.

PowerDirector displays its progress in the Preview window as it writes the output file.

DVD Authoring and Burning

The Disc Wizard mode in PowerDirector is actually an independent DVD authoring tool with a step-by-step interface. Click on the Disc Wizard button to the right of the Modes Wheel to continue working with an open project, or launch the Wizard separately to author a DVD from media files saved on disc.

When you finish authoring your production, you can burn it directly to a DVD or VCD format, or save it to hard disk as a disk image or as a DVD volume folder. You then can import a disk image or DVD folder into the Disc Wizard to burn the production at a later time. You can also save and reuse your Disc Wizard projects.

Start a Project

When you open Disc Wizard, it presents the Welcome screen. As you step through the screens, they include help for common questions that you can click for more information. You can click on the disc icon at the top left of the screen to pull down the File menu to open or save your existing project. Click on the Show Step Links icon (microscope) to display the list of steps on the left of the window.

Click on the Next button at the bottom of the screen to begin moving through the authoring steps. The Disc Wizard displays the Create a New Movie screen.

You can select Load Existing Movie File to burn a DVD from a disc that you previously saved to disc. Disc Wizard can burn a copy of a DVD saved to disk as a DVD volume folder (with the same VIDEO_TS directory and files burned to DVD) or from a disc image file (with the DVD data packed together and ready to burn).

Click on Create New Movie to start a new DVD production.

Use the next Choose Disc Type screen to select the disc format (DVD, VCD, SVCD, or MiniDVD/DVD on CD) and the television format (NTSC or PAL).

Select Videos and Slide Shows

Use the Select Media Files screen (see Figure 8.13) to select a list of individual files on disk or to import files from a PowerDirector project library.

Also use the Add Personal Photos as Slideshows screen to add up to 100 slide shows, each with up to 256 images and a background audio track. You can rotate, resize, and rearrange the slides; and set the time duration that each slide will be displayed

Next, use the Adjust Main Menu Order screen (see Figure 8.14) to finalize the order of the clips and slide shows (to be automatically laid out on one or more menus).

You then can use the Set Chapters screen to define chapter points within clips to use in the menus and to jump between with the remote control. As before, you can insert chapter points manually or use automated detection.

FIGURE 8.13

Select the media files for your production from existing PowerDirector projects or from files on disk.

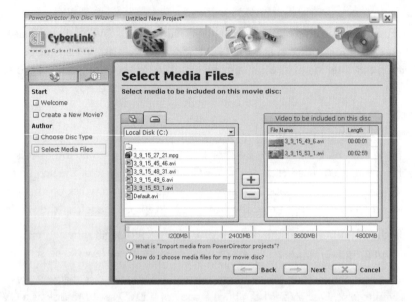

FIGURE 8.14

Adjust the order of your video and slide show elements to appear in the main menu of the DVD production.

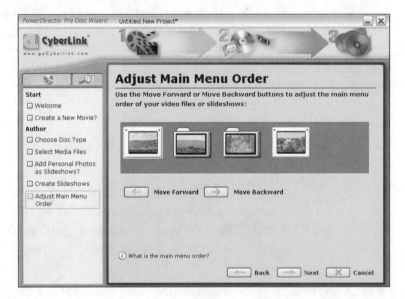

However, to create a DVD like Hollywood movies (so you can play through continuously or jump to chapter points), you must use only one long video file. Otherwise, when a DVD is created from a collection of clips, each clip plays to the end and then jumps back to the menu. Also, jumping between chapters during playback is not supported for VCD and SVCD discs.

Design the Menus

After you have defined all the content for your disc, you then use the Select a Menu Type screen to choose whether to create a DVD with or without menus. Creating a DVD without menus is much faster, but the resulting disc can only be played back; it will not have any interactive features or even chapter points so that you can skip through the content.

Select DVD/VCD/SVCD with Menus and then use the Select a Template for Your Menu screen to choose a predefined graphics template for the menu background and graphical design.

Then, use the Modify Menu Options screen to fine-tune the design (see Figure 8.15). You can add a background music clip, and click on the text boxes to type and format the menu title and button descriptions. Also use the tabs to change the number of buttons, menu style, background, framing around the buttons, navigational button style, and clip button style. Click on Next Page and Previous Page to preview and edit any other menu pages.

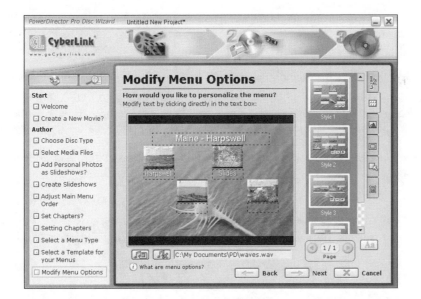

FIGURE 8.15

You can modify the design of individual menus and add title and button text.

Preview and Produce Your DVD

When your design is complete, use the Preview Movie Content screen to choose to preview the project with the Preview Movie screen (see Figure 8.16). Click in the preview window to select a DVD menu button, or use a virtual remote control to test the navigation. Click on the Full Screen button (under the 7 key) to view your DVD at full size on your display.

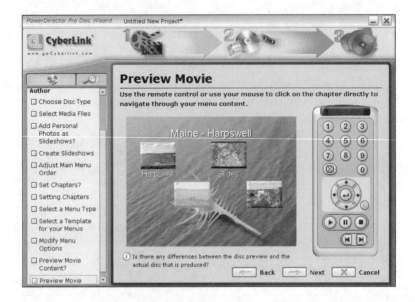

When you are ready to output your production, use the Burn Now or Save for Later screen to choose whether to burn a CD or DVD disk, or to build the project and save the result on hard disk to burn copies later.

You also can select the Include PowerDVD Runtime on the Disc option to include a version of the PowerDVD player on disc. The disc then uses the Windows auto-play feature so that it starts playing automatically on any computer, even without a DVD player application.

Choose Save to Hard Disk Drive to build the project to hard disk, and move on the Saving as a Movie File screen.

If you are creating a DVD project, you can choose Save as a DVD Folder to create a standard VIDEO_TS volume on your hard disk. You then can use a DVD player application, such as CyberLink PowerDVD, to play the DVD production from hard disk.

For a DVD, VCD, and SVD project, you can choose Save as a Disc Image File to build your DVD production, and save it as a single packaged disk "image" file on hard disk. You then can use the Disc Wizard to burn copies of the production to disc directly and efficiently from this image file. The file is in a proprietary format that only the Disc Wizard can read and burn.

Choose Burn Disc Now to record your production to disc, and move on to the Disc Burning Configuration screen. You can use the Enable Disc Burning Simulation option to test the burning process the first time you use it, and use the Include Buffer Under-Run Protection option to buffer up the data for burning to allow you to continue using your computer during the burning process.

InterVideo WinProducer

InterVideo WinProducer is a more sophisticated and customizable video editor, with a timeline instead of a clip-by-clip storyboard. For DVD authoring, instead of a separate DVD authoring component, WinProducer can create a CD or DVD directly from the production on the timeline by specifying a graphical theme for menus and defining chapter points in the production.

WinProducer 3 was released in July 2002 and added support for MPEG-4 and DivX formats. It is available in two versions: WinProducer CD for Video CD authoring (about $80) and WinProducer DVD for DVD authoring (about $80).

This section takes you on a quick tour of WinProducer to demonstrate InterVideo's approach to integrated timeline editing and DVD authoring.

Using WinProducer

WinProducer provides a familiar video-editing interface (see Figure 8.17), in which you capture and import clips in the Media panel on the left side of the window, with tabs for Video Clips, Images (and image sequences), Audio Clips, Input Sources, and Output Targets.

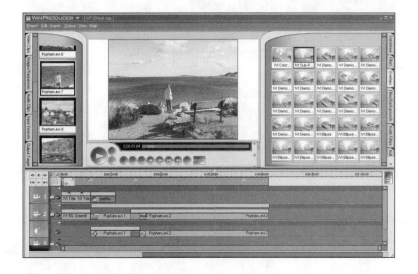

FIGURE 8.17

The WinProducer interface includes the Media panel with clips, the Player Window, the Timeline, and the Effects panel.

You then assemble and edit your production by arranging clips on the Timeline at the bottom of the window, and preview the results in the Player Window at the center of the screen. You can apply effects from the Effects panel on the right side of the window, with tabs for Transitions, Filters, Overlays, Titles, and Audio Filters.

With WinProducer's Timeline approach, you can apply effects to an individual clip, or place it in the filter track to apply it to multiple clips in a video track. You can also use key frames to dynamically change filter properties during a clip.

The WinProducer window also can be resized, and the relative sizes of the panels can be adjusted (for example, to show more rows in the Timeline or to enlarge the size of the Monitor window). WinProducer also uses a floating Properties Bar window, which is used to display and also to set properties associated with the current selection.

Capturing Video and Audio Clips

To capture video and audio clips, click on the Input Sources tab in the Media panel on the left side of the window. The Media panel displays icons for each available input device, including analog devices, such as TV tuner cards and DV camcorders (see Figure 8.18).

FIGURE 8.18

Use the Input Sources tab in the Media panel to capture clips from analog or digital devices, in the format specified in the Properties Bar.

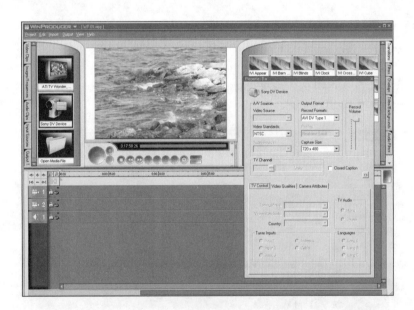

Use the Properties Bar to set input options for the A/V Sources, such as the TV channel, and to select the Output Format for recording to disk. WinProducer can capture in AVI DV Type I and II formats, or capture and convert directly to MPEG.

Click on the Record button to capture a clip, and click on Stop to end the capture. After each clip is captured, it is saved to the Video Clips tab in the Media panel.

Importing Clip Files into the Library

To use existing media files in your production, you first must import them into the appropriate tab in the Media panel. You can drag and drop files from Windows Explorer, and WinProducer will automatically place them in the appropriate tab; or pull down the Import menu and choose Media Files or Image Sequence (or use the right-click pop-up menu).

Use the Video Clips tab for AVI and MPEG-1 and MPEG-2 files, use Audio Clips for MP3 and WAV files, and use Images/Sequences for single images or a sequence of images named with sequential numbers.

Previewing and Splitting Clips

You can then review your material by clicking through the tabs in the Media panel. Click on an individual clip thumbnail to preview it playing right in the Media panel. Use the Properties Bar or pop-up menu to display properties of the clip.

When you click to select a clip in the Media panel, it is also displayed in the Player window. You then can use the play controls to play, pause, and step through the clip.

To segment a longer clip into scenes, right-click on the clip thumbnail and choose Generate Scene Cuts from the pop-up menu. You can then use the Scene Cut Settings dialog box (see Figure 8.19) to analyze the clip content and break it into scenes when the content changes (but not using DV time code). Any new scenes generated are then added to the Media panel. You also can use the pop-up menu to merge scenes back together again.

Editing in the Timeline

WinProducer provides a multitrack Timeline for editing, with the capability to overlap video and audio clips and effects.

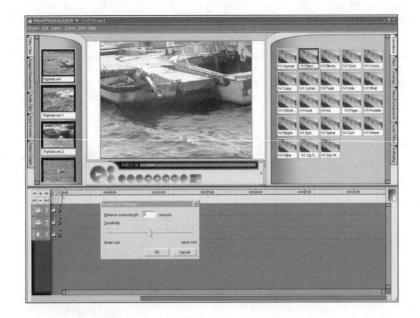

Assembling Clips

To assemble your production, drag a clip from the Media panel into the first video track of the Timeline. WinProducer displays the video and associated audio portion of each clip on individual lines, so you can edit them separately. Drag a second clip and place it in the same track after the first clip. Notice that you can slide the second clip so it immediately follows the first, or push into the first to create an overlapping area for a transition.

Click on the Shrink Time Line and Expand Time Line buttons (magnifying glass icons) at the top left of the Timeline panel to zoom in and out to see all the clips.

To rearrange clips in the Timeline, use the standard Cut, Copy, Paste, and Delete operations from the Edit or pop-up menus. Clips are pasted at the Frame Indicator line.

With the Timeline selected, use the play controls to view a real-time preview of your production in the Monitor window, or drag the Frame Slider to move the red Frame Indicator line in the Timeline. You also can right-click on the clip and use the pop-up menu to Left-Align or Right-Align a clip to the Frame Indicator or to the adjacent clip.

To trim clips in the Timeline, drag the ends of the clip, or move the Frame Indicator line and right-click on the clip and choose Mark In or Mark Out from the pop-up menu, or remove the trims by choosing Restore to Original Length.

You also can split a clip at the Frame Indicator line by selecting the clip and clicking on the Split button below the zoom controls.

Use the Properties Bar to adjust the playback speed and audio volume.

For video clips, you can adjust the playback speed by using the Time Stretching control. You also can specify how clips are Fit to Output if the size is different: Center, Stretch, Letter Box (keep aspect ratio), or Pan (crop aspect).

For audio clips, you can adjust the Volume from zero to 200 percent, and specify a Fase In and Fase Out time in milliseconds.

As you work in the Timeline, use the Lock/Unlock button (the lock icon) on the left of each track to lock the track and prevent accidentally making unwanted changes. You also can use the Enable/Disable button (the eye icon) to disable just the video or audio portion of a track, so it is no longer visible in the production. To remove an entire track, right-click on the left of the track, and choose Delete from the pop-up menu.

Inserting Transitions

To insert a transition effect between two clips, first place the clips on the same track and then slide the ends of the clips together to create an overlapped region. Click on the Transitions tab in the Effects panel to view the available transitions (see Figure 8.20). The thumbnails animate to show the effect of the transition. To insert the transition, drag from a thumbnail to the overlapped region in the video track.

Use the Properties Bar to set the video and audio transitions options. Click in the overlapped area in the video track to view the transition name, and click on Reverse to reverse the effect. Click below in the overlapped area in the audio track to set the Audio Transition effect to overlap or cross-fade.

Applying Video and Audio Filters

To change the appearance of the video clips, click on the Filters tab in the Effects panel to view the built-in video filters, including Blur, Brightness, and Monochrome. Again, the thumbnails animate to show the effect of the filter.

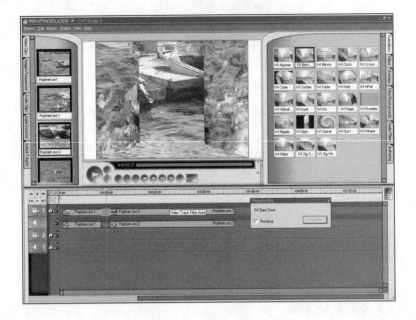

To apply a filter to an individual clip, drag it on top of the clip in the video track. With the timeline interface, you also can apply a filter to multiple clips in a track, or portions of clips, by dragging it to the Video Track Filter Area above the video track. You also can apply multiple filters by dragging another filter on to a clip or the Filter Area.

Use the trim controls to control which portions of the associated clips that the filter is applied to. Move the Frame Indicator line over the filter to show it in the Monitor window, and use the Properties Bar to set the available options for each filter. Use Enable Filter in the pop-up menu to enable or disable individual filters.

Similarly, to apply sound effects, click on the Audio Filters tab in the Effects panel to view the built-in audio filters, including Echo, EQ, Reverb, and Compress. Apply these filters by dragging them onto the audio track, and set options in the Properties Bar.

Overlaying Tracks

The Timeline can contain multiple video and audio tracks, where each track is a layer in the final production. When video tracks overlap, the layers on top (lower track numbers) are on top of lower (higher-numbered) layers. For a simple production, you can arrange all your clips in a single track. But for more complex productions, you should lay out the main production in a lower track, and add titles and overlays in the top tracks.

To add an overlay video track, right-click to the left of the track and choose Add Overlay Video Track from the pop-up menu. Then, drag a still image or a video clip into the overlay track on top of the main video production.

Click on the Overlays tab in the Effects panel to view the built-in overlay effects (see Figure 8.21). You can overlay transparent objects with Color matching for blue-screen type effects. You can also overlay picture-in-picture type inserts with various geometric shapes (diamond, ellipse, rectangle) and motions (center, side, corners).

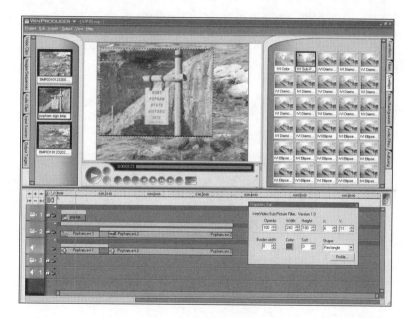

FIGURE 8.21

Use the Overlays tab to control the size and motion of image and video overlays.

Apply the overlays by dragging them onto the video track. Move the Frame Indicator line over the overlay to show it in the Monitor window, and use the Properties Bar (or the overlay rectangle in the Monitor window) to set the subpicture position and size.

You also can add additional audio-only tracks for background music, sound effects, or voice-overs. The audio tracks are at the bottom of the Timeline. To add a new audio track, click to the left of an audio-only track and choose Add Audio Track from the pop-up menu.

Titles and Backgrounds

WinProducer provides both animated titles and built-in colored backgrounds for titles or video overlays. Click on the Titles/Backgrounds tab in the Effects panel to view the built-in backgrounds and text (see Figure 8.22).

To use a colored background, drag a color thumbnail to a video track. Move the Frame Indicator line over the background to show it in the Monitor window, and use the Properties Bar to set the color and to set a second color for gradients. Use the plain Background thumbnail to position and resize a background, and you also can load and save a Profile for a specific background.

To use the simple Title, drag the Title thumbnail to a video track. Use the Properties Bar to edit the text; change its color and opacity; change the font, size, and style; and set a drop shadow. Position the tile by dragging on the Monitor window or entering coordinates in the Properties Bar. You also can load and save a Profile for a specific animated text effect.

FIGURE 8.22

Use the Titles/ Backgrounds tab to add moving text titles and colored backgrounds.

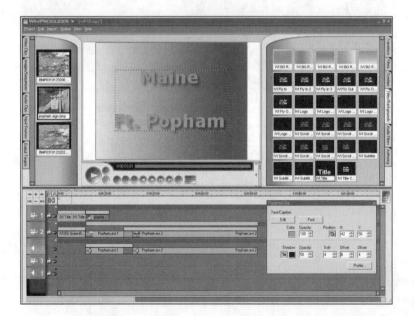

Key Frames

Another advantage of a timeline interface for video editing is the capability to set control points to dynamically change the properties of effects. With WinProducer, you can set key points along the Timeline, set different options for an effect, and then those options will be smoothly changed between the key points.

Use the Key Manager buttons in the top-left corner of the Timeline panel to work with key points: Add Key or Delete Key, move to the Previous Key or Next Key, and Move Key Forward or Move Key Back to nudge the position of a key point.

To set a key point, move the Frame Indicator line to the desired position in the effect, and press the Add Key button. Then, change the effect options for that key in the Properties Bar.

Previewing and Exporting the Production

While you are editing your production in the Timeline, you can continue to preview it in the Monitor window. Use the Property Bar to control the Preview Quality (Fast or Full Quality).

You can scan quickly through the Timeline by dragging the Frame Indicator line or click in the Time Line Ruler to jump to a specific point. You can then use the play controls under the Monitor window to preview the production from that point. The play controls include Previous Frame and Next Frame buttons to step through individual frames, and Previous Change Point and Next Change Point buttons to skip to the next key point or clip boundary.

You can then export it from the Timeline to a movie file on disk in a variety of formats.

Output Movie File

To output your production, click on the Output Targets tab in the Media panel. You can select To Hard Disk to write a video file, To Burn Device to author a DVD or VCD, or To DV Device to copy to a camcorder.

Before outputting your production, you can select the portion of the Timeline to be used. Right-click in the Output Range Track above the video tracks in the Timeline, and choose Select Entire Range. WinProducer displays a purple Output Range Bar to show the extent of the Timeline to be output. You then can trim and drag this bar to select a shorter portion of the Timeline.

Click To Hard Disk under the Output Targets tab to display the Choose Content for Hard Disk dialog box. You can select to output directly to a Video File, or as CD, or DVD Content to hard disk (for testing, or to burn later).

Select Video File and click next to choose the output file format (see Figure 8.23).

FIGURE 8.23

*Export your movie
as an AVI/DV file,
or in MPEG-1,
MPEG-2, or
MPEG-4 format.*

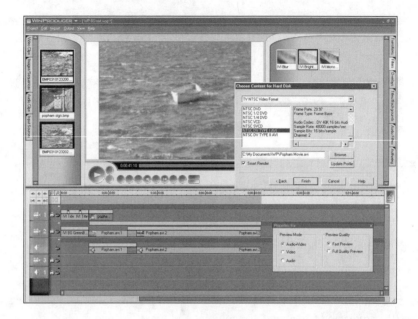

WinProducer can export to formats including MPEG-1 and MPEG-2 (VCD/SVCD/
DVD-compatible), DV as a Type I or Type II AVI, standard AVI, and MPEG-4 as
Windows Media (WMV, ASF). You can select a predefined output format profile
for the output video and audio format, or create a new profile by cloning and
modifying an existing format.

WinProducer then renders each frame in your production, saves it to disk in the
specified format, and adds it to the Media panel.

To export from the Timeline back to a DV camera, click To Burn Device under the
Output Targets tab. WinProducer will send your production over the
FireWire/1394 connection to be recorded on your DV video camera.

DVD Authoring and Burning

Instead of a separate DVD authoring mode, WinProducer can author your production directly from the Timeline to CD or DVD (depending on the version of
the application). You just select a graphical theme for the menus, set and name
chapter points in the Timeline, and WinProducer will format and burn the disc.

Design the Menu

Click on the Authoring tab in the Effects Panel and then drag a theme to Output Range Track.

In the Output Range Track, right-click on the theme and choose Theme Editor from the pop-up menu. In the Theme Editor dialog box, double-click on the title to edit the text; and to change the font color, size, and style (see Figure 8.24).

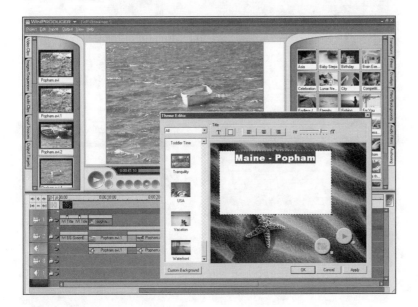

FIGURE 8.24

Use the Theme Editor dialog box to design the menu graphics and text for exporting to a DVD production.

Create a Chapter List

Next, define chapter points within the production on the Timeline to be used in the menu. Move the Frame Indicator to the desired position and right-click to choose Add Chapter Mark from the pop-up menu. WinProducer marks the chapter point with a triangle in the Output Range Track.

To name the chapter point, right-click on the chapter mark, choose Chapter Properties from the pop-up menu, and then enter a name in the Properties dialog box.

Create a Video Disc

Finally, click To Hard Disk under the Output Targets tab to burn your video production to a CD or DVD using the menu theme and chapter list (see Figure 8.25).

Depending on the version of WinProducer, you can burn your production to VCD, SVCD, DVD on CD, or DVD.

FIGURE 8.25

Select To Burn Device under Output Targets to burn your project to DVD or CD.

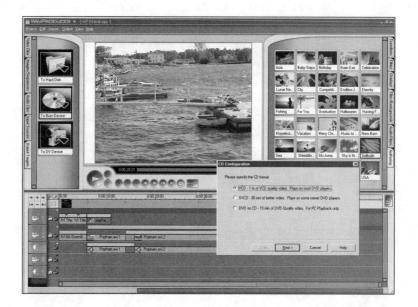

Summary

The two applications, CyberLink PowerDirector and InterVideo WinProducer, demonstrate two approaches to integrating DVD authoring with video-editing tools. Although these are new and developing products, these tools include sophisticated capabilities, including DV capture, direct capture to MPEG, extensive editing capabilities, real-time preview, and MPEG and DVD export.

Chapter 9 describes MyDVD, a dedicated tool for DVD authoring that provides more control over the DVD design while still automating the process of laying out the menu navigation.

Part IV, "Personal DVD Authoring," describes the next step in DVD authoring tools, with Apple iDVD and Sonic DVDit! These applications provide more hands-on control over the layout and design of individual menus.

Automated DVD Authoring with Sonic MyDVD

Sonic MyDVD IS A POPULAR Windows DVD authoring tool for recording, editing, and sharing video content on recordable DVD and CD discs. MyDVD allows you to easily author full DVD productions from your video, including graphical menus with thumbnail buttons to play your clips. MyDVD is based on the Sonic Solutions DVD formatting technology used throughout the Sonic product line, which also includes Sonic DVDit! (see Part IV, "Personal DVD Authoring") and Sonic ReelDVD and Scenarist (see Part V, "Professional DVD Authoring").

To create your DVD productions in MyDVD, you can import clips from media files on your hard disk, or you can capture clips directly within MyDVD. MyDVD then automatically lays out the menu structure and navigation for your clips, including a sequence of linked menu pages for a large collection of clips. As you capture long clips, you can add chapter points to more conveniently access scenes within the clip. You also can create a hierarchy of nested menus to group related clips or the chapters of a clip together in their own menu.

MyDVD version 4.0, released in July 2002, introduced a new user interface. It added the capability to create slide shows from still photos, with transitions and background audio, supports QuickTime import, and exports to Video-CD (VCD) format. The MyDVD Video Suite version of the product adds video-editing capability via the ArcSoft ShowBiz video editor.

MyDVD can burn your productions to DVD, so you can play them back on set-top DVD players. It can also burn short productions to CD in Video-CD format, so you can burn and share your productions even if you do not have a DVD burner. You can also save your production to a folder on hard disk in DVD format to test and share.

On recent PCs with fast processors (over 1GHz), MyDVD can transfer your videos "Direct-to-DVD," straight from DV to DVD with no additional editing and authoring steps: capturing the video (and audio) input from a DV camcorder, converting it to DVD format, and burning it to DVD.

Even after you burn your project to DVD (or Video CD), MyDVD 4.0 provides the capability to re-edit the contents of the disc. MyDVD creates OpenDVD-compliant discs that include project information on the disc; so you can open the disc as a new project and then add (or delete) clips, change the menus, and even change the graphical style. These OpenDVD-compliant discs can be created and edited with any application that supports the OpenDVD format.

Stepping Through a New Project with Sonic MyDVD

This section introduces MyDVD by stepping through the process of creating a new DVD project from existing media clip files. You will set up the project and design style, add some clips to the menu, edit the menu text, preview the resulting production, and then save your production to a DVD volume on hard disk.

MyDVD allows you to focus on assembling and designing the DVD production, and takes care of all the details of creating a DVD or Video CD for you. Even so, it provides quite a bit of flexibility in customizing the layout and visual design of your menus.

Step 1: Start MyDVD for a DVD Project

When you first launch MyDVD, it displays a Welcome screen that can guide you through setting for the kind of project you want to work on (see Figure 9.1). You can choose to work on a DVD-Video or Video-CD project, or choose Edit Video to launch the video editor to edit individual clips.

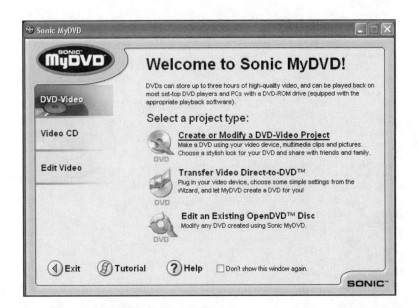

FIGURE 9.1

When you launch MyDVD, it displays the Welcome screen to set up for a DVD-Video or Video-CD project.

You can click on Tutorial or Help at the bottom of the screen to see more information on using MyDVD. When you are familiar with using MyDVD, you also can select the option to not show the Welcome screen each time you start MyDVD.

Click DVD-Video on the left side of the window to display the options for working on a DVD project. The Welcome screen displays the options for working on a DVD production: Create or Modify a DVD-Video Project, Record Direct-to-DVD, or Edit an Existing DVD Disc.

To start working on a DVD project, click Create or Modify a DVD-Video Project.

Step 2: Start a New Project

MyDVD then displays the main application window with a blank menu screen ready for you to add clips and text (see Figure 9.2). You can use the buttons on the left side of the screen to choose an activity: Capture new video clips, Get Movies from clips on disk, Add Slideshow from photo files, or Add Sub-menu with more clips.

FIGURE 9.2

MyDVD displays the main application window, configured to work on a DVD project.

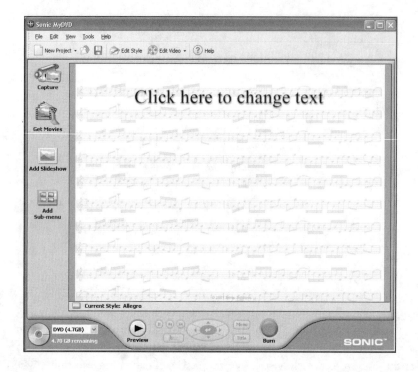

Step 3: Add Clips to the Menu

Next you can import some media clips into your project files from video files on your hard disc. MyDVD can import video clips in several formats, including Windows AVI.

Click on the Get Movies button on the left of the main MyDVD window. MyDVD displays the Add Movie(s) to Menu dialog box. By default, MyDVD shows the contents of the My Videos folder under the My Documents folder, or you can browse to another folder with video clips. Select one or more video files to add to the menu.

You can click on Get Movies again and import more clips, or you can drag and drop clip files from an Explorer window.

MyDVD adds the selected clips to the menu area, and makes a thumbnail image of the first frame of each clip to use as the button image (see Figure 9.3). As you add clips, MyDVD automatically rearranges the layout to keep the buttons centered in the menu. You also can drag and drop the buttons to arrange them in a different order. MyDVD adds up to six clips to a menu and then creates additional linked menus for more clips.

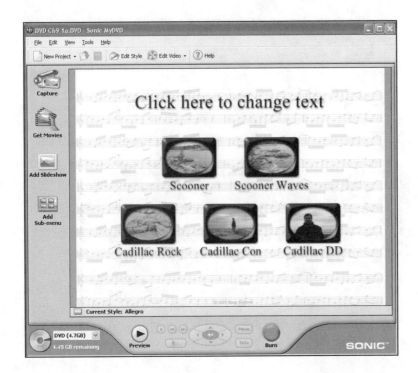

FIGURE 9.3

MyDVD automatically lays out menu buttons as you add video clips to your menu.

The disk space area at the bottom-left corner of the MyDVD window provides a pie chart indicator to show how much of the available disc space the project will use.

Step 4: Edit the Menu and Button Text

Next, you can edit the menu title and button caption text. MyDVD automatically inserts a placeholder menu title, and generates a caption for each button using the filename of the associated video clip.

Click on the menu title or a button caption, and MyDVD displays a text box so that you can edit the text (see Figure 9.4). Type the new text, and then press Enter or simply click elsewhere on the window.

To change the font style, character size, or color of the text fields in MyDVD, you can customize an existing style or create a new custom style (see "Customizing Menu Styles" later in this chapter).

FIGURE 9.4

Click on the menu title and the button captions to edit the menu text fields.

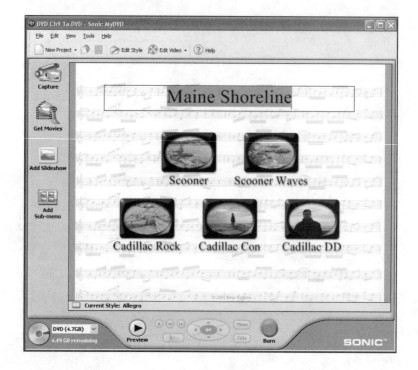

Step 5: Preview the Production

After you are finished laying out your project, you can preview how it will play back. This is pretty obvious for a simple one-menu project like you have created here. However, as you add multiple menus, and especially nested menus, it is a good idea to step through the navigational structure of your entire project to verify that it works the way you expect.

To check your project, click on the Preview button at the bottom of the main MyDVD window. MyDVD changes the window to Preview mode, with DVD control buttons at the bottom of the window, such as those on a DVD remote control (see Figure 9.5).

Click on the arrows in the center of the controls to move the button selection highlight around the current menu, and then click on the center Enter button to activate the highlighted button and play the associated clip. You also can select a button with the mouse and click to play the corresponding clip.

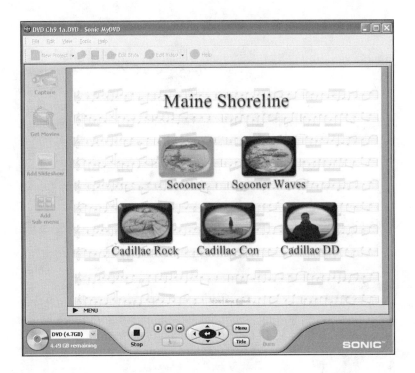

FIGURE 9.5

*Use the MyDVD
Preview mode to
navigate through
your DVD design.*

While a clip is playing, the display below the video shows the current play time
and chapter number in the clip. Also while the clip is playing, you can click the Title
button to return to the Main menu, or the Menu button to return to the previous
menu or return to playing a video clip. On projects with multiple chapters, you can
use the Previous Chapter and Next Chapter buttons to skip between chapters.

When you have previewed your project and are satisfied with it, click on the
yellow Stop button to return to the menu-editing mode.

Step 6: Save the Project

This is also a good point to save a copy of your project. Click on the Save Project
button (diskette icon) at the top of the window (or pull down the File menu and
choose Save Project).

MyDVD displays the Save dialog box. Browse to the folder where you want to
save your project, and enter a name for the project. The saved project includes
the menu layout with imported clips, and menu styles and text.

Step 7: Record Your Project

The final step in creating your project is to make a disc by recording it to DVD or Video CD. And even if you do not have a recordable DVD drive you also can make a DVD-format disc volume in a folder on your hard disk. Pull down the Tools menu and choose Make DVD Folder. MyDVD displays the Browse for Folder dialog box so that you can select the destination folder where your DVD production will be created.

MyDVD then begins building the DVD files. As it works, it displays the current operation in a status area at the bottom of the window (see Figure 9.6).

FIGURE 9.6

As it builds your DVD production, MyDVD provides status feedback at the bottom of the window.

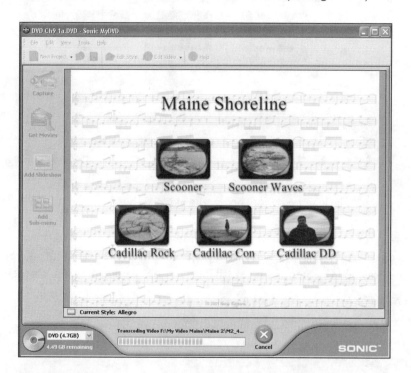

Each of your clips must be converted into DVD-compatible formats. The video and audio from each clip are processed separately; each is *transcoded* from one compressed format to another.

After all the clips are converted, MyDVD then combines, or *multiplexes*, the menu and media components into the final DVD file structure.

MyDVD writes the DVD-format data to the specified folder on the hard disk. Open the output folder in Windows Explorer to view the DVD-format files in the VIDEO_TS folder (see Part II, "Exploring DVDs on Your Computer"). MyDVD also creates an OpenDVD folder to save information that can be used to re-open and continue editing the DVD data (see Figure 9.7).

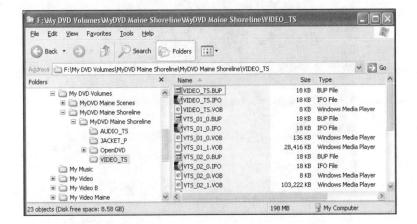

FIGURE 9.7

MyDVD writes the DVD-format data to a folder on the hard disk, along with the OpenDVD information for re-editing the DVD contents.

Step 7: Play Back the DVD

The DVD folder that you have just created is formatted in the standard DVD directory structure and media formats. You therefore can play the contents using the DVD player software installed on your machine (see Chapter 7, "Playing DVDs in Windows XP").

Use the Sonic CinePlayer application that is bundled with some versions of MyDVD, or another DVD player, to play the saved DVD folder (see Figure 9.8). Use the Browse for DVD Folder (or similar) option to open and play the saved DVD folder from hard disk (some older players do not offer this option). You then can navigate the menus and play the clips as if the DVD data was playing from a DVD disc on a set-top player.

The contents of the DVD folder also should be playable on any computer with DVD player software, including Macintosh, Windows, and UNIX systems. You can transfer the folder like any other collections of data files over a network to play on another machine.

FIGURE 9.8

*You then can play
the contents of the
DVD folder using
Sonic CinePlayer
or another DVD
player application.*

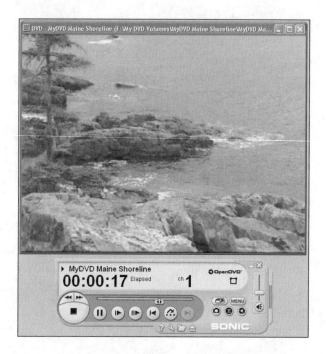

In addition, for shorter DVD productions (around 15 minutes), you also can burn the DVD data files to CD-R/RW discs to save and share with others. Because the CDs can be played on any computer with a CD-ROM drive and DVD player software, this provides a convenient and low-cost alternative for saving and sharing productions at full DVD quality. However, do not expect set-top DVD players to play CDs in this format.

Now that you have stepped through the DVD authoring process with MyDVD to create a simple disc, it is time to move on to create more sophisticated menus and navigation, and to customize the look of your DVD.

Adding and Organizing Movies in DVD Menus

Creating a DVD with "automated" DVD authoring tools, such as MyDVD, is mainly a process of importing clips and laying them out in menus. You decide how you want to group the clips and in what order, and the tools can automatically create the menu buttons and navigation to play your clips.

In MyDVD, you can add clips from media files on hard disk, or capture new clips to add to the end of the menu. As you add more clips than can fit on a menu page, MyDVD will create a linked sequence of menus to hold your clips. You can create your own additional nested menus, linked from buttons in the parent menu. You also can change the audio track associated with a clip.

Even after you create your menus, you can reorganize the menu structure by rearranging buttons, and by deleting individual clips, chapter points within clips, entire menus, and even entire hierarchies of menus.

Adding and Organizing Video Clips

In MyDVD, you author a DVD project by adding video clips to menus in the project.

When you add a video file to the menu, MyDVD adds a new button with a thumbnail of the clip. The file may contain video and audio, or just video. If you add a video-only clip file, and there is an audio clip file with the same name in the folder with the video clip, MyDVD will use both clips for the associated button.

Importing Video Files

MyDVD can import video and audio clips stored in a variety of common media file formats, including Windows AVI (.avi), Apple QuickTime, MPEG-1 (.mpg, .m1v, and so on), and MPEG-2 (.mpg, .m2v, and so on). You can prepare these files before using them in MyDVD by capturing and editing them with other applications. MyDVD can import files in compressed formats only if the associated codec (decompressor) is installed on your Windows system. (See the MyDVD documentation for more information on compatible media file types.)

Adding Clips in Linked Menus

As you add more clips to your project, you will run out of room on the initial menu page. MyDVD will then create a linked set of menus, with additional buttons chaining to the next and previous menus in the chain.

Add more clips to the MyDVD menu so that now there are more than six clips in the project. MyDVD imports the clips, and warns you that it is creating a new menu page for the additional clips.

MINIMIZE COMPRESSION WHEN
EDITING VIDEO

General media file formats, such as AVI and QuickTime, can contain video and audio material in a variety of compression formats, including raw uncompressed data. With any of these file formats, the files can have very different characteristics—including resolution, frame rate, and the amount of compression applied to the data. Compression can be very light (to preserve the best quality) to quite heavy (to squeeze the data harder, with an associated loss in quality). A lossless compressor reduces the size without removing any information, whereas a lossy compressor actually removes detail from the video or audio, but hopefully the loss is not very perceptible.

DVD-Video data is compressed in MPEG-2 format, using advanced compression techniques to significantly reduce the video size without introducing visible artifacts. DVD video uses 720×480 resolution for NTSC or 720×576 for PAL television.

When you capture and edit video files on your computer, you can control the media file format, video characteristics, and amount of compression. For the best results, you want to import files into MyDVD with lossless (or at least only light) compression, so they compress well into DVD format. Otherwise, if you use video that already has visible artifacts from previous compression, the MPEG-2 compression will make the video look even worse. Ideally, you should also capture your video at the DVD resolution (that is, from a DV camcorder), but MyDVD can resize your video as needed to fit the DVD requirements.

When MyDVD finishes importing the clips, it displays the second menu page (see Figure 9.9). The menu includes the thumbnail buttons for the additional clips, plus two additional Home and Previous navigation buttons that are automatically generated along the bottom of the menu. The Home button (house icon) jumps back to the home or Main menu, and the Previous button (pointing left) returns to the previous menu in the chain.

In MyDVD, you can use these buttons to navigate through the menus while you are editing the project by double-clicking on them.

When you double-click on the Home or Previous button to return to the first menu, you will see that MyDVD also has added a Next button (pointing right) to the home menu.

Similarly, if you add several more clips to the menu so that there are more than 12 clips in the project. MyDVD will create a third menu page. The second menu page will then have both a Previous and a Next button.

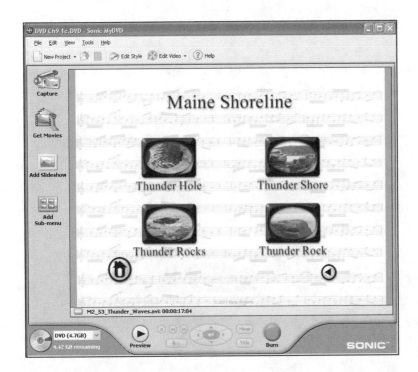

FIGURE 9.9

MyDVD creates a second menu page when you add more than six clips, and adds Home and Previous navigation buttons.

Editing Menus and Sub-Menus

Although a linked chain of menus is a useful way to page though a small number of video clips, it becomes unwieldy when creating a project with lots of clips, or different groups of clips. MyDVD helps you organize the structure and navigation of your project by creating hierarchical sub-menus to organize different groups of clips.

If you have several collections of clips, you might want to organize each group of related clips into different menus. And if you have clips that contain multiple chapters, you also might want to organize them into sub-menus. Each sub-menu then can contain a linked chain of menus, or also can be further organized into additional sub-menus. In this way, you can create a hierarchical tree structure to organize your project.

Adding Clips in Nested Menus

To create a nested or hierarchical menu in MyDVD, click the Add Sub-menu button on the left of the window. MyDVD adds a new Untitled Menu button to the project (see Figure 9.10). This menu button does not play a clip, but instead branches to another menu.

FIGURE 9.10

Click the Add Sub-menu button to add a new nested menu to the current menu.

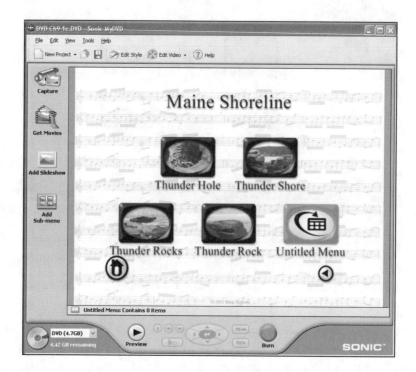

Double-click on the Menu button to edit the new menu. MyDVD displays the new empty nested menu (see Figure 9.11). The menu includes Home and Return navigation buttons that are automatically generated. The Return button (curved-arrow icon) jumps back to the next-higher parent menu. Again, while editing, you can double-click on these buttons to view and edit the menu structure.

Now if you add at least seven clips to this nested menu, MyDVD will create additional linked menus, with the Previous and Next buttons. The Return button will also appear on all the linked menus, and always jumps to the higher-level parent menu that contains the button that these menus are nested under.

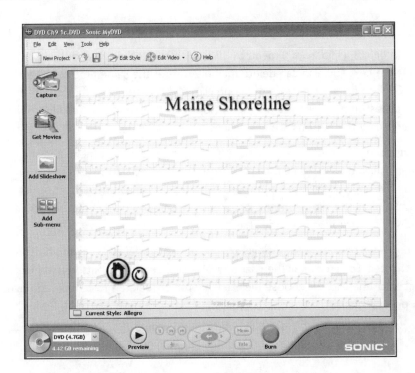

FIGURE 9.11

The new nested sub-menu is empty, except for the Home and Return buttons.

And, of course, you then can add a new sub-menu to a nested menu, so menus can be nested under nested menus, and so on. In this way, you can create quite a complex hierarchy to organize your clips. If you find yourself doing this a lot, however, it is time for you to think about stepping up to a more sophisticated DVD authoring tool that gives you better tools and more control for designing your DVD menu navigation (see Part IV, "Personal DVD Authoring").

Rearranging Menu Buttons

After adding new buttons to a menu you still can rearrange the order of the buttons. Simply click and drag a button, and then drop it into a new position before or after another button on the menu. MyDVD displays a flashing vertical line to indicate where the button will be inserted.

To rearrange buttons across different menus in MyDVD, you can delete the buttons from one menu and add the same clips to another menu.

Deleting Menu Buttons

You can delete a clip from a menu by clicking to select the clip and then pressing the Delete key. You also can delete multiple clips at the same time by using Ctrl+Click to first select more than one clip. MyDVD removes the buttons for those clips from the menu. Only the buttons are deleted; the actual media files referenced by the buttons are not changed.

When you delete clips from a menu, MyDVD rearranges that menu and the chain of menus linked to it. To fill the space from the deleted buttons in the current menu, MyDVD will fill in the menu with clips from the next menu, and so on down the chain. If all the clips from the last menu are shifted down in this way, the last menu will be removed from the chain.

If you delete the button for a single chapter, MyDVD deletes only the button for that chapter. To remove all the chapters of a clip, delete the button that links to the start of the clip. Or choose Delete Chapter or Delete Movie from the right-click pop-up menu.

If you delete a button to a nested sub-menu, MyDVD will delete that menu and all its clips, as well as any linked menus or sub-menus.

Adding Audio Tracks

Some video clips, such as MPEG-1 and MPEG-2 media files, are video-only, and do not have an associated audio track. Other clips may contain video with an associated audio track, but you still may want to remove or replace the audio.

MyDVD provides the capability to add or replace the audio track of a clip, or to delete the audio track.

Adding and Replacing Audio Tracks

To check if a clip has an associated audio track, you can click on Preview and play the clip. Even easier, just right-click on the clip (or select the clip and pull down the Edit menu), and check to see whether the Remove Audio option is available (see Figure 9.12). If the clip does not have an audio track, then Remove Audio is grayed-out. If the clip does have an audio track, you can choose Remove Audio to remove the audio track.

To add an audio track to a clip, drag and drop an audio-only media file onto the clip. If the clip already had an audio track, it will be replaced with the new track.

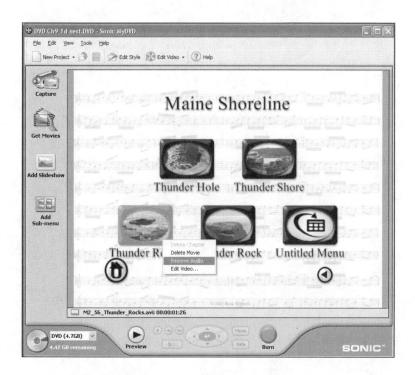

Importing Audio Files

MyDVD supports a variety of common audio-only file formats, including Windows WAVE (.wav), AIFF (.aif), MPEG-1 Layer 2 (.abs, .mpa), and MPEG-1 Layer 3 (.mp3). MyDVD can import compressed audio formats only if the associated codec (decompressor) is installed on your Windows system. (See the MyDVD documentation for more information on compatible media file types.)

The audio file should contain one audio track, which can be mono or stereo. As with video compression, it is better to use uncompressed audio formats because the audio data needs to be recompressed to DVD-compatible format.

Capturing Video Clips

In addition to using media clip files that you already have stored on your hard disk in your DVD productions, you also can capture video clips directly in MyDVD from digital or analog sources. Of course, you also can capture clips into files independently of MyDVD by using other video editing and capture software, and then import the files into MyDVD.

Depending on your system configuration and the type of capture hardware you have installed, MyDVD can capture digitally from a DV camcorder through a Firewire (IEEE 1394) interface. Some versions also can capture from analog sources, such as a TV tuner or VCR. See your MyDVD documentation and web site for information on supported configurations.

One advantage of capturing clips directly in MyDVD is that it converts each captured clip into the compressed MPEG format used for DVDs before storing it on hard disk. Clips stored in MPEG format can be much smaller than clips stored in other formats, such as analog clips captured to common AVI formats or digital clips stored in DV format.

Another advantage of capturing directly in MyDVD is that it can break the clip into chapters in the menus. Especially when capturing long clips in MyDVD, this makes it easier to skip through the clip and to jump directly from the menus to interesting points in the clip.

In MyDVD, a button to each clip that you capture is added to the end of the currently displayed menu . And if you create chapter points as you are capturing, MyDVD adds a new menu button for each chapter. As a result, you may want to create a new sub-menu to capture a clip with chapters, so the chapter buttons for the new clip are not mixed with other clips in your project.

T I P

Capturing video is an intense process for your computer, as video data comes streaming into your system, is processed and compressed, and then is written to disk. As with all video-processing applications, you should reduce the processing load on your computer while it is capturing. A high-end computer may be able to handle capturing with capacity to spare, but it is a good idea to close down other applications, especially background processing, such as system monitors, virus checkers, or networked downloads. As you experiment with how much load your system can handle, you also should avoid activities—such as playing intense 3D video games or editing huge photo files while the system is capturing.

In addition, it is a good idea to allocate separate disks for your capture folder and for an application work area. Use the MyDVD Preferences dialog box (under the File menu) to define the location for captured video files and temporary files. Also run a disk defragmenter program to ensure that the disk can accommodate writing large files.

Capturing Clips from a DV Camcorder

Before starting to capture, first navigate to the MyDVD menu to which you want to add the new clip. The new clip and any chapters will be added to the end of the current menu.

And before starting to capture from your DV camcorder, make sure it is attached to your computer using a Firewire (IEEE 1394) cable. Also, turn on your camcorder to the VCR (playback) setting, not the camera setting.

Click on the Capture button on the left side of the MyDVD window to display the Capture dialog box (see Figure 9.13).

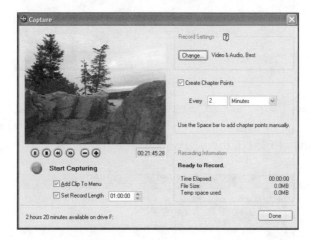

FIGURE 9.13

Use the Capture dialog box to configure your input device and capture new video clips.

MyDVD can automatically recognize your DV camcorder if it is attached and available under Windows. If necessary, use the Record Settings area to select and configure your DV device.

When capturing from a DV camcorder, use the play controls under the video window to play through the tape, and then position it to the start of the clip that you want to capture. Also use the Set Record Length field to set the maximum time for the recording, especially if you are capturing a long clip.

Before recording a clip, you can click the Change button in the Record Settings area to display the Change Device Settings dialog box (see Figure 9.14). Use the Record Settings drop-down box to choose to record both Video & Audio or just Video, and to select the desired video quality (Good, Better, Best). (See the MyDVD documentation for more details on trading off the visual quality and the size of the files that will be recorded.)

Finally, to start recording, click the red Start Capturing button at the bottom of the Capture dialog box.

FIGURE 9.14

*Use the Change
Device Settings
dialog box to select
the input device
and set the
recording quality.*

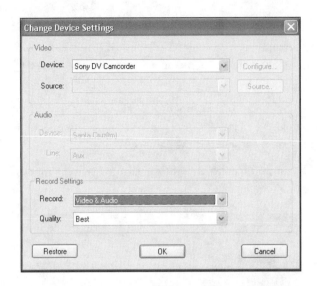

MyDVD displays the clip in the Capture dialog box as it is being captured (see Figure 9.15). Click on the red Stop button to stop capturing when the playback reaches the end of the clip that you want to record.

FIGURE 9.15

*MyDVD displays the
clip as it is captured
from the DV
camcorder and
saved to a video file
on disk in MPEG-2
video format.*

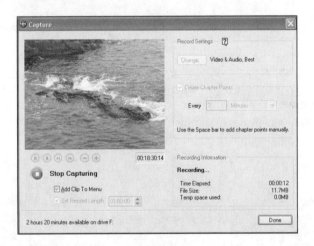

MyDVD then displays a Save As dialog box. Browse to the folder in which you want to save the file and type a name for the clip file. By default, MyDVD saves your captured clips in the My Videos folder under the current user's My Documents folder.

MyDVD saves the clip file in the specified folder, compressed in MPEG-2 (.mpg) format, and adds the new clip to the current menu. Because the clips are saved to your hard disk, you also can use the Get Movies button to add them to other menus and other projects.

You then can use the Capture dialog box to capture additional clips. When you have finished capturing clips, click on Done to close the Capture to Disk window.

Capturing Clips with Chapters

Especially when capturing a long clip, it is useful to mark chapter points at various points in the clip and add the individual chapters as separate buttons to the DVD menu. In this way, instead of having to play through the long clip to see its contents or to find a specific event, you can browse through a group of buttons with thumbnails of different points in the clip, and use them to jump directly to the corresponding point in the clip.

For example, when recording an hour-long tape to a DVD disc, creating a chapter every two minutes results in 30 chapters. At six chapter buttons per menu, MyDVD will create five menus of thumbnails for your disc.

To help organize your DVD production, especially when a clip contains many chapters, you might want to use the Add Sub-menu button to first create a new nested menu, and move to that new menu before you start capturing (see "Editing Menus and Sub-menus" earlier in this chapter).

To automatically create chapters during capture with MyDVD, click on the Create Chapter Points option on the Capture dialog box see (refer to Figure 9.13). Then, specify how regularly you want to insert chapter points—from every few seconds to a number of minutes. If the clip contains several very different scenes or several important points within a long scene, you also can insert chapter points manually by pressing the Spacebar while watching the material.

When you finish capturing a clip with chapters, MyDVD adds a series of buttons to the current menu, one for each chapter. The buttons are labeled with the name of the clip, followed by the chapter number (see Figure 9.16).

When you play back the DVD and select one of the chapter buttons, the clip will play starting at that chapter and continuing through the end of the clip—past any other following chapters.

FIGURE 9.16

When you capture a clip with chapters, MyDVD creates a menu button and thumbnail for each chapter.

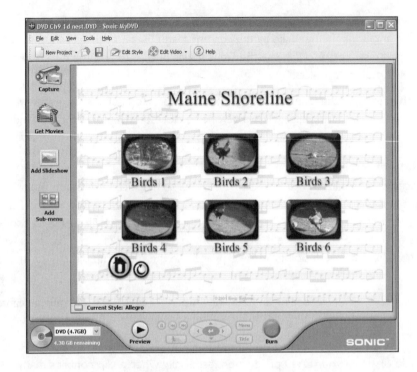

CLIPS AND CHAPTERS

A Hollywood movie DVD typically contains two kinds of menus to access the content on the disc: a clip index for different kinds of clips, such as a "Making Of" documentary or a movie trailer; and a chapter index to logical chapter points within the main movie itself.

A movie chapter index typically looks much like the menus that you are designing here, with groups of thumbnails representing the starting point of each chapter in the movie. In the movie chapter menus, however, when you select a chapter button, you jump to that point in the movie, play through the clip, and then continue playing to the end of the movie—through any other following chapters.

When designing menus for individual clips, as you are doing here, the navigation of the DVD is different. When you select a button, you jump to the beginning of the corresponding clip and play through that clip. At the end of the clip, however, the navigation jumps back to the menu again instead of continuing on through the rest of the clips on the DVD. This is similar to the way a "special features" menu works on a movie DVD. In that case, when you select a movie trailer, the DVD plays that specific program clip and then returns to the menu.

DVD authoring tools, such as MyDVD, can provide the capability to create both types of menus. When you add a list of individual clips, by default each clip plays to the end and then returns to the menu (although you can change this option in MyDVD). When you capture a long clip and mark chapter points within it, the chapter thumbnail plays from that point in the clip and continues to the end of the entire clip, continuing past any other chapter points.

More-advanced DVD authoring tools can give you more control over this behavior, with the capability to split and merge clips, add new chapter points, and explicitly specify whether a clip returns to the menu or continues playing.

Trimming and Editing Clips

DVD authoring tools, such as MyDVD, are designed to import existing media files that you have already edited, or to capture clips directly. You can use a separate video-editing tool, if desired, to create a polished video production with titles, transitions, and other effects. You then can use a DVD authoring tool to format the edited clip onto a DVD.

However, it is still useful to be able to perform some simple editing on the clips that you use in your DVD productions. MyDVD provides a Trimming window to remove unwanted material from the beginning or end of your clip.

Trimming Clips

To trim a clip that you have added to a menu in MyDVD, double-click on the clip's thumbnail button in the MyDVD window. MyDVD displays the Trimming dialog box (see Figure 9.17).

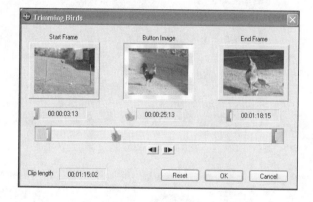

FIGURE 9.17

Use the MyDVD Trimming dialog box to select a section of the clip, and to specify the image for the button thumbnail.

The Trimming dialog box displays thumbnails of the Start Frame and End Frame of the clip, along with the current timecode of each frame and the duration of the clip.

To adjust the start frame, click and drag the green slider on the left side of the time bar at the bottom of the window. As you drag the slider, MyDVD displays the new start frame, and updates the timecode and duration. Similarly, click and drag the red slider to adjust the end frame of the clip.

When you trim a clip, the original clip remains unchanged, but MyDVD uses only the portion between the start and end frames in your production. If you specify a new start frame, that frame is used as the thumbnail on the clip's button. This is particularly useful when a clip begins with black or a fade-up effect.

Because the entire original clip is still available even after you have trimmed it and closed the Trimming dialog box, you always can adjust the trim again, and you can even set the start and end points back to the ends to show the entire clip.

The middle Button Image displays the frame in the clip that is used as the thumbnail on the associated menu button. To choose a different thumbnail image, click and drag the thumbs-up icon along the slider, or click the Nudge Left or Nudge Right buttons under the slider.

Editing Clips

The MyDVD Video Suite version of the MyDVD product includes the ArcSoft ShowBiz video-editing application (see Figure 9.18). You can run ShowBiz directly, or from the initial MyDVD Welcome screen by clicking Edit Video.

FIGURE 9.18

MyDVD Video Suite includes the ArcSoft ShowBiz video editor for editing video clips and adding transitions and effects.

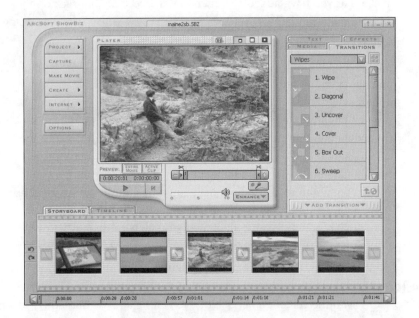

As you are authoring within MyDVD, you also can edit clips on the current menu. You can send the clips to ShowBiz, edit the clips, and then export them back to MyDVD as new clips (the original clips will not be changed).

To edit clips on the current MyDVD menu, click the Edit Video button at the top of the MyDVD window, and choose to send one selected clip to ShowBiz, a group of clips, or to send all the clips in the menu to be edited. If you send multiple clips, they will be combined together and exported back to MyDVD as a single clip. Also, if you edit a clip with chapters, the new clip will not contain chapter points.

To then export the new edited clip from ShowBiz back to MyDVD, pull down the Export menu and choose To MyDVD Project. ShowBiz will prompt for a filename to save the new clip, and then add it to the project in MyDVD.

T I P

Be careful when editing compressed video clips, such as the MPEG files that you capture in MyDVD. When you edit clips that have already been significantly compressed and then compress them again, you will start to see noticeable compression artifacts, such as blockyness. If you need to edit such clips, apply all the edits at once, and then save and compress the final result once.

Creating Photo Slide Shows

Although we tend to think of DVDs for playing video, you also can use them to present photo slide shows. With MyDVD, you can create a slide show from a collection of images, add an audio soundtrack, and even add transition effects between the slides.

Adding a Slide Show

To create a slide show on the current menu, click the Add Slideshow button on the left of the MyDVD window. MyDVD displays the Create Slideshow dialog box to add photos and set the display options.

To add images to your slide show, click the Get Pictures button on the left of the dialog box. Then select one or more still image files to add to your slide show. MyDVD displays thumbnails of the images in the Create Slideshow dialog box (see Figure 9.19).

FIGURE 9.19

Use the MyDVD Create Slideshow dialog box to import still images and set options for a photo slide show.

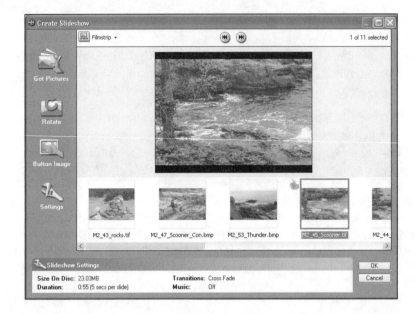

Use the drop-down menu at the top left of the dialog box to alternate between different views of the slide show: Filmstrip, smaller Thumbnails, or file Details. As you preview the images, you can use the Rotate button to flip slides upright.

When you finish creating the slide show, MyDVD adds a new button to the current menu to play the slide show. As you edit the production, you can change the slide show again by clicking on the button. Use the Button Image button to select the image that will be used for the slide show thumbnail in the MyDVD menu (as indicated by the thumbs-up icon).

Setting Slide Show Display Options

The current options for displaying the slide show are summarized in the Slideshow Settings area at the bottom of the dialog box. To change these options, click the Settings button to display the Slideshow Settings dialog box (see Figure 9.20).

Use the Basic tab in the Slideshow Settings dialog box to select a background Audio track to be played with the slide show. Also set the Duration of time that each slide is displayed, from one to 60 seconds, or choose to fit the slides to the music so that they change at equal intervals as the music plays.

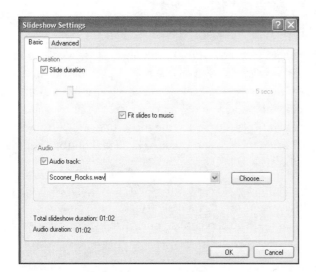

FIGURE 9.20

Use the Slideshow Settings dialog box to set options for displaying the slide show.

Use the Advanced tab in the Slideshow Settings dialog box (see Figure 9.21) to choose a Transition effect to be used between each image, including various wipes and fades. You can select the background color for the Slide Display, which is used when the shape of the slide does not fill the screen so that they are letterboxed. And you can choose to Archive the images by having MyDVD include the original image files on the disc that you create.

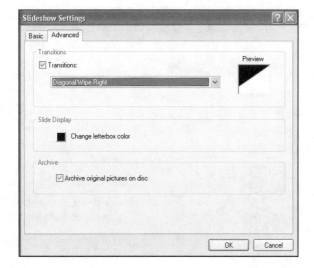

FIGURE 9.21

Use the Advanced tab of the Slideshow Settings dialog box to specify the transition and background color, and to copy the images to the output disc.

Customizing Menu Styles

DVD authoring tools, such as MyDVD, typically provide a collection of predefined menu styles or design templates to define the graphic look of the menus. The menu styles are based on a graphical theme which is applied to the various menu elements, including the background graphic image, the framing around the buttons, and the text fonts and colors used for the menu title and button caption text. The clip thumbnails, nested menus, and other navigational buttons are then laid out on the menu using the style.

In MyDVD, the style that you select is used for all the menus in the project. You can choose a style when you start a new project, but you also can change to a different style at any time. You can choose one of the styles included with MyDVD, or you can design your own custom styles.

Changing the Menu Style

While you are editing your DVD project, you can change the graphical look of your menus by clicking on the Edit Style button at the top of the MyDVD window.

MyDVD displays the Edit Style dialog box (see Figure 9.22). To choose a style, scroll through the list of styles on the left side of the dialog box to see examples of the look of each style.

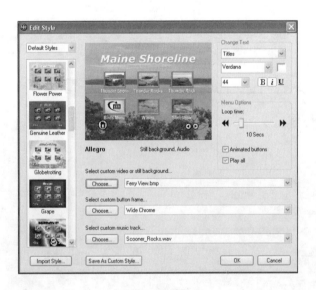

FIGURE 9.22

Use the Edit Style dialog box to select the graphical and text styles for your menus.

Setting Text Style Options

Use the Change Text area at the top right of the Edit Style dialog box to set the text attributes for your menus. Pull down the drop-down menu to select the menu field to change: Titles, Buttons, or All Text. Then choose the font, font size, and style (bold, italic, or underlined). Click the color chip to select the font color from a color palette.

Setting Menu Style Options

Use the Menu Options area on the right side of the Edit Style dialog box to set the display options for the menus. Select Animated Buttons to have MyDVD create motion menu buttons, with short video sequences of each clip playing as the button thumbnails instead of just showing still images. You can change the starting point for this animated sequence by setting the Button Image in the Trimming dialog box. Set the Loop Time for the motion buttons, from one to 60 seconds.

Select Play All to have your DVD play through all the clips, one after another, instead of returning to the main menu at the end of each clip.

Setting Background Style Options

Use the area at the bottom of the Edit Style dialog box to customize the menu background image, audio, and button frames.

Use the first Custom Video or Still Background option to choose a still image or even a video clip file to be used as the background for your menus.

Use the second Custom Button Frame option to select the style for the frame around the menu buttons, including different colors, shapes, and transparency.

Use the third Custom Music Track area to select an audio file to be played while the menu is displayed. This can be the audio part of the selected background video, or a separate audio clip, or you can choose to have no audio with the menu.

T I P

Be warned that motion menus require significant processing to create, so MyDVD displays only still images while you are editing, and even in Preview mode. To see the motion menus in Preview mode, click the Build Motion Menus button (the running person icon under the play controls). MyDVD then builds the motion menus so that you can preview them. Similarly, projects with motion menus require more processing to create the final DVD. You can reduce the processing time by limiting the Loop Time duration for the moving sequences.

Using Custom Menu Styles

After you have edited the menu style you can save it to use later to create your own collection of common themes for different productions.

Click the Save as Custom Style button at the bottom of the dialog box to save your settings as a new style. MyDVD adds your new style to a new Custom category, accessible from the drop-down menu at the top left of the dialog box.

You also can use Adobe Photoshop to create new graphical styles by downloading the Sonic Style Creator plug-in. Then click the Import Style button to import the styles into MyDVD.

When you finish editing the menu style, click the OK button to close the Edit Style dialog box. MyDVD will then change the style of all the menus in your project (see Figure 9.23). The name of the current style also is displayed at the bottom left of the MyDVD window.

FIGURE 9.23

MyDVD applies the new style to all the menus in your project.

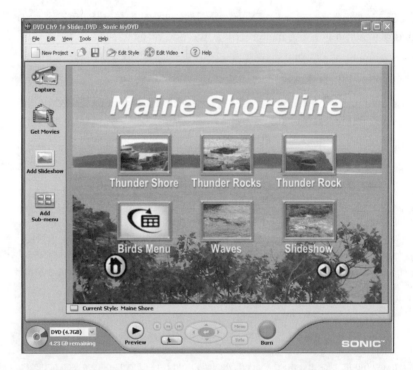

Burning DVDs

After you finish authoring a DVD project, you probably want to burn it to a disc to save and share it. You have several options for how to deliver your final production. You can burn your production to DVD, of course, if you have the necessary DVD burner hardware. You also can create a Video-CD project with the same material, which you can burn on a CD recorder and play on many set-top DVD players, albeit at a lower quality.

Instead of burning your DVD or VCD production to a removable DVD or CD disc, you also can save the output DVD- or VCD-format disc volume in a folder on your hard disk (see "Stepping Through a New Project with Sonic MyDVD" earlier in this chapter). Because the DVD (or VCD) volume on hard disk contains exactly the same files in exactly the same folder hierarchy, you then can play back your production directly from hard disk using DVD player software.

Disc Capacities: DVD and VCD

MyDVD provides three quality settings when capturing video: Good, Better, and Best. You can fit approximately 60 minutes of video on a DVD at the Best quality setting, and up to 180 minutes at the Good setting. MyDVD uses the Best setting when converting video files from other formats.

For Video-CD projects, MyDVD always uses a Good quality setting to fit around 60 minutes on a 650MB CD, or 65 minutes on a 700MB CD.

Burning a DVD Disc

Burning a DVD disc requires that you have a compatible recordable or rewritable DVD disc drive installed on your system. (See the MyDVD documentation and Sonic web site for more information on compatible drives.) If the necessary Windows drivers are installed for your disc drive, MyDVD can write to the full compliment of recordable DVD formats (including DVD-R, DVD+R, DVD-RW, and DVD+RW). (See Chapter 3, "Consumer DVD Recorders: Recordable Formats," for more information on DVD disc formats and drive hardware.)

To start recording your production to DVD, click on the red Burn button at the bottom of the MyDVD window.

MyDVD displays the Make Disc Setup dialog box (see Figure 9.24). If more than one recordable DVD drive is available on your system, then select the destination DVD recordable drive from the drop-down menu. You can set the Copies option to burn your production to multiple discs. You also can set the Write Speed when creating a VCD.

FIGURE 9.24

Use the MyDVD Make Disc Setup dialog box to start burning your production to a DVD disc.

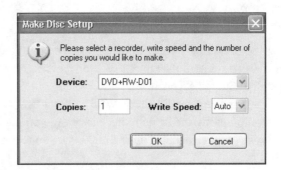

Insert a DVD recordable disc into the drive, and click on OK. MyDVD will build any slide shows, import and transcode (compress) your media files, organize and build the DVD navigation and file system into DVD format, and then format and write the files to the disc.

Depending on the format, you then can play the disc in compatible set-top players, as well as on computers with DVD drives.

Editing an Existing DVD

When you record a DVD project to disc, the individual clips, menu navigation, and various graphical elements in the menus are all combined together into the monolithic DVD volume format. As a result, the individual elements are no longer visible, and cannot be retrieved directly from the DVD contents. In addition, the video and audio clips on the DVD have been compressed to significantly reduce their size. As a result, it is often a good idea to save a copy of the original DVD authoring project, along with all the associated original media files so that you have them available if you want to use them again in another project.

On the other hand, if all you want to do is to update a project by adding or deleting clips from the menus (or even trimming the ends of some clips), then it would be very useful to be able to open and edit an existing DVD. The new DVD Video

Recording (VR) format used in some set-top DVD recorders provides some of this capability for updating existing discs. The VR format also is beginning to be supported in DVD authoring tools, providing the capability to edit the same disc on both set-top recorders and on computers.

MyDVD goes a step further to create discs using the Sonic OpenDVD format, which includes project information as additional data on the disc. OpenDVD-compliant discs can be created and edited with any application that supports the OpenDVD format. You can open the disc as a project in MyDVD and then add (or delete) clips, change the menus, and even change the graphical style. You also can save the results directly back to a DVD+RW disc, without needing to copy the project to hard disk first.

Editing an OpenDVD Disc

To edit an existing DVD (or VCD) disc in OpenDVD format using MyDVD, first insert the disc in a drive on your computer. Then, choose Edit an Existing OpenDVD Disc from the MyDVD Welcome menu, or pull down the MyDVD File menu and choose Edit DVD.

Use the Browse dialog box to select the DVD or CD drive in which you installed the MyDVD disc that you previously recorded. MyDVD opens a new project using the information saved on the DVD. You then can edit the project as usual.

If some of the clips you used in the project were trimmed, only the trimmed portion of the clips were burned to DVD, so you cannot now remove the trimming to see more of the ends of the clip. If you want to use the entire clip, you need to add the original clip file to the project again.

When you finish editing, you can save the project as usual to the hard disk. MyDVD will transfer the project information to the hard disk (including the media clips), so you do not need the DVD disc any more to continue editing the project. If you are editing a full DVD, this will take a while to transfer 4GB or more of data back to your hard disk. You then can burn the new project to another DVD (or CD), or write the DVD volume to hard disc.

Even better, if you are using a DVD+RW rewritable disc, you can burn the new project back to the same disc, without having to transfer it to hard disk first. Of course, this changes the contents of the disc, so make sure you did not want to save the original disc.

Editing an Existing DVD Volume on Hard Disk

With MyDVD, you also can open and edit DVD volumes that you have stored on your hard disk. Pull down the File menu and choose Edit DVD. Use the Browse dialog box to select the folder on hard disk that contains the DVD volume that MyDVD previously recorded (the folder named for the project that has the VIDEO_TS folder in it). MyDVD then opens a new project using the information saved with the DVD volume. Because you are working from hard disk, this is much faster than editing from a DVD or CD drive.

Again, you can edit the project as usual. However, when you save the project, use Save As to save the project to a different directory, instead of replacing the original project information saved in the DVD volume folder. In this case, MyDVD does not create a copy of all the media files in the new project, so when you edit the new project, MyDVD will reference the clips contained in the previously recorded DVD volume folder.

Recording Direct-to-DVD

The DVD format provides significant advantages over videotape for viewing a program because it is much faster to search and skip through a disc than to wait for a tape to rewind. Even better, DVDs can have index menus to allow you to visually search through thumbnails of clips and scenes, to understand what is on the disc, and to then jump directly to the clip that you want to watch.

As a result, one obvious use for DVDs is to simply make copies of your videotapes. Not only do you get the advantage of being able to access them much more easily, but you also can play them back on any set-top DVD player or DVD-equipped computer. As a bonus, you also get digital backups of your tapes, which you can even edit again later.

Copying an entire tape, with one or more hours of material, can be a pain, however. In traditional DVD authoring, you would first capture the entire contents of the tape to a file on hard disk, use a DVD authoring tool to design the menus and chapters, convert all that material to DVD format (including compressing the video into MPEG-2 format), and then finally burn the result to a DVD disc. That is a lot of work, and requires a lot of time and spare disk space.

If you want to simply copy a tape to DVD, it would be wonderful if you could just press one button and have the copy made automatically. Of course, as described in Chapter 3, you can do this with a set-top DVD recorder designed to work as a digital VCR: You feed the recorder a video signal, and it records the video to DVD.

Computers are becoming quite powerful these days, with processors faster than 1GHz, and with internal bus speeds fast enough to process full-rate video and audio. So it is now actually feasible to automate the recording process on a computer, to capture video and burn it directly to DVD. This tape-to-DVD conversion works well with DV camcorders because with the availability of DV camcorders and FireWire/IEEE 1394 connectors on computers, you now can capture and process full-quality DV digital video. Plus, the DV-video format conveniently matches the DVD resolutions, and can be efficiently transcoded (recompressed) into MPEG-2 format.

Setting Up MyDVD for Direct-to-DVD Recording

MyDVD can automatically convert live video to DVD or VCD, complete with menus in a selected style. While it is capturing, MyDVD can add chapter points automatically at fixed intervals, or you can add them yourself at interesting points. It is a really good idea to add chapter points while you are capturing to DVD because otherwise you will not be able to index or skip through the DVD as you play it.

Before you start the process, connect your video source to your computer, and insert a recordable disc in the recorder that you will use. If you will be recording from DV, turn on your camcorder to the VCR (not camera) mode.

Also, do what you can to reduce the load on your computer from other applications during the Direct-to-DVD processing. Your system needs to move lots of data in real-time: in from the video capture device, processed on the hard disk, and then out to the recording device. Besides needing to keep up with these external devices, your system also does some intensive processing while it compresses video and audio and then combines the data into DVD format. As a result, you should close down any extra applications (especially background processing like system or virus checkers or networked downloads). Until you have experimented with how much load your system can handle, you should also avoid using other processing-intensive applications at the same time.

Setting Up MyDVD for Direct-to-DVD Recording

To start a direct-to-disc recording with MyDVD, select DVD-Video on the initial Welcome screen, and then click Transfer Video Direct to DVD. Or in the main MyDVD application, pull down the Tools menu and choose Direct-to-DVD.

MyDVD displays the Sonic MyDVD Wizard screen, with a three-step process to create the DVD (see Figure 9.25).

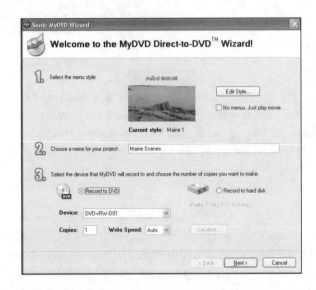

Use Step 1 to select the menu style (see "Customizing Menu Styles" earlier in this chapter). You can click Edit Style to display the Edit Style dialog box to choose or edit a style, or select No Menus to create a disc without menus to just play the recorded video.

Use Step 2 to enter a name for your project. MyDVD will use this name for menu titles, menu button labels, or the disc name.

Use Step 3 to choose the DVD recording options (see "Burning DVDs" earlier in this chapter), or to record to a DVD volume on hard disk (see "Stepping Through a New Project with Sonic MyDVD" also earlier in this chapter).

After selecting the options for your recording, click the Next button.

MyDVD first checks the selected drive and your disc to verify that the media is ready for recording.

MyDVD then displays the Recording Wizard (see Figure 9.26). As described earlier in "Capturing Clips from a DV Camcorder," make sure that Record Settings are set to record both video and audio from your DV device. Also, enable Create Chapter Points to create chapter points at regular intervals to create thumbnail menus of the tape contents.

If you are recording from a DV camcorder, use the play controls under the video window to position the tape to the start of the material you want to capture. Otherwise, position your input tape and start it playing.

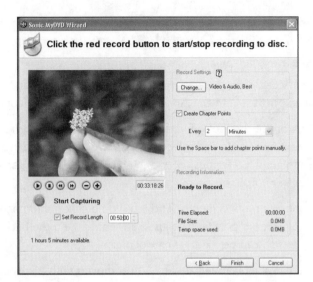

FIGURE 9.26

Finally, use the Recording Wizard to start and stop the direct-to-disc capture.

Set Record Length for maximum time to capture if desired, and then click on the red Start Capturing button.

MyDVD then begins capturing your video (and audio) material. You can monitor the progress in the video window.

MyDVD continues capturing until it reaches the capacity of the type of disc that you selected. As it is capturing, it creates chapter points at the specified regular intervals, and you also can insert chapter points manually at key points by pressing the Spacebar. You also can stop the recording by clicking on Stop.

MyDVD compresses the video as it is being captured. When capture is completed, it then processes the clips and menus, combines the elements into DVD format, and then burns the result to the selected DVD recorder. When MyDVD completes the Direct-to-DVD process, your videotape has been transferred to DVD, complete with menus, and is ready for viewing.

Summary

As you have seen in this chapter, even introductory DVD authoring tools, such as MyDVD, can offer a wide range of capabilities.

MyDVD can capture video clips, or import existing clips from hard disk. It automatically lays out clips with thumbnail buttons in linked menus, but also gives you the capability to rearrange the buttons and organize them in linked sub-menus. It also can create photo slide shows, timed to a background audio clip, and with transition effects.

To fine-tune your video clips, you can trim them directly in MyDVD, or the MyDVD Video Suite can export them to the ArcSoft ShowBiz video-editing application.

You then can customize the look of your menus by using the built-in styles, or by selecting a different front style and selecting your own background image, background audio, and graphical frames around the buttons. You even can create your own menu styles in PhotoShop.

MyDVD also supports motion menus. The clip thumbnail on the menu buttons can be a short moving video clip instead of just a still image. And the background behind the menus also can be a repeating video clip.

Even better, you can start learning about DVD authoring with MyDVD even if you do not have a DVD burner. With MyDVD, you can create Video-CD productions, and burn them to CD to share with others. VCDs can be played on any computer with just a CD drive and DVD player software, and also can be played on set-top DVD players. MyDVD can also save your DVD and VCD productions to hard disk, so you can test them before burning. You can then share them by copying the data over the network, or even burn short DVD productions to a CD to play on another computer.

To make creating DVDs even easier, MyDVD provides the Direct-to-DVD option to transfer your videotapes to DVD with a minimum of fuss. Just pick a style and MyDVD does the rest—capturing and compressing the video, building the DVD menus, and then burning the resulting project to disc.

And writing a DVD is not the end of your possibilities. With its OpenDVD format, MyDVD and other tools add project information to the discs they create. This means that you can re-open an existing disc to edit and update it, maybe to add new clips or even to change the menu style.

Even as an introductory "automated" DVD authoring tool, MyDVD packages an impressive array of technology to both simplify the authoring process and still offer you the ability to customize your creations. For even more control over the look, layout, and navigation of your DVD projects, check out the tools in Part IV, "Personal DVD Authoring."

Part IV

Personal DVD Authoring

Part IV introduces the next level of sophistication in DVD authoring, "personal" DVD authoring tools that provide more control over designing and customizing your DVDs, while still greatly simplifying the complexity of the full DVD specification.

Chapters 10 and 11 describe Apple iDVD and Sonic DVDit!, two tools designed to import clips, provide significant capability to customize the menu layout and design, and then burn the result to DVD. Unlike the automated tools, these applications do not provide built-in video capture, nor do they provide much video editing. They do provide automated assists for building DVD menus, as well as the capability to override and customize the design.

The workflow for these tools assumes you are not just quickly transferring video to DVD, but instead that you are first using a separate video-editing tool, such as iMovie, to edit your raw material into various movie clips, which you will then present as part of your DVD production. These productions can also include more use of background audio, and slide shows with accompanying audio.

chapter 10

Personal DVD Authoring with Apple iDVD

WITH THE NEW POWER MAC SYSTEMS introduced in 2001, Apple delivered a complete digital video solution, including the capability to create and record full-quality video productions to DVD using the iDVD authoring application and the SuperDrive CD-R/RW and DVD-R burner. At the same time, Apple also transitioned to the next-generation Mac OS X operating system with a UNIX-based core operating system.

Current DVD-enabled Macintosh systems, such as the new iMac, include all the necessary hardware components plus a full suite of bundled applications, so that you can capture DV video over FireWire (IEEE 1394) cables, edit video and audio clips in iMovie, author your movies into a production in iDVD, and then burn the result to a DVD-R disc. And these DVDs are not just for viewing on computers; you also can watch your movies on set-top DVD players.

This chapter shows you how to use iDVD to author DVD productions. It begins by stepping you through the entire process of using iDVD and then explores additional features for customizing your productions.

About iDVD

iDVD is a consumer-level application intended to compliment the Apple iMovie editor by shielding users from the complexity of DVD authoring. It provides drag-and-drop simplicity along with professionally designed graphical themes for creating menus to turn iMovies, QuickTime files, and pictures into DVDs that can be played on consumer DVD players.

The second version, iDVD 2, introduced in October 2001, was the first tool in its class to support "motion menus" with motion video for buttons and menu backgrounds. It can record up to 90 minutes of material on a DVD (up from 60 minutes). It requires Mac OS X because it can take advantage of OS X multiprocessing support to perform MPEG video encoding in the background while you are working. Thus, by the time you are ready to build your production, you no longer have to wait for all your clips to be encoded.

Stepping Through a New Project with iDVD

This section steps through the process of creating a new DVD project in iDVD from existing QuickTime movie files. iDVD has a straightforward workflow. First, you use iMovie to capture and edit your video into the clips you want to show on your DVD. Then, you drag and drop the clips into iDVD to create new buttons on the current menu. You can then design the graphical look and the menu navigation of your DVD production, using themes and customization options. Finally, you preview your DVD to test the navigational links, and burn your DVD to the SuperDrive.

iDVD's simplicity comes from what Apple left out. You do not capture or edit clips in iDVD; that's what iMovie is for. There is no clip shelf for importing and organizing your clips as in iMovie; instead you just drag and drop clips from the Finder straight to the menus. There are no multiple views, such as a storyboard and a timeline; instead, you just add folders and navigate the links directly in the main window as you edit.

Step 1: Launch iDVD

As soon as you launch iDVD 2, you notice that something is seriously different. Yes, there is a Project window with a large work area and editing buttons along the bottom. But instead of a blank or static screen, you are greeted with a moving and revolving globe with music playing in the background (see Figure 10.1). This is a motion menu; the menu background is actually a video clip instead of just a still image. That is a sure way to jazz up even a quick DVD of some vacation clips.

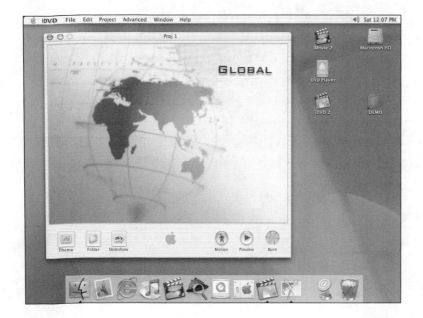

FIGURE 10.1

iDVD has a single Project window that you use to design your DVD.

> **TIP**
>
> *If you find the motion menus and background audio distracting as you are working, you can click on the Motion button at the bottom of the iDVD window to pause them.*

Step 2: Add Clips to the Menu

To add clips to the DVD menu for your new project, open a Finder window with some QuickTime movie clips, and drag and drop a clip onto the menu. iDVD creates a button for the clip using a thumbnail of the clip (see Figure 10.2).

FIGURE 10.2

Drag and drop QuickTime movie files from a Finder window to create menu buttons.

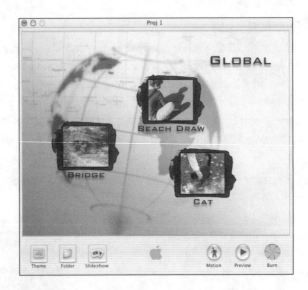

Even better, the thumbnail is not a still image; it is a motion menu with moving video of the clip. As you can see, iDVD actually provides two kinds of motion in motion menus: The background image can be in motion, and the clip thumbnails used for the menu buttons also can be in motion.

Next, drag more clips onto the menu, one by one. As you add the additional clips, iDVD automatically repositions them on the menu.

T I P

iDVD is designed for assembling an interactive DVD production from a collection of finished clips, not for capturing or editing video clip footage. You can use iMovie to capture video and audio scenes from DV camcorders or other sources; you can then edit them into a polished movie clip, with titles, transitions, and other effects. When you export the final movie from iMovie, use the Export for iDVD option to ensure that the material is ready to import into iDVD. See Chapter 4, "Digital Media and DVD on the Macintosh," for an introduction to iMovie.

Step 3: Select a Menu Style

You can change the graphical style of your DVD by choosing a different theme. Click on the Theme button to open the slide-out drawer on the left side of the iDVD window. Then, click on the Themes tab at the top of the drawer. (To close the drawer, click on the Theme button again.)

You then can use the controller to navigate through your menus and check the design and links, or just click directly on the menu buttons. Click on the Preview button again, or press the Exit button on the controller to close the window and continue editing your DVD.

> **T I P**
>
> *While you are editing your menu, you also can play an individual clip by double-clicking on its button without needing to preview the entire DVD.*

Step 6: Save the Project

Before you continue, this is a good time to save your project. Pull down the File menu and choose Save Project. iDVD saves all the project information and data in a file with the project name and the suffix dvdproj.

> **T I P**
>
> *You also can use Save Project As to save copies of your work in progress as you make changes to your project, or start a new version of a project under a new name. However, these DVD project files can get very large because they contain the media assets used in the project (see the section later in this chapter called "Setting Up iDVD Preferences").*

Step 7: Check the Project Status

One of the most useful features of iDVD happens behind the scenes while you are working. iDVD takes advantage of the multiprocessing capabilities of Mac OS X to encode the video clips that you imported into your project in the background, even as you are editing the menu and previewing the disc. Instead of having to wait for all the clips to be encoded when you finish authoring the design, iDVD may well have finished with them while you were working.

In the Themes drawer, click on the Status tab to see the list of clips in your project and check the progress of the encoding (see Figure 10.6). You can also pull down the Project menu and choose Project Info to see more detail.

iDVD can record up to 60 or 90 minutes of material on a DVD. Check the Status tab to see how much material you have imported into your project of the available duration. iDVD specifies an available duration of 60 minutes for up to the first hour of material, or a duration of 90 minutes if you import more material. In order to fit 90 minutes on a DVD, however, iDVD does use slightly lower video quality.

FIGURE 10.6

Use the Status tab in the Themes drawer to see the progress of encoding your clips in the background.

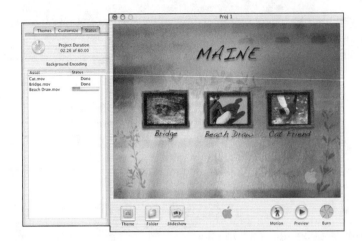

> **TIP**
>
> *Because iDVD encodes your video and audio clips in the background while you work, it is a good idea to import all your clips into the project right away. That way, you can give iDVD as much time as possible to encode the clips while you continue to edit the menu design.*

Step 8: Record Your Project

Finally, it's time to burn a disc. On the new Power Macs and iMacs, iDVD uses the SuperDrive to record your project to a DVD-R disk.

Click on the Burn button at the bottom left of the iDVD window to open and enable it, and click on it again to start the burning process. If you disabled your motion menus (by clicking the Motion button off), iDVD will warn you so that you can turn them on again.

Insert a blank DVD-R disc in the DVD drive, and iDVD will step through the various stages of the recording process (see Figure 10.7). Even though iDVD can encode your video clips in the background, it still must prepare and encode the menu graphics. It then combines, or multiplexes, all the DVD material together, and finally burns the DVD disc.

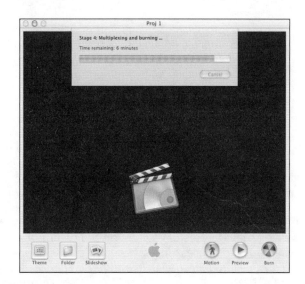

FIGURE 10.7

iDVD steps through the process of burning your project to disk, including preparing the menu graphics, combining all the material into DVD format, and actually recording to disc.

Step 9: Play Back the CD

When iDVD completes the recording process, your presentation has been burned to DVD with your movie clips organized into menus with professionally designed graphics. Now you can play it back on the Macintosh with the DVD Player application, or insert the disc in a set-top DVD player, and enjoy it on television.

Setting Up iDVD Preferences

iDVD does not require much in the way of setting up before starting to work with it. The general program options are defined in the iDVD Preferences dialog box (see Figure 10.8).

Use the Video Standard section to select the target video format for your DVD, either NTSC (for North America) or PAL (for much of Europe).

You can also select Delete Rendered Files to reduce disk space usage when you close a project. iDVD saves all the DVD format data that it creates for your project in the dvdproj data file, including the encoded video clips. Because a DVD can contain up to 4.7GB of data, these project files can get rather large.

Finally, you can select or deselect Show Watermark to choose whether to show the Apple logo watermark on your menu screens.

FIGURE 10.8

Use the iDVD Preferences dialog box to set general program options and especially to free up disk space.

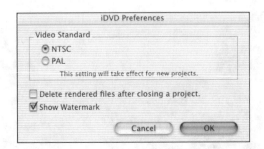

Organizing Clips in DVD Menus

iDVD offers the capability to reorganize the order of clips on your menus, and to organize groups of clips into folders of multiple nested menus of clips. You also can easily copy and move clips between menus.

Reorganizing Menu Buttons

As you add new clips to a menu, iDVD automatically lays them out according to the design defined in the current menu style. To change the order of the clips, simply click and drag them on the menu into a new position (see Figure 10.9). As you drag the clips, iDVD slides the others around into their corresponding new positions.

FIGURE 10.9

Regoranize the order of the clips on the menu by dragging the buttons to a new position.

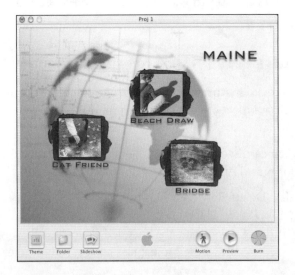

T I P

Although most of the themes use a simple layout with two rows of three clips each, others use a more irregular layout, different thumbnail sizes, or even plain text with no thumbnail image. However, iDVD also offers complete control over the look and layout of the buttons under the Customize tab in the Themes drawer. You then can turn off the automatic grid structure, and position the buttons anywhere on the menu.

Adding Clips in Nested Menus

As you add more clips to your project, you can organize them into subfolders to create nested hierarchical menus. Click on the Folder button at the bottom left of the iDVD window to create a new Folder button on the current menu.

To edit the nested menu, double-click on the associated button on the menu, and iDVD displays the empty menu for the new folder. You can now import new clips into the new menu, and change its theme. iDVD also adds a Back button to the nested menu so that you can navigate back up to the original menu (see Figure 10.10).

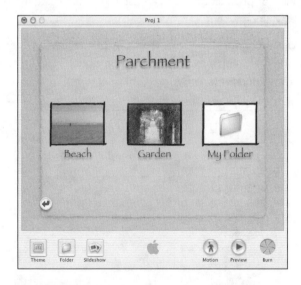

FIGURE 10.10

Use the Folder button to organize your clips into nested folders. iDVD adds a Back button to the nested menu to move back up the hierarchy.

Copying, Moving, and Deleting Menu Buttons

To copy and move buttons between menus, simply use the standard Macintosh Cut, Copy, and Paste operations.

To delete a button from a menu, click on the button to select it and then press the Delete key. iDVD deletes the button from the menu with a cute animated cloud of dust. If the button is a folder, the entire nested contents of the folder are also deleted.

You can click to select an individual button to act on or choose Select All from the Edit menu to act on all the buttons on a menu at once.

T I P

iDVD provides both an Undo and a Redo option under the Edit menu, so you can experiment and then undo your changes, and even recover from accidentally deleting entire menus.

If you save your work as you go, you also can revert back simply by closing the project without saving the latest changes and then reopening it back to its previous state.

Creating Slide Shows

For a different kind of production, you can use iDVD to create a slide show with a soundtrack to play along with it.

Click on the Slideshow button at the bottom left of the iDVD window to create a new button on the menu for the slide show. Then double-click on the button to show the Slideshow window (see Figure 10.11).

FIGURE 10.11

Use the Slideshow window to organize a slide show of still images with a background audio track.

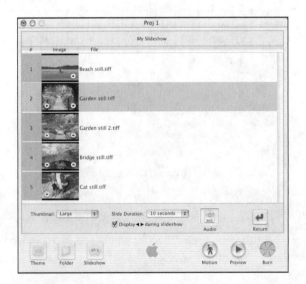

To add images to your slide show, open a Finder window, and drag image files into the window. You can click and drag as usual to change the order of the slides. Use the Thumbnail menu at the bottom left of the window to adjust the size of the image thumbnails as you edit your slide show.

To add a background audio track to the slide show, drag a QuickTime audio file from a Finder window to the Audio well below the list of slides. To remove the background audio, drag the file icon out of the well.

Select the Display arrows option to display left and right arrows as a reminder to the user to click on the left and right navigation buttons on their remote control to advance to the previous or next slides. The arrow icons themselves are not clickable.

Use the Slide Duration menu to set the length of time each slide is displayed before advancing to the next. Select Fit to Audio to match the slide show to the duration of the audio clip, or choose Manual to require that the viewer explicitly click to advance to the next slide.

You can click on the Preview button at the bottom of the iDVD window at any time to preview your slide show timing and audio.

When you have finished creating your slide show, click on the Return button at the bottom right of the window to return back to the menu that contains the slide show.

Customizing Menus

iDVD provides a predesigned collection of themes or menu design templates to define the graphical look of the menus. The themes are based on a common graphical style, which is applied to the various menu elements—including the background graphic image, the framing around the buttons, and the text fonts and colors used for the menu title and button caption text.

These themes are great for getting started and creating your first DVDs, but iDVD also gives you the flexibility to override each individual element of a theme, and apply changes to a single menu or throughout the project.

To customize your menus, click on the Customize tab at the top of the Themes drawer.

Customizing Button Motion

When you click on a button in a menu, iDVD pops up a small slider and check box (see Figure 10.12). Use the Motion check box to specify whether the button thumbnail for a video clip is to be motion video or just a still image.

Use the Motion Duration slider at the top of the Customize drawer to set the length of the all the motion sequences in the menu, including the background and video buttons. The motion menus can be up to 30 seconds long.

Customizing Button Images

Each button on the menu is represented with an image thumbnail or icon. Buttons for video clips use a thumbnail image of the first frame of the clip, and buttons for folders and slide shows use default icons.

To use a different frame of a video clip, drag the slider above the button to select another poster frame to represent the clip when the button is not in motion (see Figure 10.12). For folder and slide show buttons, the slider will display the clips in the folder or the images in the slide show.

You can also use your own custom image for a button. Simply drag and drop a still image file from a Finder window onto the button. The image will be resized to fit the button. You can then select the custom image by moving the slider above the button all the way to the right.

FIGURE 10.12

Use the pop-up button menu to control the button motion and to select a poster frame. You can also drag and drop custom images to use for buttons.

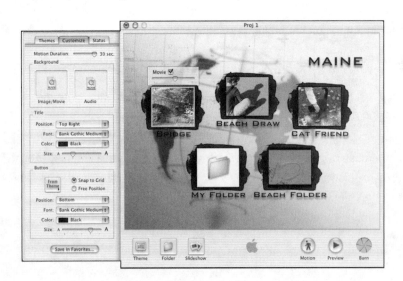

Customizing Menu Backgrounds

Use the Background controls at the top of the Customize drawer to select a different background scene and background audio track to show with the menu (see Figure 10.13).

To change the menu background graphic, drag a still image or QuickTime movie file to the Image/Movie well (or just drop it on the background of the main window).

To change the background audio, drag a QuickTime audio file to the Audio well. To remove the selected files, just drag the associated icon out of the well, and iDVD will revert to the style of the selected theme.

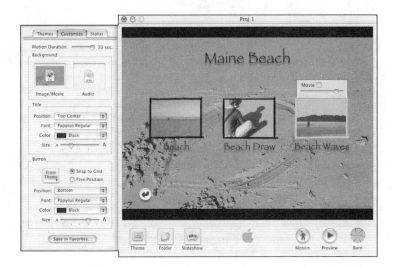

FIGURE 10.13

Use the Background controls under the Customize tab to add your own background image or video and background audio to the menu.

Customizing Menu Titles

Use the Title controls in the middle of the Customize drawer to change the position and text attributes of the menu title (see Figure 10.14).

Use the Position pop-up menu to position the title in predefined locations or to have no title, or choose Custom to drag the title to any location on the menu. Use the Font, Color, and Size fields to adjust the look of the title text.

FIGURE 10.14

Use the Title controls under the Customize tab to adjust the position and look of the menu title text.

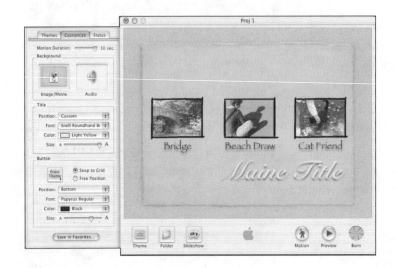

Customizing Menu Buttons

Use the Button controls at the bottom of the Customize drawer to change the position and text attributes of the buttons (see Figure 10.15).

Use the From Theme pop-up menu to select whether the button frame design should be set from the current theme or to choose a different design from the menu.

Use the Snap to Grid or Free Position check boxes to select whether the buttons should automatically be laid out according to the grid design of the theme or whether you can freely move the buttons to any position on the menu.

The remaining controls affect the button labels. Use the Position pop-up menu to select the location of the label text relative to the thumbnail image; you can also choose that the buttons be Text Only, or that they have No Text and just graphics. Use the Font, Color, and Size fields to adjust the look of the label text.

T I P

If you choose to manually position your menu titles and buttons, and to use a custom background, be careful to keep the important elements within the safe area, the center portion of the display. When you display a DVD on a television set by playing it on a set-top DVD player, the edges of the DVD images may not be visible on the TV screen.

To protect against this problem, pull down the Advanced menu and select Show TV Safe Area. iDVD then displays a shaded area around the screen to approximate the safe area in which you can place your elements.

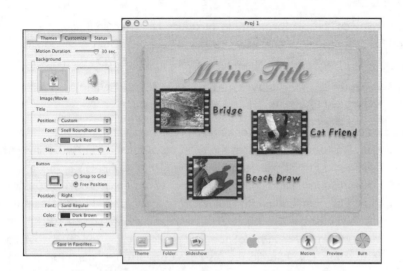

FIGURE 10.15

*Use the Button
controls under the
Customize tab to
adjust the positions
of the buttons, their
graphical frame, and
the location and
look of the button
label text.*

Applying Menu Themes

When you use the Themes drawer to select a new theme or to customize a menu, those changes apply only to the currently displayed menu. However, after you have changed the design of a menu, you also can apply that design to other menus in your project.

To apply the design of a menu to all the menus in a project, pull down the Advanced menu and choose Apply Theme to Project. This way, your entire project can share a common graphical design.

To apply the design of a menu to all other folders nested below it, choose Apply Theme to Folders. You can then use different graphical designs for different sections of your DVD. Just edit the design of a higher-level folder and then apply the changes to the lower-level folders under it.

Summary

Apple's iDVD provides the best of both worlds for personal DVD authoring: a simple interface with automated assistance for laying out great-looking DVD menus, plus the ability to customize the graphical look and explicitly control the layout. The addition of motion menus, in particular, can make your DVDs visually stunning.

With the Power Mac platform, Apple introduced a convenient and effective end-to-end DVD authoring system even for personal use—from DV video capture and editing with iMovie to DVD creation and burning with iDVD and the SuperDrive.

The next chapter ("Personal DVD Authoring with Sonic DVDit!") describes DVDit!, a personal DVD authoring tool for Windows.

Apple also offers DVD Studio Pro, a more professional and full-featured DVD authoring tool, as described in Chapter 12, "Professional DVD Authoring with Apple DVD Studio Pro." DVD Studio Pro complements Apple's Final Cut Pro tool for video editing, effects, and compositing. It provides professional encoding of video into MPEG-2 and audio into Dolby Digital formats, and supports up to 99 video tracks and multiple language tracks. You can include slide shows, still or motion menus from layered PhotoShop files or video clips, and interactive links directly to the web. DVD Studio Pro also can output to DLT tape for mass duplication or DVD-RAM to inexpensively test projects.

chapter 11

Personal DVD Authoring with Sonic DVDit!

THE PRECEDING CHAPTER, "PERSONAL DVD AUTHORING WITH APPLE iDVD," showed how Apple's iDVD transforms DVD authoring into a simple drag-and-drop experience. Just drag clips onto a menu to make buttons, select a menu style, edit the menu and button text, create nested menus, and then preview and burn your production.

Sonic DVDit! begins with a similar drag-and-drop approach as a Windows DVD authoring tool, but also provides access to more advanced controls for creating arbitrary links between menus, adding text and graphic designs, setting chapter points in clips, and giving explicit control over the compression. Like iDVD, DVDit! is not a video capture or video-editing tool. It is designed to import finished clips that you have already prepared, and then combine them into an interactive production. As a Windows application, it offers compatibility with a wider range of media formats, including Windows AVI and Apple QuickTime video files. It also can output your production as a DVD volume on hard disk to then use to test and burn copies.

With this additional control, however, comes more complexity in the interface, and the need for you to manually define some of the layout and navigation that is automatically created in simpler tools. For example, you must explicitly position buttons on the menus, create links to nested menus and back again, and add and edit text for menu titles and button labels.

To support this level of control, DVDit! also has more elements in the user interface. Instead of dragging clips directly from disk folders, in DVDit! you first import them into a Palette window. This is used to organize all your media assets, including video, background audio, images, buttons, and text fonts. The DVDit! interface also makes the components of your design visible by providing the Menus/Movies list so that you can review all the menus and clips that you have created and used in your project—and so that you can more easily link between them. You then can create your menu design separately from preparing the clips, and create the navigational links between the two.

This chapter shows you how to use DVDit! to author DVD productions. It begins by stepping you through the entire process of using DVDit! for quick drag-and-drop authoring. It then provides more details on importing media clips, customizing the design, working with menus and movies, building the interactive navigation, and creating the final DVD production.

About DVDit!

Sonic DVDit! (www.dvdit.com) is a leading DVD authoring application for videographers and corporate video producers, and is bundled with major video editing, capturing, encoding, and media production systems.

The Sonic product line shares a common underlying DVD authoring technology, called AuthorScript, which has been used to create millions of Hollywood, professional, and consumer DVD titles. It also offers wide compatibility among set-top and PC playback devices. Sonic has licensed its authoring technology to companies ranging from InterVideo to Adobe to Microsoft.

DVDit! is a powerful yet accessible application for publishing video productions on DVD. It offers drag-and-drop ease for creating simple productions with nested menus via links to video and still image clips, and automatic conversion from AVI and QuickTime movie formats.

DVDit! then provides access to more sophisticated DVD designs with custom buttons and titles, a video timeline for setting chapter points, explicit control of navigational links, and the capability to play unattended by automatically linking between menus and clips. It also supports advanced DVD features, including control over compression bit rates, widescreen video format, Dolby Digital stereo audio, and writing the final production to DLT tape for professional mastering.

DVDit! version 2.5 from early 2002, as described here, is available in several versions, both as a retail product and bundled with computer systems, DVD peripherals, and other software tools.

DVDit! LE, the light or limited edition, is often used as a bundled product; and provides drag-and-drop menu creation, real-time preview, and integrated support for burning to CD and DVD discs. DVDit! SE, the standard edition, adds support for background audio with menus, the video timeline for setting chapter points, integrated transcoding to DVD video and audio format, and a bundled DVD player application. DVDit! PE, the professional edition, adds support for widescreen video, Dolby Digital audio, and mastering to DLT tape. The following sections focus on the standard DVDit! SE product, and discuss the more professional features in the PE version.

Stepping Through a New Project with DVDit!

To show how easy it is to use DVDit! for drag-and-drop DVD authoring, the following sections step through the entire process, from starting a new project, importing assets, creating menus, adding titles and navigation, through previewing your production and creating the output DVD.

Step 1: Start a New Project

Each time you start up DVDit!, it displays the Project Planner dialog box, which is the beginning point for either setting up a new project or opening an existing project (see Figure 11.1).

To begin working on a new project, click on Start a New Project.

FIGURE 11.1

Choose Start a New Project from the Project Planner to begin setting up a new project.

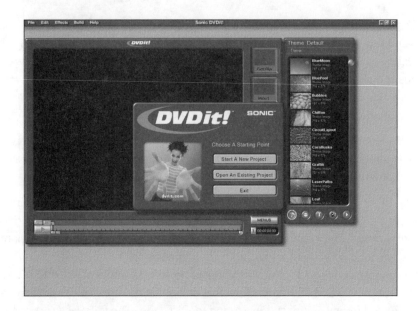

Step 2: Select the Output Format

Use the next screen of the Project Planner to specify the output format that you will use when you generate your DVD production (see Figure 11.2). Select the desired television format (NTSC or PAL) to determine the display screen resolution to be used for the project. Select the video compression format (MPEG-1, or MPEG-2 for DVD or cDVD) to determine the video resolution and compression format.

> **TIP**
>
> *These project settings determine the type of video files that you can import into your project. You can import AVI and QuickTime files into any project because DVDit! will convert them to the required format. However, the DVD specification has strict requirements for video resolution and compression data rates. So, for example, you cannot import PAL material into an NTSC project or import MPEG-1 video into an MPEG-2 project. If you intended to create a CD disc containing DVD format data (what Sonic calls a "cDVD" disc), then some of the compression-format requirements can be relaxed so that any file in the specified MPEG format can be imported.*

Step 3: Select the Output Format

Use the final screen of the Project Planner to specify the screen aspect ratio—typically 4:3 for normal television display (see Figure 11.3). Then, click on Finish to start your new project.

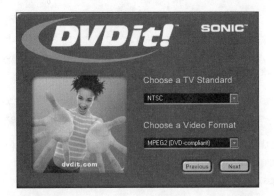

FIGURE 11.2

Select the output television standard and compression format to determine what kind of material can be imported into the project.

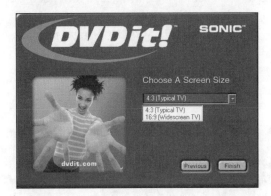

FIGURE 11.3

Finally, select the screen aspect ratio for the project.

Step 4: Import Clips into Your Project: The Palette Window

DVDit! opens a new empty project for you to work on. On the right side of the display is the Palette window, which contains collections of media assets that you can use to create your project. The assets include still image files, video and audio clip files, and text fonts. On the left side is the Video Monitor window, in which you edit and preview your production.

With DVDit!, you can organize your assets into different groups, or themes, in whatever way is useful for you—perhaps by project, by different sources of material, or by graphical design style. The name of the current theme being displayed in the Palette window, the Default theme, is shown at the top of the window. This theme contains graphical images that are included with DVDit! when it is installed.

Click through the first three Palette window buttons at the bottom of the Palette window to review the different collections of assets. Backgrounds contain menu background images, Buttons contains graphical menu button images, and Text contains available font styles.

The text fonts displayed in the Palette window are the fonts currently installed on your Windows system, and therefore they are available in all themes.

Click on the fourth Palette window button to display the list of Media files installed in this theme, including video and audio clips and still images. The Default theme has no media clips, so the list has no entries.

To add media clips to the Theme window, select a few video clip files in a Windows Explorer window, and drag-and-drop them into the Palette window (or pull down the Theme menu in the window or right-click in the window, and choose Add Files to Theme).

DVDit! adds each of the files to the Palette window, and displays each with a thumbnail of the first frame and summary information about the clip file (see Figure 11.4).

FIGURE 11.4

Drag-and-drop a few video files into the Media section of the Palette window.

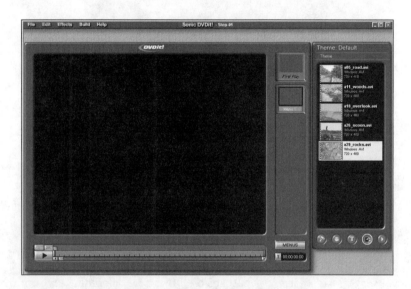

Step 5: Create the Main Menu: The Menu/Movie List

Next, you can create the main menu that will be used to link to these clips. As you add menus and movies from the Palette window to your project, DVDit! keeps track of them in the Menus/Movies Placeholder area to the right of the main

Video Monitor window. These lists contain placeholders for the menu and movie clip assets in your project, and are used as containers for creating and editing menu and movie objects and links.

The top entry, shown in both lists, is the *First Play* placeholder. The First Play is the menu or video clip that starts playing automatically when you load the final disc into a DVD player. You can select any menu or movie clip to be the First Play simply by dragging it onto the First Play placeholder.

Click on the Menus/Movies button at the bottom of the Placeholder area, and choose Menus from the pop-up menu. DVDit! displays an empty placeholder for adding a menu.

Click on the first Backgrounds button to scroll though the list of available background images for your menu. Click to select an image, and drag-and-drop it on the First Play placeholder.

DVDit! adds the new menu to the Menus placeholder list, and also shows the menu as the First Play (see Figure II.5). Again, the First Play placeholder is not a separate object; it simply is showing which of the other menus or movie clips will be shown as the First Play.

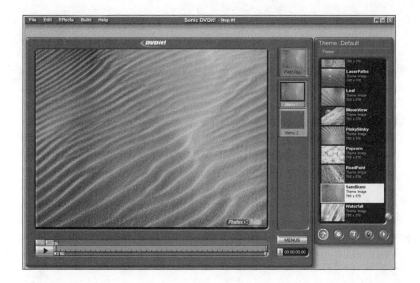

FIGURE 11.5

Drag-and-drop a background image from the Menus list to the First Play placeholder. The project now has one menu, which is also the First Play.

Step 6: Add Movie Clips to the Menu

Next, add some movie clips to the blank menu in the Video Monitor window. Click on the Media button below the Palette window to display the clip thumbnails, and drag-and-drop two clips onto the menu. DVDit! creates buttons for the clips using a thumbnail image of the first frame of each clip.

DVDit! adds the clips to the menu thumbnail in the Menus placeholder list (see Figure 11.6). You can also click on the Menus/Movies button to see that the clips have been added to the Media placeholder list.

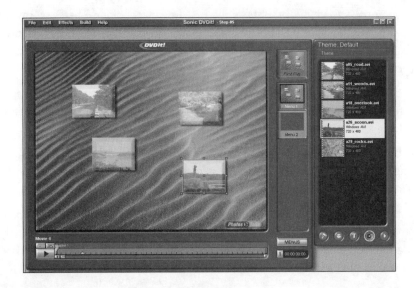

> **T I P**
>
> *This is the first big difference between DVDit! and the automated DVD authoring tools: DVDit! does not automatically lay out the buttons. Instead, it gives you full control over the layout and design of your menu buttons. You can click and drag the buttons to different locations. You can resize the buttons by dragging the red handles that are displayed on the frame around the currently selected buttons.*

Step 7: Add a Title and Adjust the Text Properties

Similarly, DVDit! does not automatically generate titles for the menus, or labels for the buttons.

To add a title to the menu, click on the third Text button below the Palette window to see a list of the available fonts. Then, drag-and-drop a font name onto the menu. DVDit! creates a text area on the menu that you can then type into.

To adjust the text size and style, click to select the title text, pull down the Effects menu, and choose Text Properties.

DVDit! displays the Text Properties dialog box to the right of the window (see Figure 11.7). You can change the font, size, and effects; and use the sliders above and below the color bar to adjust the text color and brightness.

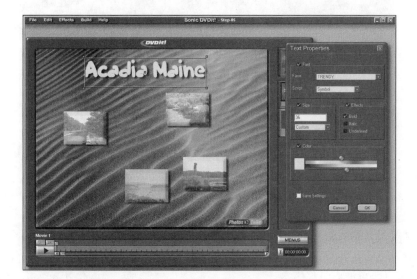

FIGURE 11.7

Add a title to the menu using the selected font. Then, adjust the properties of the menu text.

Step 8: Create a Linked Menu

To create another menu, click on the first Backgrounds button below the Palette window, and choose a different background image to drag onto the empty Menu 2 placeholder.

DVDit! displays the second empty menu in the Video Monitor window (see Figure 11.8).

> **T I P**
>
> *Unlike the automated DVD authoring tools, this menu is not automatically added to the DVD navigation. Instead, you have full control over the navigation, as well as the responsibility to link menus and clips together. This means you need to add a link from the main menu to this menu, and add another link from this menu back to the main menu.*

Step 9: Add a Button Back to the Main Menu

Add another video clip or two to this menu from the Media palette and then click on the second Buttons button below the Palette window. The Buttons list is simply a collection of image files that are the appropriate size to use as menu buttons.

FIGURE 11.8

Add a second menu to the project by dragging a background into the empty Menu placeholder.

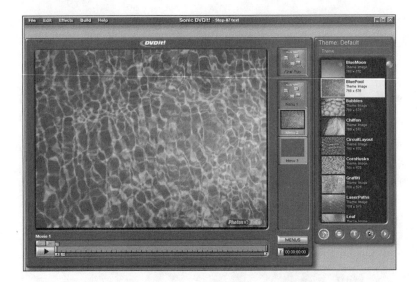

Drag the Up arrow button to the menu in the Video Monitor window to be used to link back to the main menu. You can resize the button by dragging on the red handles (see Figure 11.9).

However, this button is just a graphic image; it is not yet linked to anything. To link the button back to the main menu, drag and drop the Menu 1 placeholder onto the button. The button is now linked to the main menu.

FIGURE 11.9

Add a graphic button to the menu, and link it back to Menu 1.

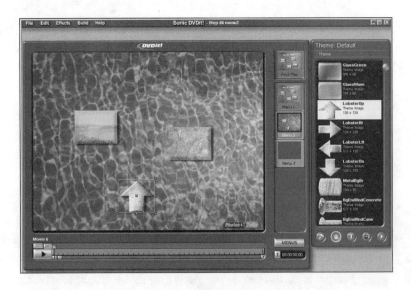

> **T I P**
>
> *As you add more menus and buttons to your project, it can become difficult to remember how they are linked together. You can test the links by previewing the DVD and clicking through the navigation (see Step 11), but DVDit! also lets you review the link structure directly (see the section, "Creating Navigation Links," later in this chapter).*

Step 10: Link from the Main Menu to the Second Menu

Next, you need to add a link in the opposite direction, from the main menu to this menu.

Click on the Menu 1 placeholder to select it, and DVDit! displays the first menu. Drag-and-drop the Menu 2 placeholder that you just created onto the menu in the Video Monitor window.

DVDit! adds a button with a thumbnail of the second menu and with a link to the menu (see Figure 11.10).

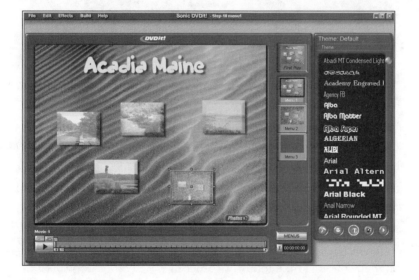

FIGURE 11.10

Select the first menu, and add a button linking to the second menu.

Step 11: Preview the DVD Presentation

You have created a complete DVD presentation with two menus, each with several video clips and with navigation links between the two menus.

This is a good time to save your work in progress. Pull down the File menu, and choose Save to save your project to hard disk as a DVDit! project file (.dvdit).

Now, you can preview your DVD by clicking on the right-most Play button (right arrow icon) below the Palette window.

DVDit! displays the Remote Control so that you can simulate playing back your presentation (see Figure 11.11). When you start the playback, the menu that you selected as the First Play is displayed in the Video Monitor window.

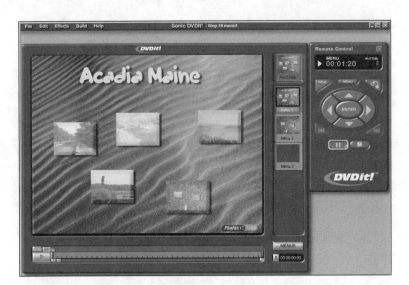

Use the arrow buttons on the Remote Control to move between the various buttons on each menu page, or click on Enter to play the selected clip. You also can click directly on the menu buttons to activate them.

Click on the Stop button at the bottom right of the Remote Control to return to editing the menu (while the Remote Control continues to be displayed). Click on the Play/Pause button to return to previewing the production, and to pause and play video clips.

Click on the X button at the top-right corner of the Remote Control to close it and return to editing your production.

> T I P
>
> *Although you must explicitly create the navigation links between different menus and clips;*
> *DVDit! automatically generates the links between the buttons on each individual menu. As*
> *you lay out the buttons on a menu, DVDit! creates the appropriate up, down, left, and*
> *right links for navigating between the buttons as you have positioned them.*

Step 12: Burn the Production to a DVD Volume

After you have completed authoring your DVD production, you can build the final DVD. DVDit! gives you a wide variety of options for how to share your production: you can burn it directly to a DVD disc or to a CD disc (if it is small enough), or you can save it to hard disk (see the section called "Creating a DVD" later in this chapter).

Saving the DVD volumes to a local hard disk is useful for testing your project before you commit to burning it to disc. You can then burn copies to DVD (or CD) discs directly from the DVD volumes on hard disk.

To start creating your DVD, pull down the Build menu, and choose Make DVD Folder.

If the project contains AVI or QuickTime files that need to be converted to DVD format, DVDit! displays a dialog box that asks whether you want to convert the files using the current settings or change the conversion settings.

Click on Convert Files Using Current Settings to continue with the default settings.

DVDit! displays the Make DVD Folder dialog box (see Figure 11.12). The Source section under the General tab shows the current project. Click on Browse in the Path section to specify the output directory for your project. Click on OK to start building your DVD.

DVDit! then works through the process of converting your project to DVD format, transcoding (recompressing) the video and audio sequences, and writing the final files to hard disk.

The data that DVDit! writes to disk is in the same DVD volume folder structure that is used on DVD-Video discs, with the data in files under a VIDEO_TS folder. You can view the contents in an Explorer window (see Figure 11.13).

FIGURE 11.12

Use the Make DVD Folder dialog box to specify the source project and destination folder for the DVD volumes to be created.

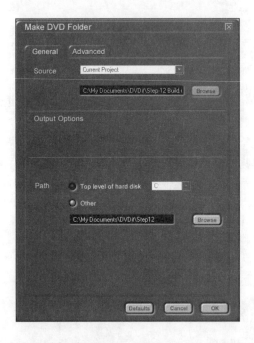

FIGURE 11.13

DVDit! can create DVD volumes on your hard disk with the same folder structure and data files burned to DVD disc. You can then test your production and burn copies to DVD (or CD) disc.

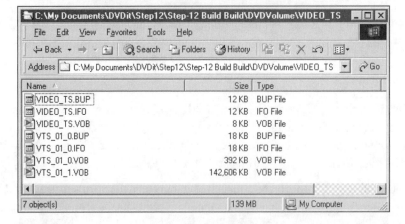

You can now play your project from hard disk with a software DVD player. However, some software players cannot play DVD content from a hard disk unless the VIDEO_TS folder is at the root (top) level of the hard disk. See the DVDit! documentation for information on using the included DVD player, or use one of the DVD players (as discussed in Chapter 7, "Playing DVDs on Windows").

Importing Media Clips into Themes

DVDit! uses the Palette window to help you organize different categories of assets that you may want to import into your projects. The buttons at the bottom of the window select the different types of assets you need to use: Backgrounds, Buttons, Text, and Media.

In DVDit!, you use images in the Backgrounds list for menu backgrounds; graphics images in the Buttons list to add buttons to menus; the Text list to add titles, labels, and text buttons to menus; and the Media list to link buttons to video clips, still image slides, and background audio clips.

To help manage all these types of media assets, you can create new themes to use like folders in whatever way is helpful to you—perhaps organized by project or by a common design theme. You can then access these themes from any DVDit! project you are working on.

T I P

DVDit! PE, the Professional Edition, provides support for widescreen video projects. Instead of working with traditional video, such as DV with a 4:3 aspect ratio, widescreen projects use 16:9 video (although the menus are still 4:3). When displayed on a normal television, widescreen video is letterboxed, with black bars at the top and bottom. When displayed on a widescreen television, the video fits the screen, and the menus have bars on the two sides. See the DVDit! documentation for more details about preparing files for widescreen display.

Working with Projects

Each menu design that you author in DVDit! is saved as a project, which includes the menu design, navigation, and media elements used in the design. Each time you start up DVDit!, you can choose to start a new project or open an existing project. You can also pull down the File menu, and choose New or Open to start working on a different project.

As you are working on a project, pull down the File menu, and choose Save to save your work in progress. You can also choose Save As to make a copy of the current project, as a backup, or to modify for a new design. However, these DVDit! project files (.dvdit) are necessarily quite large (multiple megabytes), so do not save extraneous copies of your projects.

Working with Themes

As you saw in the preceding section, DVDit! provides a Default theme with a selection of background and button images that you can use in your projects. To help you manage your own media assets, it is useful to create your own themes to store different collections of assets.

Pull down the Theme menu in the Palette window, and choose New Theme. In the Select a Name dialog box, enter a name for your new theme (see Figure 11.14).

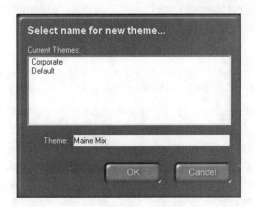

DVDit! opens the new theme, and displays its name at the top of the Palette window. The new theme is empty; there are no entries under Backgrounds, Buttons, or Media. (Text always contains the available fonts on your system.)

To switch between themes, pull down the Theme menu, and choose Open Theme; or choose the name of the theme from the list at the bottom of the menu.

Importing and Viewing Movie Clips

After you create new themes as folders to organize your assets, you can add asset files to the different categories.

To add media clips to your theme, click on the Media button and then drag and drop some video files from an Explorer window.

You can preview the clips in the Palette by playing them in the Video Monitor window. Position the cursor over a clip thumbnail, right-click to display the pop-up menu, and choose Play. The clip then plays back in the main window (see Figure 11.15). To stop playback, click on the Stop button control at the bottom left of the window.

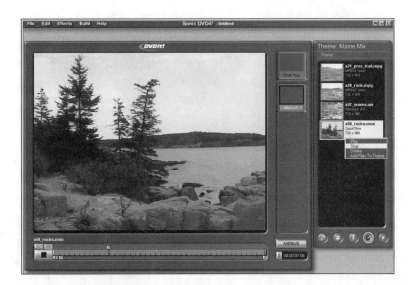

FIGURE 11.15

Use the pop-up menu to preview your clips by playing them in the Video Monitor window.

To delete clips from the Media list, click to select the clip, right-click on the clip, and select Delete from the pop-up menu.

O R G A N I Z I N G   F I L E S   I N   T H E M E S

When you add a file to the DVDit! Palette window, DVDit! actually only keeps a link or a short-cut to the actual file on disk. When you delete a file from a theme, you actually are deleting only the shortcut; the original file is left unchanged on the disk.

But if you rename, move, or delete media files on the hard disk that are referenced in your DVDit! themes, the links will be broken, and the shortcuts in DVDit! will no longer be valid. The next time you access that theme, DVDit! will warn you about the lost shortcuts.

DVDit! actually stores your themes as folders with Windows shortcut files under the DVDit! pro-gram directory (typically C:\Program Folders\Sonic Solutions\DVDit). As a result, you can reor-ganize the DVDit! themes by changing the associated folders in an Explorer window.

Video File Formats

DVDit! is designed to import media files in a variety of formats and (if required) to convert them to an appropriate format to be used on DVD. DVDit! assumes that you have used separate tools to prepare the media you will use in your project, including a video capture tool for acquiring clips from analog or digital sources, a video-editing tool to trim and enhance the clips into movies to show on DVD, per-haps an audio editor to prepare background audio clips, and even an image editor to prepare menu backgrounds and button images.

DVDit! can import video (and audio) files in the common Windows AVI and Apple QuickTime Movie (.MOV) formats. However, these formats are just a wrapper for video and audio data, and can contain video and audio compressed in a wide variety of formats. Although your system may be able to play some files, it may not be able to play others if your system does not have the appropriate codec (coder/decoder software) installed.

In general, if you can play an AVI file with the Windows Media Player or a QuickTime movie file with the QuickTime Player, then you should be able to use the file in other Windows applications, such as DVDit! If the file does not play, you need to find out how it was created and then install the appropriate codec.

DVDit! also can import files with standard MPEG-1 and MPEG-2 video compression. Unfortunately, MPEG files can have a variety of file extensions, including the same type for both formats (.MPG), and with explicit numbers for MPEG-1 and -2 (for example, .M1P, .M1V, .M2P, and .M2V).

T I P

If you will use a video clip more than one time in a DVD production, it's a good idea to compress it first to DVD-compatible MPEG-2 format. Because the file is ready to go, DVDit! does not need to convert (transcode) it to MPEG each time you use it in a project. You not only save the compression time, but you also save disk space because the MPEG-2 is significantly smaller than even a DV-format AVI or QuickTime file.

Many capture tools can now transcode from DV or analog to MPEG-2 as part of the capture process, and most video-editing tools can export productions in MPEG-2 format. Just be sure to do a test run of the end-to-end process to verify that the formats are compatible with what DVDit! is expecting. See the DVDit! documentation for more details on compatible formats.

Importing and Viewing Audio Clips

Similarly, you can organize audio files to use in your project for background music when the menus are displayed. Click on the Media button, and add your audio files in with the movie files or create a new theme to contain just the audio files.

To preview an audio clip, right-click over the clip thumbnail, and choose Play from the pop-up menu (see Figure 11.16).

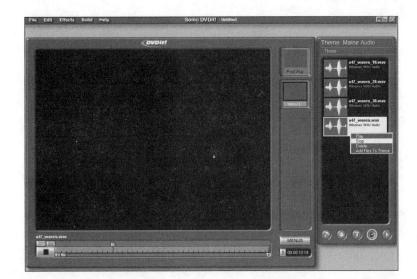

FIGURE 11.16

You can also preview audio clips by playing them from the Palette window.

DVDit! supports the standard Windows Wave (.WAV) audio format, as well as MPEG-1 Layer II audio. Depending on the project settings, DVDit! converts Wave and MPEG-1 audio files to PCM or Dolby Digital format.

The PE version of DVDit! also can import Dolby Digital audio files (.AC3) directly.

Importing and Viewing Images

DVDit! uses still images in three different ways: as image slides to display in response to a menu button press, as background images behind menus, and as graphical images for menu buttons. When you import image files, you must place them in the different categories in the Palette window, depending on their intended use: stills under Media, menus under Backgrounds, and buttons under Buttons. Import some background and still images to the Background and Media lists. You can preview them like the other media types by right-clicking and choosing Play from the pop-up menu (see Figure 11.17). DVDit! then displays the image in the Video Monitor window for five seconds.

DVDit! can import image files in a wide variety of formats. DVDit! resizes the images you import as needed to display on the DVD, but it is best to use images that match the final resolution and aspect ratio. Because menus and clips are displayed at different aspect ratios, the recommended sizes for menu backgrounds and stills are different: 640×480 for images used as menus and 720×540 for images displayed as stills.

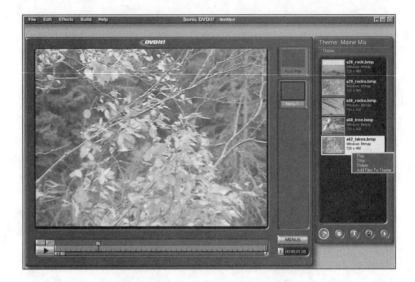

Images used for buttons can be smaller. The recommended size is at least 72×60 pixels, or 300×80 for larger buttons. You also can resize button images in DVDit!, especially to make them smaller, but enlarging small buttons will make them look blocky. You also can create irregularly shaped buttons by creating images with transparent regions. DVDit! can import Photoshop files with background transparency and with multiple layers—with one button in each layer.

Customizing the Design

DVDit! makes it easy to create navigational links by dragging media clips onto a menu. It automatically creates a default rectangular button with a thumbnail of the clip, and links it to the clip. Although you can create all the navigation in a DVD production this way, including links to other menus, you also can use DVDit! to customize your menu design by using graphical images for buttons—and by using text for menu titles, button labels, and even as links.

In DVDit!, buttons and text are just graphical objects that you can use any way you want. You can use them to decorate and annotate the menus, or use them to create links to menus and movies. For example, if you put some large text at the top of a menu, you can use it as the menu title. Or, you can design the title as a graphic image, and import it through the Buttons list. You can position smaller text near or on top of a linked button to use as a label for the button link, or you can create a link directly from text—with no button image.

As you design the menus for your production, you can edit them by moving and resizing the button and text objects, and also use Copy and Paste to duplicate the button design and layout between different menus.

You can then create links from the buttons or text to media clips and other menus by simply dragging and dropping them onto the menu objects.

Customizing Buttons and Text

DVDit! provides a second collection of built-in images under the Corporate theme. Pull down the Theme menu in the Palette window, and choose Open Theme to select the Corporate theme (or select Corporate if it already appears on the list of recently used themes). DVDit! opens the new theme in the Palette window.

Click on the first Backgrounds button under the Palette window to show the background images in the theme, and drag a background image into the empty Menu placeholder in the Menus list to create a new menu.

Next, click on the second Buttons button to display the button images. Drag several of the button images to the menu background. Unlike the rectangular buttons created for media clips, these button images can be defined with a transparent background, and therefore appear irregularly shaped.

Also, drag one of the video clips onto the menu from the Media list that you have imported into another theme. DVDit! creates a default rectangular button for the clip.

To add text to the menu, click on the third Text button to display the available text fonts. Scroll in the Text list, and drag a font name to the menu. DVDit! adds the word Text to the menu in that font style. You can position the text against the menu background as a title or annotation, place it near or on top of a button as a label, or use it as a link instead of a button.

To edit the text, double-click on the word Text. DVDit! highlights the text field so that you can edit the text (see Figure 11.18). When you are finished editing, click in another area of the menu.

To change the properties of the text, click to select it, pull down the Effects menu, and choose Text Properties.

DVDit! displays the Text Properties dialog box to the right of the window. You can change the Font, Size, and Effects. Use the Color sliders above and below the color bar to adjust the color and brightness. Select Save Settings to remember the settings the next time you open the dialog box.

FIGURE 11.18

You can also create a menu in DVDit! by first designing the buttons and text, and then adding the navigation and links to media clips.

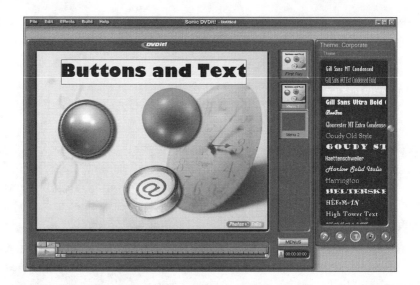

In DVDit!, the menu design can be done independently from linking to the media content. You can add or change the button and text links at any time by dragging a video or image clip to the menu object from the Media list in the Palette window, from the Movies list, or even from a chapter point in the timeline. After you have linked a button to a video or image clip, you can add a background audio clip to it. Or, you can link a button to another menu by dragging a Menu placeholder from the Menus list.

> **T I P**
>
> *DVD players are not designed to support overlapping buttons and text links on a menu. DVDit! will not permit you to create a DVD in which menu buttons with links overlap.*

Editing Menu Buttons and Text

After you have created button or text objects on your menus, you can easily move, resize, and cut and paste them.

To select an individual object on a menu, click on it to select it. DVDit! then displays a frame around it with red handles. You also can select multiple objects by Ctrl-clicking on them.

To move the selected objects, simply click and drag them. To nudge them one pixel at a time, press the Up, Down, Left, or Right arrow keys. To move them in 10-pixel increments, hold down the Shift key while pressing the arrow keys.

To change the size of a menu object (or group of selected objects), click and drag one of the red handles (see Figure 11.19). Hold the Shift key while dragging to maintain the same shape while resizing.

You also can use the Edit menu's Cut, Copy, and Paste options to copy menu objects, including between different menus. You can delete the selected objects by pressing the Delete key.

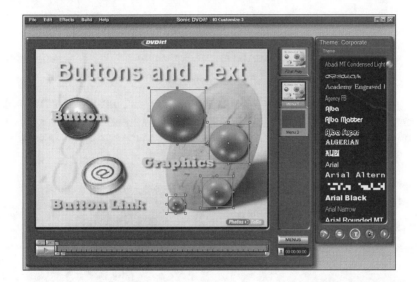

FIGURE 11.19

You then can move, resize, and copy the button and text objects on your menu.

> **TIP**
>
> *To undo an editing operation, pull down the Edit menu, and choose Undo. You can actually undo a sequence of editing operations in this way, or choose Redo to apply them again.*

Customizing Menus

DVDit! provides color adjustment and drop shadow effects for customizing menu backgrounds and button and text objects. The effects can be applied to the menu background, an individual object, a group of selected objects, or to all elements of a menu.

To adjust the menu colors, select the objects to be changed, pull down the Effects menu, and choose Adjust Color. DVDit! opens the Color Adjustment dialog box.

Use the Apply To drop-down list to select whether the adjustment is applied to the background image of the current menu, the selected menu items (if you have selected one or more objects), or to the entire menu (including the background and all objects).

Then use the sliders to adjust the menu colors: Hue (color), Saturate (gray to pure color), and Brighten (dark to light).

To adjust the drop shadows for menu buttons and text, select the objects to be changed, pull down the Effects menu, and choose Drop Shadow. DVDit! opens the Drop Shadow dialog box.

Use the Apply To drop-down list to select whether the adjustment is applied to the selected menu buttons and text, or to all the objects in the entire menu.

Then use the sliders to adjust the drop shadow effect: Distance (from the background), Blur (sharp to diffuse edges), Opacity (dark to subtle), and Color (hue and brightness). Also rotate the Light Source sun icon to change the angle of the shadow under the object (see Figure 11.20).

FIGURE 11.20

Use the Drop Shadow dialog box to change the distance, color, sharpness, and angle of the drop shadow under menu objects.

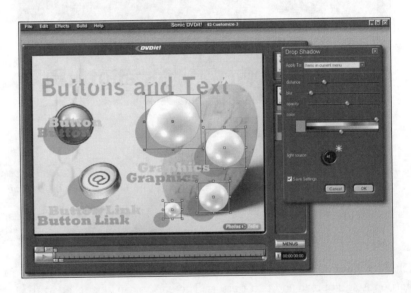

Select Save Settings before you close these dialog boxes to keep the current defaults when you reopen the dialog box. You can then apply the same settings to other objects and other menus.

Working with Menus and Movies

You can use DVDit! to create a simple production by creating a few menus, dragging clips from the Media list onto them to create linked buttons, and then dragging cross-links to the other menus.

You also can design a more sophisticated production by first designing your menus, organizing the clips that you want to play, and then creating links between them. When you drag a clip directly to a menu, DVDit! automatically adds it to the Movies list in the Menus/Movies placeholder area.

You also can drag video or still image clips directly to the Movies list and then prepare them for use on the menus. You can add background audio, preview the clip in the timeline under the main Video Monitor window, set clip playback properties, and even define multiple chapter points in the clip to link from the menus.

Working with Menus

To create a new menu in your presentation, click on the Menus/Movies button at the bottom of the Menus/Movies placeholder area on the right of the Video Monitor window, and select Menus. Click on the Backgrounds button in the Palette window, and drag a background image for the menu into the empty Menu placeholder at the end of the Menus list.

DVDit! creates a new Menu placeholder with the thumbnail for the menu, and shows the empty menu image in the Video Monitor window. To change the menu background, drag a different image to the placeholder or to the menu displayed in the Video Monitor window.

To add background audio to a menu, click on the Media button, and drag an audio clip into the Menu placeholder or to the menu displayed in the Video Monitor window. DVDit! plays a tone to indicate that the audio has been added to the menu, and displays a speaker icon above the right end of the timeline when displaying the menu in the Video Monitor window.

To change the background audio, drag a new clip to the Menu placeholder (or the Video Monitor window). To delete the background audio, right-click on the Menu placeholder (or in the Video Monitor window), and choose Clear Audio from the pop-up menu.

To review the current settings for a menu, right-click on the Menu placeholder (or in the Video Monitor window), and choose Properties from the pop-up menu. DVDit! displays the Menu Properties dialog box (see Figure 11.21), with the file-name of the background image and audio files, and the duration of the audio clip (which repeats by default as the menu is displayed).

FIGURE 11.21

Add a background audio clip to play when the menu is displayed. Use the Menu Properties dialog box to see the files used in the menu.

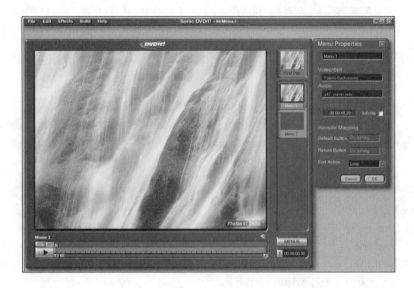

To delete a menu in the list, click on the Menu placeholder to select it, and press the Delete key (or pull down the Edit menu, and choose Clear Menu/Movie). DVDit! displays a warning to confirm the deletion.

T I P

As you add multiple menus to the Menus list, the Menus list becomes scrollable. You can rearrange the list by dragging the entries into a different order.

Working with Movies

The whole point of menus is to include buttons with links to material that you want to play on your DVD. Menu buttons can be links to video clips or still images, or links to other menus.

To edit a menu, click on the thumbnail for the menu in the Menus/Movies placeholder area. DVDit! then displays the menu in the main Video Monitor window so that you can edit it.

The easiest way to add button links from the menu to a movie or still image is to simply drag the clip onto the menu. Click on the Media button below the Palette window, and drag a couple video and image thumbnails from the Media list onto the menu. DVDit! automatically generates a button for each clip, with a thumbnail image of the first frame in that clip.

If you drag the thumbnail onto an existing button, DVDit! changes that button to link to the new clip.

DVDit! also adds the clips to the Menus/Movies placeholder area. Click on the Menus/Movies button, and choose Movies to view the list of movies in use for this project.

You also can add videos or images to your project before using them in menus. To do this, drag the clip from the Media list directly to the empty placeholder at the bottom of the Movie list. You can then link to this movie from your menus (see the section, "Building the Interactive Navigation," later in this chapter). You can click on the placeholder label to change the name of the clip in the Movies list (see Figure 11.22).

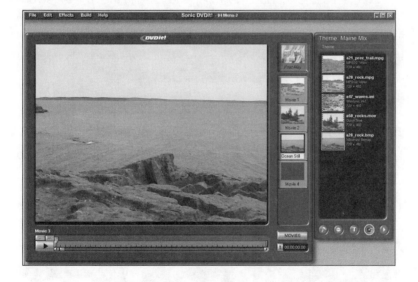

FIGURE 11.22

Prepare and view the clips used in your production in the Movies list.

As with the Menu placeholders, you can add an audio soundtrack to a movie by dragging an audio clip onto the placeholder, or remove the audio clip by right-clicking and choosing Clear Audio from the pop-up menu.

To change the movie in the Movies list, drag a different video or image onto it from the Media list. To delete the movie, click to select it, and press Delete. This deletes the movie from your project and from any menus that link to it.

Viewing Movies and Images on the Timeline

When you click on a Movie placeholder in the Movies list, DVDit! displays the clip in the main Video Monitor window. You can then use the play controls and time-line below the main window to play back the clip. Or, click on the move name label above the left side of the timeline to select a different movie in your project from the pop-up menu.

Click on the Play button to the left of the timeline to start and pause playback. While playback is paused, click and drag the playhead slider to jump to a different point in the movie. To jump to a specific point in the movie, click in the timecode area to the right of the timeline, type a timecode (***hours:minutes:seconds:frames***), and press Enter.

You also can zoom the timeline display in and out by clicking on the Zoom buttons (with the mountain icons) above the Play button. When the timeline is zoomed all the way out (using the small mountain icon on the left), you can see the entire length of the clip, from the green starting point on the left to the red finish point on the right. When the timeline is zoomed-in (using the large mountain icon on the left), the tick marks on the timeline get closer together, and you can then use the scrollbar below the timeline to move from one end to the other (see Figure 11.23).

FIGURE 11.23

Use the timeline below the main Video Monitor window to preview clips on the Movies list.

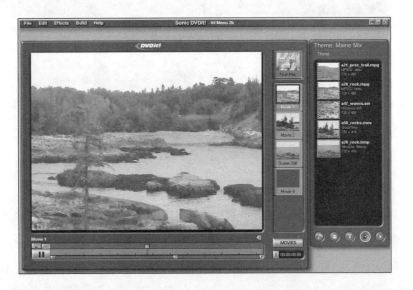

The Movie list, like the Media list in the Palette window, can contain both video clips (possibly with audio) and still images (possibly with a background audio soundtrack). By default, still images will be displayed for five seconds.

To review an item on the Movie list and to change the length of time that a still image displays, right-click on the Movie placeholder, and choose Properties from the pop-up menu. DVDit! displays the Movie Properties menu, listing the Video/ Still clip and the associated Audio clip (if any). To change how long a still image is displayed, click in the Duration field and type a new time.

Setting Chapter Points

You also can add chapter points within the movie to mark different scenes within an individual clip. You can use these chapter points in two ways: You can create a scene selection menu by linking menu buttons to different chapter points within a clip, and you can permit the user to skip through the clips with the Next Chapter and Previous Chapter buttons on the DVD Remote Control.

To add a chapter point, double-click on the timeline. DVDit! adds a triangular chapter point icon at that point, and moves the playhead to that point to display the corresponding frame. You can then play from a chapter point by clicking on it to move the playhead and then clicking on the Play button.

To add more chapter points, double-click on the timeline again. You can also add a chapter point at a specific timecode by clicking on the "T" (timecode) button to the right of the timeline to change it into "C" (chapter). Then type the timecode at which you want to add a chapter point and press Enter (see Figure 11.24).

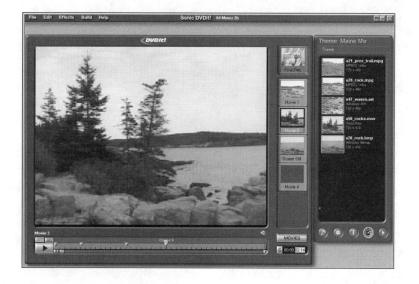

FIGURE 11.24

Insert chapter points into your clip by double-clicking on the timeline, or by typing a specific timecode.

To move a chapter point, click on the triangle icon and hold down the Ctrl key as you drag it to a new position on the timeline. Or click to select a chapter point, and then hold down Ctrl and press the Left/Right arrow keys to jump the chapter point in one-second increments.

To delete a chapter point, hold the cursor over the triangle icon, right-click, and choose Delete from the pop-up menu.

By default, DVDit! names the chapter points in numeric sequence: "Chapter 1" and then "Chapter 2," and so on. As you add new chapters between existing ones, it renumbers the chapters appropriately to keep them in sequence. You also can use your own names for chapter points; right-click on the triangle icon, choose Rename from the pop-up menu, and then type the new name.

T I P

Chapter points cannot be set too close together. DVDit! requires that chapter points be at least 15 frames apart. In any case, it is not particularly useful to mark major scene points less than a second between each other.

Building the Interactive Navigation

With DVDit!, you can build the interactive navigation between your menus and movies by first designing the menus and preparing the clips (in the Menus/Movies placeholder list) and then dragging and dropping between them to create the links.

DVDit! also provides several tools to review your navigational links, including viewing the properties for individual menus and movies; displaying all the links in a menu in text form; and, of course, using the Remote Control to preview the playback of your DVD production.

You can control whether your DVD waits for the user to press a button after showing a menu or playing a clip, or whether it automatically continues on to another link. In this way, you can create a production that automatically plays several clips one after another, or even displays title slides between them.

Setting the First Play

The First Play for a DVD is the first thing that happens when you insert and start playing a DVD. DVDit! provides a variety of choices for defining the First Play. You can immediately show a main menu, from which the user can access the rest of the material on the DVD. Or your DVD can start with a still image slide as a title or copyright notice, or can even play an introductory video sequence.

The First Play placeholder in the Menus/Movies list is used to show which menu or clip will be used as the First Play. To define the First Play, drag any menu from the Menus list, clip from the Movie list, or video or still image file from the Media list to the First Play placeholder.

The top First Play entry in the list always remains fixed at the top of the list, whether you are displaying the Menus or Movies list. It simply lists the current item from the Menus or Movies list that has been selected as the First Play.

If you specify a video or still movie as the First Play, it plays to the end and then steps to the first menu on the Menus list.

To clear the First Play, right-click on the First Play placeholder, and choose Clear First Play (see Figure 11.25). When it first plays, the DVD then waits for the user to press Play on the Remote Control.

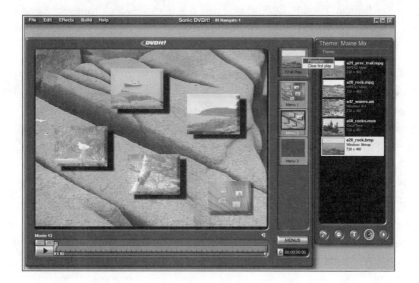

FIGURE 11.25

Use the First Play placeholder to select a menu or clip to be the first thing displayed when you play the DVD.

> **T I P**
>
> *You can get more creative with the First Play by linking several slides or movies to be played one after another using the Menu and Movie Properties dialog boxes (see the following section, "Setting Menu Properties"). You can also have the DVD play through menus and clips automatically if the user is not using the Remote Control.*

Creating Navigation Links

As you have seen previously, you can create a button to a video or a still image simply by dragging the clip thumbnail from the Media list in the Palette window to the background of a menu. DVDit! then automatically creates a rectangular button with a thumbnail image from that clip.

You can create a button from a clip in the Movie list or from a chapter point. Select the menu from the Menus/Movie list to display the menu in the main Video Monitor window. Then, click on the movie name above the timeline Play button, and select the movie from the pop-up menu. DVDit! displays the timeline for the movie, which may include multiple chapter points. Finally, click on a triangular chapter point icon in the timeline, and drag it to the menu background to create a new button. To link to the entire movie, simply drag the default Chapter 1 point at the start of the movie.

To change the video frame used for the thumbnail on the default rectangular buttons, click to select the button, right-click at a different point on the timeline, and choose Set Button Thumb. DVDit! updates the button with a thumbnail of the selected frame and marks the thumbnail frame with a triangle icon on the bottom of the timeline.

As described previously, instead of creating these rectangular buttons automatically from clips, you also can create buttons from images in the Button list in the Palette window and from fonts in the Text area. You can then drag a thumbnail from the Media list or a chapter point from the timeline on top of the button to link to that clip (plus a background audio clip), or you can drag a placeholder from the Menus list. To clear links created in this way, right-click on the button; you can then choose Clear Video, Clear Audio, or Clear Menu Link, respectively, from the pop-up menu.

As you add more buttons and menus, it is useful to be able to review all the links in a menu. Right-click on the menu, and choose Show Button Links from the pop-up menu. DVDit! changes the menu display to show the names of the links for each button.

To quickly check which clip an individual button is linked to, click on the button (so it is highlighted with the red resizing handles). DVDit! then updates the timeline to show the associated movie name and highlights the chapter point within that movie that is linked to the selected button. You also can right-click on the button, and choose Link Properties from the pop-up menu to display the media files' names and other information about the movie linked to that button (see Figure 11.26).

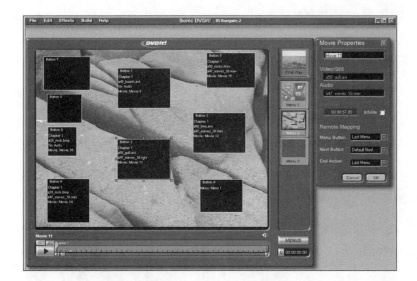

FIGURE 11.26

Use Show Button Links to review all the links on the menu, and select Link Properties to check the links for the selected button or text.

A button may be linked to another menu or clip on the Movie list. For menus, the button shows the name of the menu in the Menus list. For movies, the button shows the name of the movie in the Movie list, with the name of the associated video or image file in the Palette window Media list (and chapter point within the clip), and the name of a background audio clip, if any.

T I P

You also can test the links in your production by using the Remote Control to click through the menus. On each menu, move the cursor over the buttons to check that DVDit! highlights each button that should be linked. You also can click on the Left, Right, Up, and Down buttons on the Remote Control to step through each active button on the menu. Notice that DVDit! automatically manages this navigation between buttons on a menu.

Setting Menu Properties

Besides defining the navigational links between menus and clips, you can also set menu and movie properties with DVDit! to control the default and automatic navigation. This includes how the navigation flows when a menu is first displayed (which button is selected by default); what happens when a movie finishes playing; and whether a menu or still displays indefinitely, or it times out and continues on with the presentation. It also determines how your DVD responds when the user presses the optional navigation buttons on the DVD Remote Control.

To set the defaults for each menu, right-click on the Menu placeholder in the Menus list, and choose Properties in the pop-up menu; or right-click on the menu background, and choose Show Properties. DVDit! then displays the Menu Properties dialog box (see Figure 11.27).

FIGURE 11.27

Use the Menu Properties dialog box to control how the menu is displayed, and how it responds to the keys on the Remote Control.

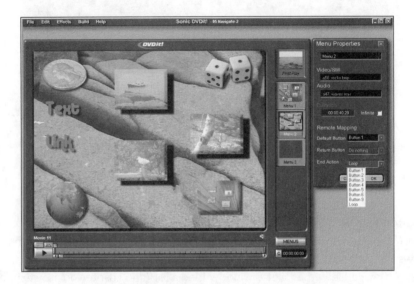

The top of the Menu Properties dialog box shows the current name of the Menu placeholder in the Menus list, and the Video/Still and Audio files used for the menu background. Use the Remote Mapping section to specify the Default Button that will be selected when the menu is displayed and the Return Button action to take if the user presses Return on the Remote Control.

By default, the menu displays continuously until the user selects an option with the Remote Control, so the Duration field is empty and Infinite is checked. You also can have the menu display for only a fixed period of time: Uncheck Infinite, enter a Duration, and then choose the End Action to be performed after the duration ends. Either Loop again (the default) or take the action defined by the selected button (which can be to play a clip or to jump to a different menu).

T I P

You can create a self-running DVD production by explicitly setting the Duration and End Action for menus and movies. You can step through a series of menu slides with background audio and play a series of linked movies. The user still can interrupt the playback at any time by using the Remote Control to explicitly press menu buttons to jump to different menus or clips; or use Return, Menu, and Next to navigate through the production directly.

Setting Movie Properties

Similarly, to set the defaults for individual buttons (and the associated movie), right-click on the button, and choose Link Properties in the pop-up menu; or right-click on the Movie placeholder in the Movies list, and choose Properties. DVDit! then displays the Movie Properties dialog box (see Figure 11.28).

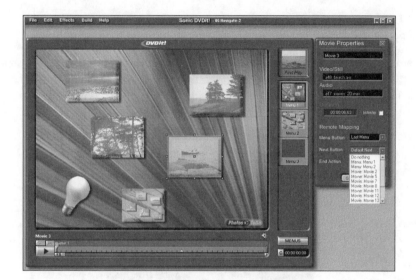

FIGURE 11.28

Use the Movie Properties dialog box to control whether the movie plays and stops, loops, or automatically links to another movie or menu.

The top of the Movie Properties dialog box shows the current name of the Movie placeholder in the Menus list and the movie files. Use the Remote Mapping section to specify the actions to take if the user presses the associated buttons on the Remote Control: the Menu Button (Do Nothing, jump to a specified menu, or return to the Last Menu by default), and the Next Button (Do Nothing, jump to a specified menu or movie, or take the Default Next action).

By default, video clips play to the end, and still images are displayed for five seconds. You then can specify an End Action to be performed when the clip finishes (Same As Next, jump to a specified menu or movie, Loop, or return to the Last Menu by default). You can change the Duration of a still image, or check Infinite to have the display freeze at the end of a video or image until the user presses a button on the Remote Control.

Creating a DVD

After you have finished your project, DVDit! lets you burn it to DVD or CD discs, create a DVD volume on your hard disk, or write a DVD master tape (with the PE version). You also can include computer data (DVD-ROM data) on the disc with your DVD video.

Choosing Project Settings

To set up the project settings for the type of DVD you plan to create, pull down the File menu, and choose Project Settings. DVDit! displays the Project Settings dialog box (see Figure 11.29).

FIGURE 11.29

Use the Project Settings dialog box to set the output disc size and to check that the current project size is still within the target size.

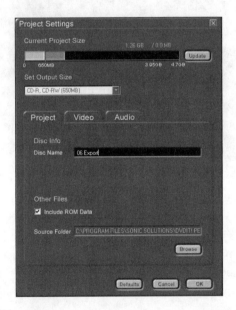

Use the Set Output Size drop-down menu to select the output disc size: CD-R, DVD-RAM, or DVD-R. Then, click on Update to see how the new setting changes the Current Project Size indicator. It displays how much of the space on the target disc is used and how much is still available (or overrun).

Under the Project tab, type a Disk Name, if desired.

To add additional computer-readable files to the DVD, set Include ROM Data, and then select the Source Folder containing the files.

Choosing Video Settings

To override the default video compression settings to use when converting AVI or QuickTime files, click on the Video tab in the Project Settings dialog box (or pull down the Build menu, and choose Video Settings; see Figure 11.30).

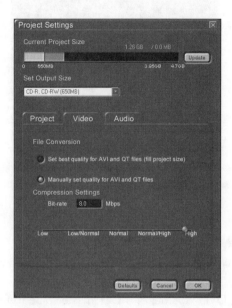

FIGURE 11.30

Use the Video Settings tab to manually control the video compression bit-rate.

DVDit! normally attempts to use the best quality compression possible to fit the project to the specified size disc. You can also set the Compression Settings manually. The amount of compression is specified in terms of the bit-rate available to store the video, measured in millions of bits per second.

Choosing Audio Settings

To override the default audio format (in the PE version of DVDit!), click on the Audio tab in the Project Settings dialog box (or pull down the Build menu, and choose Audio Settings; see Figure 11.31).

DVDit! normally converts the audio to PCM format at a fixed bit-rate. With Dolby Digital, you can change the bit-rate and select mono or stereo format.

FIGURE 11.31

Use the Audio Settings tab to select Dolby Digital audio format and manually control the compression bit-rate.

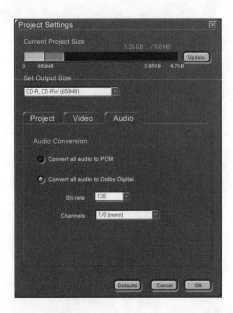

Creating a DVD Disc

To create your DVD production on a DVD or CD disc, pull down the Build menu, and choose Make DVD Disc. The general build process is the same, whether you are creating a disc, a DVD volume, or a DLT master tape (refer to the previous section called "Step 12: Burn the Production to a DVD Volume").

No matter what type of DVD you are creating, if the project contains AVI or QuickTime files that need to be converted to DVD format, DVDit! first displays a dialog box that asks whether you want to convert the files using the current settings or whether you want to change the conversion settings.

You can then click on View or Modify Conversion Settings, which displays the Project Settings dialog box to review the project and media compressing settings (refer to the previous section); or you can click on Return to Project to cancel the build and continue authoring.

If the project is done, and the settings are correct, click on Convert Files Using Current Settings to continue with the default settings. DVDit! then displays the Make a DVD Disc dialog box.

Under the General tab (see Figure 11.32), you can select the Source for the DVD to be the Current Project that you are editing, a DVD Volume that you previously built on hard disk, or a DVD Disc Image file from another authoring tool. Under Output Options for a CD-R, you can choose Include DVD Player to create a cDVD disc with a DVD player included on the CD with the DVD content, so the CD can be played back on any Windows machine. Finally, select the CD or DVD Recorder and the Write Speed and Options for your burner. You can also choose to burn multiple copies of your disc.

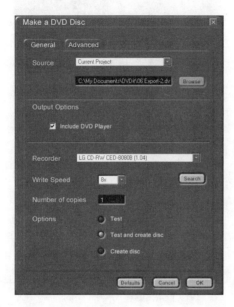

FIGURE 11.32

Use the General tab of the Make a DVD dialog box to choose the input source and the output recorder and burning options.

Under the Advanced tab (see Figure 11.33), use the File System options to make your disc compatible with more systems. Deselect Use Joliet if your project does not contain any computer-readable DVD-ROM files, and deselect Use Long File Names to allow the disc to be playable on MS-DOS machines. Use the Temporary Storage options to control where and how DVDit! uses temporary storage when converting your media content and building the final disk format. It is useful to have DVDit! use a different large scratch disk for these large files.

Then click on OK to start building your DVD. DVDit! works through the process of converting your project to DVD format, transcoding (recompressing) the video and audio sequences, and creating the final DVD format data.

When prompted, insert a blank CD or DVD disc to burn.

FIGURE 11.33

*Use the Advanced
tab of the Make
a DVD Disc dialog
box to specify File
System options for
compatibility and to
control temporary
storage use.*

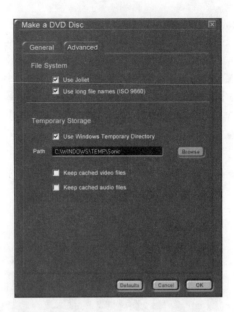

Creating a DVD Volume

As described in "Step 12: Burn the Production to a DVD Volume," you can also
write your DVD production to hard disk as a DVD Volume, in the same folder
structure and data format that it would be written to a DVD disc. You can preview
it on hard disk using a DVD player application, and then later burn copies to disc.

Create your production as a DVD Volume on hard disk, pull down the Build
menu, and choose Make DVD Folder.

DVDit! displays a dialog box, asking whether you want to convert any AVI or
QuickTime files in your project. DVDit! then displays the Make DVD Folder dialog
box. Use the General tab to select the Source project and Path to the output
directory. Use the Advanced tab to set options for Temporary Storage.

Creating a DVD Master

With DVDit! PE, you can create a master tape in DLT format to be used at a professional mastering facility to replicate your DVD. To create a tape, pull down the
Build menu, and choose Make DVD Master. Use the dialog box to select the output tape drive and options, and DVDit! works through the process of creating the
DVD on tape (as described previously).

Summary

Automated DVD authoring tools, such as Sonic MyDVD, are great for quickly laying out a collection of clips into DVD menus, as described in Chapter 9, "Automated DVD Authoring with Sonic MyDVD." These automated tools also prove an end-to-end solution, directly from video capture to burning a DVD. But the trade-off for this simplicity, of course, is limited control over the graphic design and navigation of your productions.

Apple iDVD, described in Chapter 10, "Personal DVD Authoring with Apple iDVD," is a drag-and-drop tool with some automated layout and navigation. It also offers the capability to disable the automated defaults and customize the design.

Sonic DVDit! goes further, combining drag-and-drop design with access to more professional DVD design and navigation features. With a little more manual work, it can be used to quickly create nested menus, such as iDVD, or with more pre-planning it can be used to organize and design more sophisticated menu designs and navigational flow.

Beyond these personal DVD authoring tools are the more sophisticated tools described in Part V, "Professional DVD Authoring." These provide access to more capabilities of the DVD-Video specification, including multiple video, audio, and subtitle tracks, and precise control over button and highlight graphics.

Part V

Professional DVD Authoring

Part V describes the final group of DVD authoring tools—"professional" applications priced in the thousands of dollars: Apple DVD Studio Pro on Macintosh, and Sonic ReelDVD and Sonic Scenarist on Windows. These tools expose almost the full range of the functionality in the DVD format, including custom button graphics, and multiple video, audio, and subtitle streams with multilingual support. But to provide this functionality, these tools no longer perform automated format conversion and layout. Instead, you are responsible for creating all the menu graphics and converting all the assets to DVD-compatible format before importing them into the tools.

chapter 12

Professional DVD Authoring with Apple DVD Studio Pro

Chapter 10, "Personal DVD Authoring with Apple iDVD," showed how Apple's iDVD tool simplifies DVD authoring by automatically laying out buttons on menus linked to video clips. It also provides the capability to customize the graphical style, text, and layout.

This chapter introduces DVD Studio Pro, Apple's professional DVD authoring tool that authors DVD productions with menus and navigational links from a group of pre-prepared media assets. DVD Studio Pro provides access to almost the full range of features of the DVD format—especially multiple streams, button highlights, scripting, and explicit control of button actions.

The DVD Studio Pro interface is built around a graphical view of your project's navigational structure. It has tools for constructing menus, tracks, slide shows, and scripts; and gives extensive support for examining the project, from item-specific properties to project-wide viewers.

This chapter reviews the capabilities of DVD Studio Pro by using the sample Tutorial project provided with the product. It begins by exploring each element of the DVD Studio Pro interface. It then provides more details on specific advanced DVD authoring features, including menu and button design, video chapters and linked story clips, multiple alternate streams, slide shows, scripts, and web links. The chapter concludes with tools for visualizing the project, information on importing assets, and help with building and exporting a project.

About DVD Studio Pro

Apple's DVD Studio Pro (www.apple.com/dvdstudiopro) is Apple's full-featured DVD authoring tool that includes almost the full range of features of the DVD-Video standard. It is priced at around $1,000.

DVD Studio Pro supports the following advanced features:

- Unlimited menus with up to 36 buttons per menu, and motion menus (with video buttons and backgrounds)

- Buttons over video tracks

- Up to 99 video tracks per project, with up to nine different video angles per track, with chapter markers and multiple stories, and up to eight audio streams and 32 subtitle streams per track for multilingual titles

- Web links using Apple DVD@CCESS for computer playback

- 16:9 widescreen format support

- Support for DVD-5 and DVD-9 (dual-layer) discs

DVD Studio Pro 1.0 was introduced with iDVD in January 2001, running only under Mac OS 9.2. The version 1.2 update, released in January 2002, added support for external DVD-R/RAM Firewire drives, and improved the output of DLT tapes.

DVD Studio Pro version 1.5, introduced in April 2002, is available under both Mac OS 9 and OS X. It supports MPEG encoding and compilation of projects in the background and provides better integration with Final Cut Pro by importing chapter markers.

The DVD Studio Pro product also includes an MPEG plug-in for QuickTime to convert QuickTime video files (that is, from Final Cut Pro) to DVD-compliant MPEG-2, and a Dolby AC-3 encoder application for creating full surround-sound DVD audio.

Exploring the Tutorial Project with DVD Studio Pro

The easiest way to understand DVD Studio Pro is to use it to explore an existing DVD project. This chapter uses the Tutorial project Apple includes with the product, which includes examples of each major feature of DVD design. This section introduces the components of the DVD Studio Pro interface by using them to explore the Tutorial project and understand its structure.

Launching DVD Studio Pro

To start exploring DVD Studio Pro, first launch the application. DVD Studio Pro opens with the default interface arrangement (see Figure 12.1).

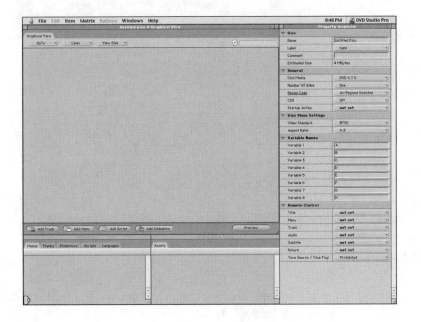

FIGURE 12.1

The default DVD Studio Pro interface fills the screen.

DVD Studio Pro provides four main windows for viewing the components of your project onscreen: the main Graphical View window on the left, the Project View window and Assets window along the bottom, and the Property Inspector window on the right.

You can enlarge, reposition, and resize these windows as desired while you are working on your project, or use the Windows menu to open and close them.

Opening the Tutorial Project

The DVD Studio Pro CD-ROM includes a DVD Studio Pro Tutorial folder that contains a sample Tutorial project and the assets used to create it (see Figure 12.2). If you have not done so already, copy this folder to your hard disk.

FIGURE 12.2

Copy the Tutorial project provided with DVD Studio Pro to a folder on your hard disk.

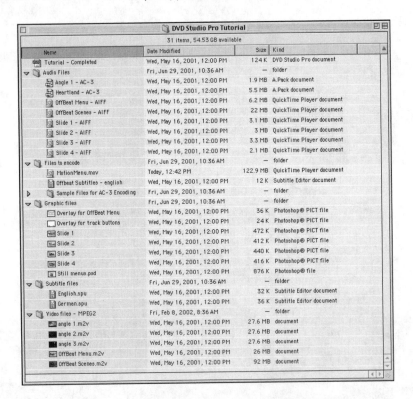

Pull down the File menu, choose Open, and then navigate to the DVD Studio Pro Tutorial folder. Double-click on the Tutorial—Completed file to open this saved project in DVD Studio Pro.

This project contains at least one example of each component of the DVD Studio Pro interface to demonstrate the corresponding DVD capability (see Figure 12.3).

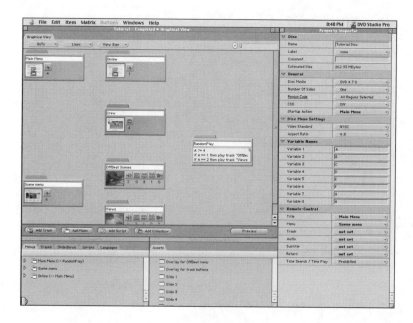

FIGURE 12.3

The Tutorial project provided with DVD Studio Pro provides an example of each major component of a DVD design.

Exploring the Graphical View

The main Graphical View window on the left contains different colored tiles for the different kinds of project elements: Menus (blue), Tracks (green), Slideshows (grey), and Scripts (orange). The different types of tiles contain a thumbnail of their contents (video track, menu, or slide show image; and even script contents) and one or more icons for the different kinds of elements they contain (that is, buttons or streams), with the count below the associated icon.

While editing the project, you can use the corresponding Add buttons along the bottom of the window to add new tiles of the associated type.

You can drag the tiles around to rearrange them to help you visualize the design. Click on the Lines menu button at the top of the window, and choose Always from the pop-up menu to display lines and arrows between the tiles to visualize the links between them. The lines are color-coded for different kinds of links. You can use choose Customize to display lines for only Jumps, Menu Buttons, or Remote Control Bottoms.

Reorganize the tiles to help understand the navigational structure of the project (see Figure 12.4).

FIGURE 12.4

Reorganize the project element tiles, and display the navigation lines to help visualize the project design.

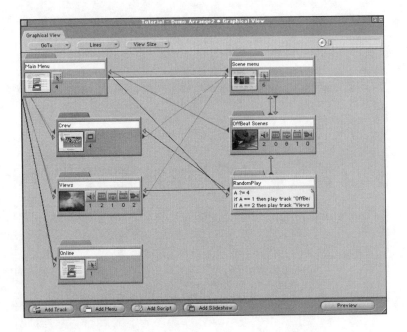

The Main menu links to four other menus:

- Scene menu, which then links to the Offbeat Scenes track
- Crew slide show
- Views track
- Online menu

There is also a RandomPlay script that links to all the other elements.

> **T I P**
>
> *To help visualize the project as it gets larger, you can click on the View Size menu button at the top of the window, and choose Small to zoom out to view more tiles in the window; or you can click on the Goto menu button to jump to a specific tile.*

Previewing the Project

An even better way to explore the project is to run it by using the Preview mode built in to DVD Studio Pro.

You preview an individual item by selecting it. To preview the full project as it would play on a DVD, first click on the background of the Graphical View window to select the disc project and then click on the Preview button at the bottom right of the window. DVD Studio Pro displays the Preview mode.

The first menu displayed is the Main menu, which is a static menu with four buttons. Click on the Debugging button at the top left to display additional information about the current item, script variables, and a playback log (see Figure 12.5).

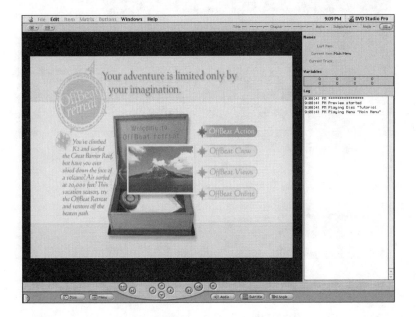

FIGURE 12.5

Use Preview mode to review your project design and DVD navigation. Display the Debugging window to see a log of the DVD actions.

The menu buttons at the top of the screen provide further control of the preview. Use the Monitor pop-up menu (monitor icon) at the top left to choose the Main Screen or an external monitor, if available. Use the adjacent Aspect Ratio menu button (arrows in a square icon) to choose Square or Rectangular pixel dimensions for a computer or TV monitor, respectively.

Use the DVD remote control keys at the bottom of the screen to navigate the DVD. Click on the four Arrow keys (triangle icons) at the center to cycle through the menu buttons.

Select the first Offbeat Action menu button, and click on OK to activate the selected button and perform the associated action; in this case, a new menu. These buttons are highlighted by using different graphics when selected and activated.

The new Offbeat Action menu is a motion menu, with moving video in the background (see Figure 12.6). The video rectangles serve as buttons to jump to the associated clips, and the menu includes the Main and Next buttons to jump back to the Main menu and to play a different set of clips. The buttons are highlighted by outlining them in yellow.

FIGURE 12.6

The Offbeat Action menu is a motion menu with moving video for the clip buttons.

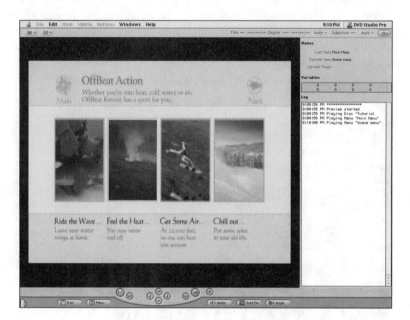

Select the second Heat clip, and click on OK to play it. The video has Action and Main menu buttons overlaid over it.

While playing the video clips, click on Previous Marker and Next Marker (triangle and line icons) to skip back or forward to the next marker point, if defined in the current track.

DVD Studio Pro also displays information about the currently playing streams at the top right of the window, including the Title and Chapter time; and the Audio, Chapter, and Subpicture stream number.

As you explore the DVD navigation further, notice that when a clip finishes playing, it does not necessarily need to return to the menu that it started playing from. This is a design decision when the disc is authored. Similarly, try clicking on Return on the left (arrow and circle icon) to go back to the previously active menu. Again, this action must be explicitly specified in the navigational design.

Use the Disc and Menu buttons at the bottom left of the screen to jump back to the Main and closest menu, respectively.

Click on the second Offbeat Crew button on the Main menu to view a slide show with still images and background audio.

Click on the third Offbeat Views button on the Main menu to play a video sequence. This and some of the other tracks contain alternate streams. Use the buttons at the bottom left to cycle through the available Audio languages, Subtitle text, and video Angle.

Finally, click on the Stop remote control key (square icon) above the Audio button to exit Preview mode and return to the DVD Studio Pro editor (or press the Esc key on the keyboard).

T I P

You might be disconcerted to discover that the project starts playing automatically if you do not make a selection from the Main menu. This feature is provided by the Random Play script (see the section, "Working With Scripts" later in this chapter).

Another surprise awaits if you select the Offbeat Online button on the Main menu. This not only displays the Online menu, but also launches a web browser to display a corresponding web link (see the section, "Creating Web Links" later in this chapter).

Viewing Properties

The Property Inspector window on the right side of the screen is used to display information and change settings for the currently selected item.

Click on the background of the Graphical View window to select the disc information for the overall project in Property Inspector window (see Figure 12.7). Click on the triangles, if needed, to expand nested items.

The Disc section includes the Name and Estimated Size of the disc.

The General section specifies characteristics for building the disc, including double-sided media, region code, and CSS copy protection. It also specifies the Startup Action menu to be shown when the DVD starts to play.

You can also check the current size of the project by using the bar next to the disc icon at the top right of the Graphical View window. It shows the estimated size of the project on the specified disc media.

FIGURE 12.7

The Property Inspector window displays information about the entire project or a selected project element.

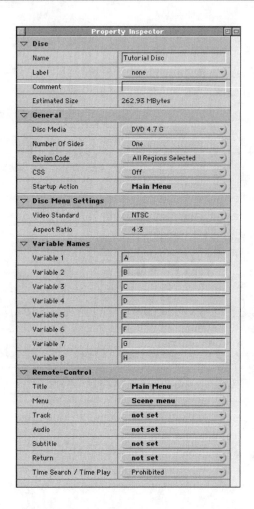

The Disc Menu Settings specify the Video Standard (NTSC or PAL) and Aspect Ratio (4:3 or 16:9 widescreen).

The Variable Names section lists programming variables used in scripts.

The Remote Control section specifies the action to be taken when the user presses various buttons on the Remote Control, including jumping to the main Title menu.

Using the Project View Window

The Project View window at the bottom left of the screen provides an alternate view of the components of the project (see Figure 12.8).

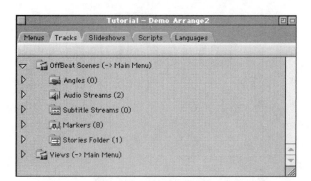

FIGURE 12.8

The Project View window organizes information about different project components into tabbed windows of hierarchical information.

Click through the tabs—Menus, Tracks, Slideshows, Scripts, Languages—to see containers for each type of item displayed with a hierarchical, folder-like organization.

Click on the triangle to the left of each folder to expand it and see the individual items. An arrow with an item name indicates a link to that item, and a number in parentheses is the count of assigned items. Items shown in italics are incomplete and still need some properties to be set.

Click on an individual item to examine and change its properties in the Property Inspector window.

The Project View is not just for viewing items and properties. You can also edit the project by creating new items (with the Item menu) and linking items by dragging them between windows.

T I P

To work more efficiently with multiple windows, you can drag a tab out of the Project View window as a separate container window.

To reassemble the Project View back to the default arrangement, close the windows and then re-open the Project View from the Windows menu.

Using the Assets View Window

The Assets View window at the bottom center of the screen contains all the asset files imported into the project, including video and audio streams, layered menu and button stills, and subtitles (see Figure 12.9).

FIGURE 12.9

The Assets View window lists all the assets imported into the project.

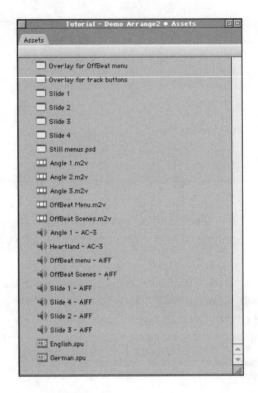

To add new assets, pull down the File menu and choose Import, or simply drag-and-drop files from a Finder window. Choose Merge to merge the assets and navigational structure of an existing project into the current project.

You can organize the assets by dragging them; or pull down the Item menu and choose Sort Assets, By Usage, By Name, or By Type.

Click on an individual asset to view and edit information about it in the Property Inspector window. You can also pull down the File menu and choose Get File Info to display information on a file before it is imported.

Each asset in DVD Studio Pro is associated with a file on disk. But files can be moved or even deleted, or you might want to use a different file for a menu or track. To review the association between the current project assets and disk files, pull down the Item menu, and choose Asset Files. DVD Studio Pro displays the Asset Files dialog box (see Figure 12.10), with sortable columns for the project assets; and associated volumes, folders, and filenames.

Click on Show Missing Files Only check box to view only assets that are not linked to a disk file. Select an item and then click on Locate to select a file for that item, or choose Assign to assign a new file.

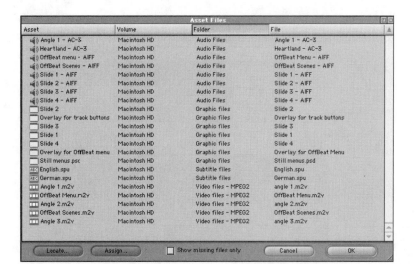

FIGURE 12.10

The Asset Files window lists all the project assets and the associated disk files.

Working with Menus and Buttons

DVD Studio Pro provides a Menu Editor window for assembling and laying out the components of a DVD menu, including the background (still or video), button hot spots, button graphics for selection highlights, and button and default actions.

Menu graphics are designed to be imported as layered Photoshop files, with the background elements and different selection states for each button in separate layers. This process is much more efficient if you maintain a consistent structure and naming convention for the layers.

Creating Still Menus

Click on the Main menu tile in the Graphical View window to select it (see Figure 12.11). Menu tiles include a thumbnail of the menu and a button icon (cursor over a square) to the right of the thumbnail, with a number under the icon to show the count of buttons used in the menu.

Click on the button icon, and DVD Studio Pro displays the Menu container window (see Figure 12.12). The container lists the name of each button, and shows its associated link. You can also review and change the button properties by clicking on them.

FIGURE 12.11

The Main menu tile shows four buttons in the menu.

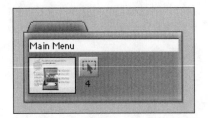

FIGURE 12.12

The Menu container window shows the button elements used in the menu.

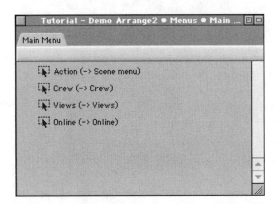

Double-click on the menu thumbnail (or pull down the Item menu, and choose Edit) to open the Menu Editor (see Figure 12.13).

FIGURE 12.13

Use the Menu Editor to construct the menu background and buttons.

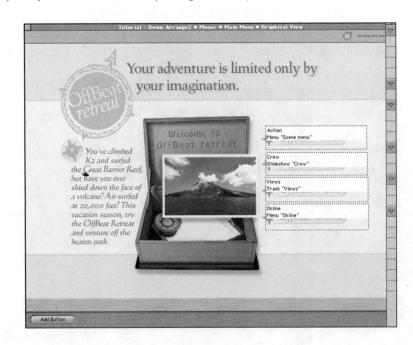

The menu is constructed from a layered Photoshop file, including the background elements and separate layers for the button graphics. Click on the menu background to select the entire menu, and review its settings in the Property Inspector (see Figure 12.14).

The Picture setting includes the still image asset file used for the menu background.

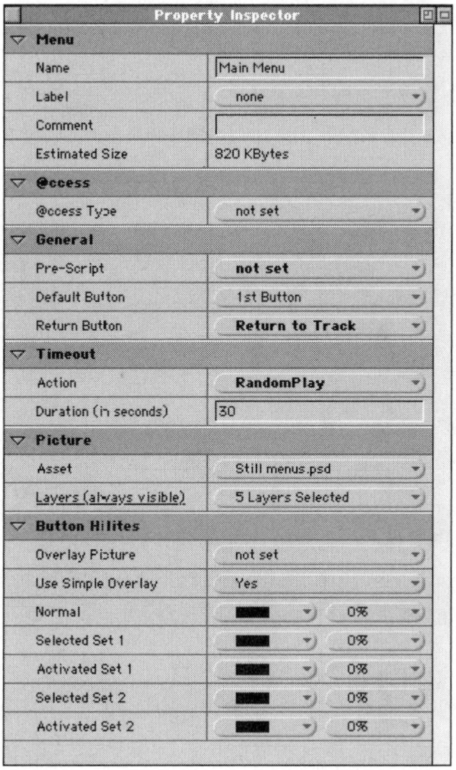

FIGURE 12.14

The menu properties include the background and button graphics.

Click on the Layers (always visible) button to display the Layers dialog box that shows all the layers in the Photoshop file (see Figure 12.15). The selected bottom layers are composited together for the menu background, and the top layers contain graphics for the different button selection states.

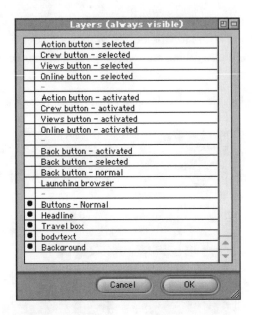

Creating Button Layers

In the Menu Editor, the hot spots for the four buttons are outlined over the menu background, with their names and associated actions. Click on a button to review or change its settings in the Property Inspector (see Figure 12.16). The bottom Buttons Links section is generated automatically by DVD Studio Pro for navigation with cursor control arrows within the menu screen.

The Display section shows how individual layers in the Photoshop file are assigned as the graphics to be displayed when the button is in each selection state: Normal, Selected, and Activated.

This is the Photoshop layer method for showing selection states. The motion menu used for the Scene menu uses a different technique—the standard highlighting method.

To exit the Menu Editor, click on the close box in the upper-left corner.

To preview the menu design and button selections, click on the Main menu tile in the Graphical View window to select it, and click on the Preview button. You can then cycle through the button states in Preview mode.

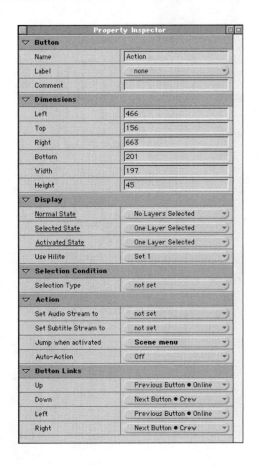

FIGURE 12.16

The button properties include the graphics used to display selection states.

Creating Motion Menus

The Scene menu contains a motion menu background, with buttons that are highlighted.

Select the Scene menu tile to select it (see Figure 12.17). It contains six buttons.

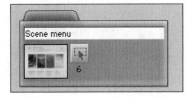

FIGURE 12.17

The Scene menu tile contains six buttons.

Review the Scene menu settings in the Property Inspector (see Figure 12.18).

FIGURE 12.18

The Scene menu properties show that the background is a motion video clip. The menu properties also specify the high-lighting colors for the buttons.

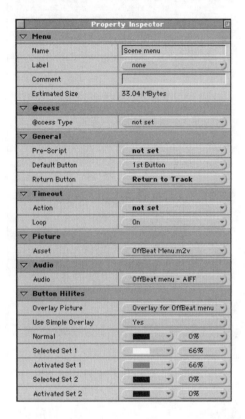

In the Picture section, the asset is a video clip—Offbeat Menu.m2v—not just a still image. The menu also includes an audio asset to play as background audio with the menu. The Timeout section is set to loop the playback if the user does not make a selection.

You can find the original video for this clip with the DVD Studio Pro Tutorial files in the Files to Encode folder. If you play the Motion Menu.mov file (with the QuickTime player), you see that the video file contains the menu background, all four composted motion video clips, and even the Main and Next button graphics.

To open the Menu Editor, double-click on the thumbnail in the Scene menu tile. As before, the hot spots for each button are outlined (see Figure 12.19).

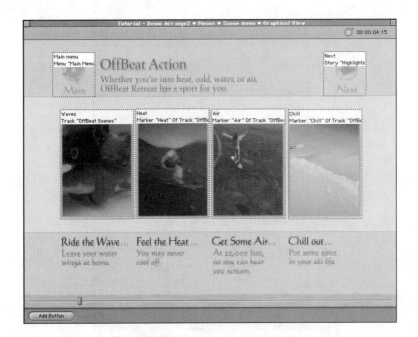

FIGURE 12.19

The Menu Editor shows the button hot spots around the video clips in the Scene menu.

Click on the Waves button, click on the Heat button, and review the settings in the Property Inspector. In the Action section, Jump When Activated is set to the OffBeat Scenes track for the Waves button and to a marker point within the track for the Heat button (see Figure 12.20).

Creating Button Highlights

Unlike the Main menu buttons, the Display section in the Property Inspector for each button does not specify layers in a Photoshop file for selection graphics. Instead, the buttons all specify Use Hilite, and the selected highlight is Set 1.

Click on the menu background to display the menu properties. The Button Hilites section specifies that the Normal highlight is nothing (0%); the Selected Set 1 highlight is yellow, blended with the background; and the Activated Set 1 highlight is red (refer to Figure 12.18). This provides a simple method of highlighting button areas on a menu, which is often more responsive than the Photoshop layer method.

FIGURE 12.20

The button proper-ties use highlighting for selection states.

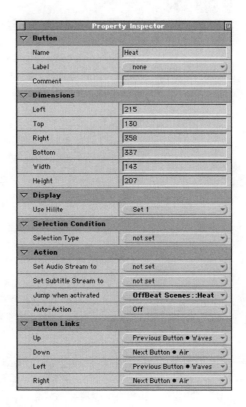

Working with Video Tracks and Markers

The Graphical View window displays the elements of the DVD design as a series of tiles. The most complex tile is the track tile, which defines not only the base video track, but alternate streams and chapter markers. Marker points can also be used to construct a story, a collection of video clips that can be played in a select-ed order, thereby reusing the tracks on the disc to present alternate paths.

Click on the Offbeat Scenes track tile in the Graphical View window to select it (see Figure 12.21). Track tiles include a thumbnail of the video clip and five icons for the additional material in the track, with the count of items under the icon. The icons are for alternate Audio streams, Subtitle streams, Markers, Stories, and multiple video Angles.

Viewing Chapter Markers

The Offbeat Scenes track tile shows that the track has markers points set in it (the number 8 under the third Markers icon with a marker on the filmstrip).

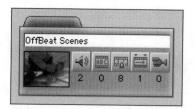

FIGURE 12.21

Track tiles include icons and counts for alternate Audio streams, Subtitle streams, Markers, Stories, and multiple Video Angles.

Click on the Markers icon to display the Marker container for this track (see Figure 12.22). The container has a list of the marker points, including the Start of Track, three subclips (Heat, Air, and Chill), and End markers for each. Click on each marker to review and change its properties of each item. To create new marker points, pull down the Item menu, and choose New Marker.

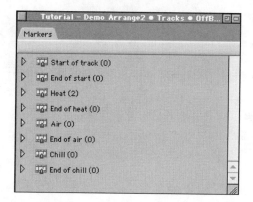

FIGURE 12.22

The Marker container includes the marker points defined in the track.

Using the Marker Editor

To set or view a marker point, click on the Heat marker in the container to select it, and pull down the Item menu, and choose Edit (or Option double-click on the marker name in the container). DVD Studio Pro displays the Marker Editor at that marker point (see Figure 12.23). (You can also double-click on the video thumbnail in the title tile to display the Marker Editor.)

The Marker Editor provides an interface for setting marker points while viewing the associated video frame. It is not intended for previewing the clip and then setting marker points; instead, you first select the marker point you want to set, and then move the video to the associated point.

FIGURE 12.23

*Use the Marker
Editor to review
current marker
points in the video
track and to select
the frame for new
markers.*

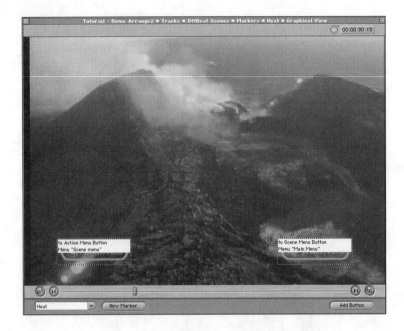

First, use the pop-up menu at the bottom left of the window to select a named marker point. You can also use the outer play control buttons on each side of the slider to move to the next or previous marker. DVD Studio Pro updates the display to show the associated video frame, moves the slider below the video to the corresponding point, and displays the timecode for that frame in the top left of the window.

To experiment with the Marker Editor without changing any existing markers, click on the New Marker button at the bottom of the window (you could also have added a marker in the Marker container window). To set the position for the new marker, drag the slider; or click on the Time Code button at the top left, and type a timecode value. You can also use the play controls on each side of the slider to move to the next or previous frame.

Due to the way the DVD video is compressed, it is not possible to start play at any arbitrary frame. Instead, DVD Studio Pro automatically adjusts the marker point to the closest possible frame.

When you are done experimenting, you can remove any new markers and undo any changes by pulling down the Edit menu and choosing Undo. Or, delete the new marker in the Marker container window by selecting it and pressing the Delete key.

To see how the marker points are used in a DVD production, select the Offbeat Scenes track tile in the Graphical View window, and click on Preview. DVD Studio Pro starts playing the track. Click on the Previous Marker and Next Marker buttons to skip through the marker points. DVD Studio Pro displays the corresponding marker names in the Log section of the Debugging information on the right side of the display.

Using Interactive Marker Buttons

The Heat marker also has one other feature: buttons that appear while the video track is playing. These interactive markers are set like menu buttons, with a hot area outlined over the button graphic. The Button Hilite section of the Property Inspector for the marker includes the settings for these buttons, including the Overlay Picture image and the selected and activated button colors (see Figure 12.24).

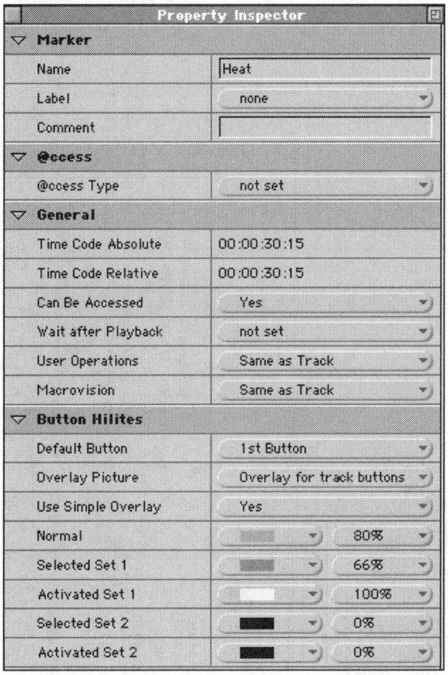

Property Inspector	
▽ **Marker**	
Name	Heat
Label	none
Comment	
▽ **@ccess**	
@ccess Type	not set
▽ **General**	
Time Code Absolute	00:00:30:15
Time Code Relative	00:00:30:15
Can Be Accessed	Yes
Wait after Playback	not set
User Operations	Same as Track
Macrovision	Same as Track
▽ **Button Hilites**	
Default Button	1st Button
Overlay Picture	Overlay for track buttons
Use Simple Overlay	Yes
Normal	80%
Selected Set 1	66%
Activated Set 1	100%
Selected Set 2	0%
Activated Set 2	0%

FIGURE 12.24

The Marker properties include settings for the interactive buttons overlaid on the video track.

These button definitions can be shared with other markers. Move to the Air marker to review its properties: The Button Hilites section is set to Use Button of the Heat marker.

When you play this track in Preview mode, you can click on the left and right menu navigation buttons to select between these two buttons while the video is playing, and click on the OK button to jump to the corresponding menu—even while the video is playing.

> **TIP**
>
> *The button highlights for interactive markers are created using the DVD subtitle feature, so they cannot be combined with subtitles on the same track.*

Defining a Story Sequence

The Offbeat Scenes track tile also shows a count under the Stories icon (with in and out points set on a filmstrip). A story is a sequence of clips, to be played in a specified order. This lets you reuse the video clips that are already used in your DVD production, but play them back in a different sequence.

Click on the fourth Story icon on the Offbeat Scenes track tile to display the Stories Folder. One story, Highlights, is defined. Click on the triangle icon to expand the story definition, a list of markers to be played in the specified order (see Figure 12.25).

FIGURE 12.25

The Stories Folder defines a list of markers in the track to be played in the specified order.

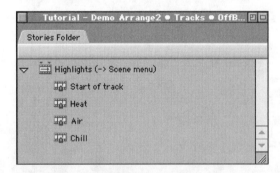

This is why each marker defined for the track also has a corresponding End marker: each clip to be played for the story is defined by a marker for its starting point, and it then plays until the corresponding End marker is reached.

You can add more clips to the story by opening the Tracks tab in the Project View window and dragging more entries from the Markers list.

To play a story, it must be linked from your DVD production. The Highlights story is linked from the Next button on the Scene menu. Double-click on the thumbnail of the Scene menu tile to display the Menu Editor, and click on the Next button in the top left to display its properties. In the Action section, the Jump When Activated field is set to the Highlights story (see Figure 12.26).

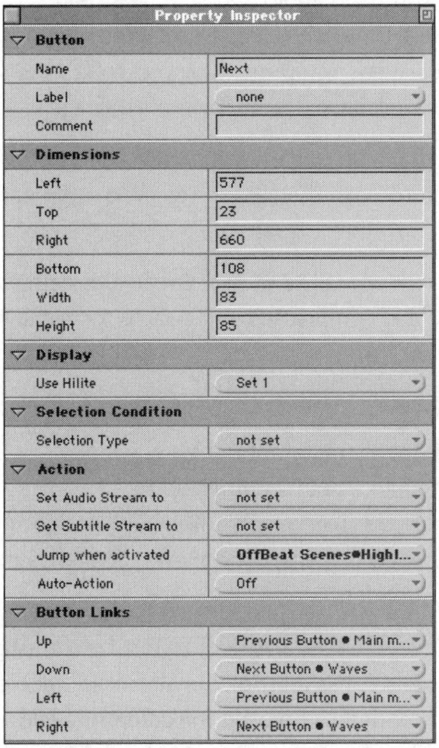

FIGURE 12.26

The Next button in the Scene menu is linked to the Highlights story.

Working with Alternate Streams and Languages

One of the most interesting features of the DVD-Video format is the capability to provide multiple streams of content—video, audio, and subtitles—to augment a video track. These can be used to provide additional options for the viewer, to select alternate video cameras angles to view a music concert, to hear the soundtrack in a different language or with commentary by the director, and to view text subtitles in various languages.

Even better, the DVD format provides the flexibility to go beyond these specific uses. For example, you can script a DVD to respond to user input and automatically select specific alternate streams, or you can use the subtitles (which are graphics overlays) for other uses, such as Interactive Marker Buttons over video streams.

In addition, the DVD specification provides explicit support for multilingual productions. Alternate menus, and audio and subtitle streams, can be tagged with a language identifier. Users then can select a preferred language for their set-top DVD player from the player's setup menu, and each DVD disc they play can then automatically play the available material for that language.

The Languages tab in the Project View window is used to define the languages to be used in the project. You can then associate alternate menu graphics, audio streams, and subtitles with the languages.

For the DVD player to dynamically switch between alternate streams, the associated media must be created and compressed in the same format and structure.

Using Multiangle Video Streams

Select the Views track tile in the Graphical View window (see Figure 12.27). Track tiles contain icons for audio streams (with a speaker icon), subtitle streams (ABC text on a filmstrip), markers (marker on a filmstrip), stories (in/out points on a filmstrip), and angles (video camera). The Views tile shows that it contains two video angles and two subtitles.

Click on the last Angle icon (video camera) to display the Angles Container (see Figure 12.28). The container has a list of the alternate video streams available with this track. These are intended to be used for different angles of a scene, such as a music concert. To add another video clip, you can pull down the Item menu and choose New Angle.

Click on each video asset to review its properties. The General section lists the Asset video file (see Figure 12.29).

Select the Views track tile, and click on the Preview button to preview this track. While the track is playing, click on the Angle button under the Preview window to switch between the video streams. The corresponding stream number is also displayed at the top right of the window.

In this production, the different angles were designed to switch between distant, closer-up, and more interior views to illustrate the spoken description in the audio track.

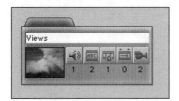

FIGURE 12.27

The Views track tile contains one audio stream, two subtitles, one marker, no stories, and two alternate video angles.

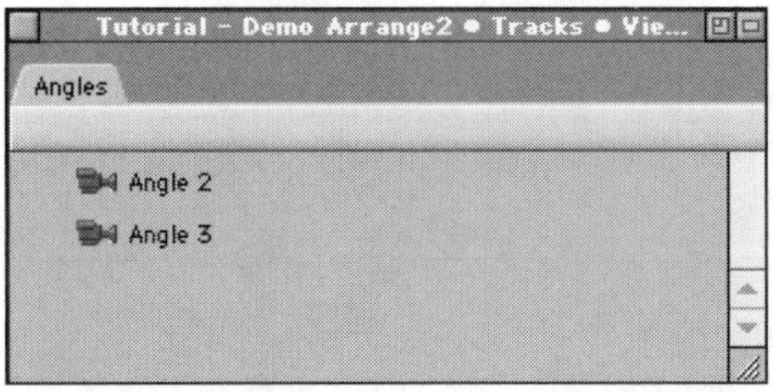

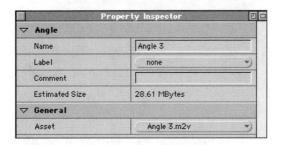

FIGURE 12.28

The Angles container lists the alternate video streams available with this track.

FIGURE 12.29

The Angle properties show the alternate video stream file.

Using Subtitle Streams

A DVD track can have subtitle streams, which are typically used for text subtitles in multiple languages.

The Views track tile shows a count of two subtitle streams under the second Subtitle icon (with ABC text on a filmstrip). Click on the Subtitle icon to display the Subtitle container. The container lists two subtitles, in English and German (see Figure 12.30).

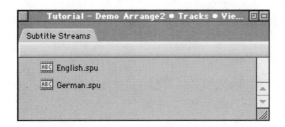

FIGURE 12.30

The Subtitles container lists the subtitle streams available with this track in various languages.

DVD Studio Pro includes a separate Subtitle Editor application that you can use to type and format subtitle text, and synchronize its display to a video track. You can also import a list of subtitles from a plain text file, which defines the lines of text and associated times codes when it is to be displayed.

When you finish editing the subtitles, you then use the Subtitle Editor to compile it into a subtitle stream, which then can be linked to a video track in DVD Studio Pro.

Click on the German subtitle in the Subtitle container to examine its properties (see Figure 12.31). In the General section, the Asset entry specifies the subtitle stream. The Language entry must also be specified, so the DVD player can automatically display the appropriate subtitles.

FIGURE 12.31

The properties for a Subtitle stream includes its language.

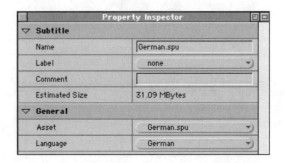

Preview the Views track to see the subtitle text. Click on the Subtitle button at the bottom of the Preview window to switch between the available subtitles. The current subtitle stream number is also displayed under Subpicture in the top right of the window.

Using Audio Streams

A DVD track can have multiple audio streams, which can be used for different voice-over narration, soundtracks, and languages.

The OffBeat Scenes track tile shows a count of two audio streams under the first Audio icon (with a speaker). Click on the Audio icon to display the Audio container. The container lists two audio streams (see Figure 12.32).

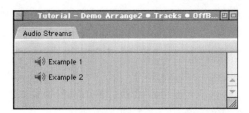

FIGURE 12.32

The Audio container lists the audio streams available with this track.

The audio stream properties show the associated audio file and language (see Figure 12.33).

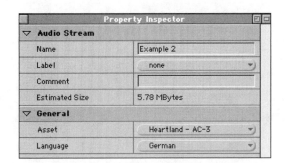

FIGURE 12.33

The Audio Stream properties include the audio file on disk and the associated language.

Preview the OffBeat Scenes track to hear the audio tracks. Click on the Audio button at the bottom of the Preview window to switch between the streams. The current subtitle stream number is also displayed under Audio in the top right of the window. In this production, the first stream includes music and voice-over, and the second stream has just music.

Working with Slide Shows

Although DVD presentations typically consist of motion video clips, they also can include slide shows: a series of still images with accompanying audio.

The Crew tile in the Graphical View is a DVD Studio Pro slide show (see Figure 12.34). The Crew tile shows a count of four slides under the Slide icon.

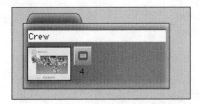

FIGURE 12.34

The Crew slide show tile shows that it contains four slides.

Click on the Slide icon to display the Slideshow container. The container lists the four slides, along with their accompanying audio tracks (see Figure 12.35).

Double-click on the thumbnail in the slide show tile to display the Slideshow Editor. The Editor shows the slide show elements, in order, with their elapsed times (see Figure 12.36). On the right, it displays suitable assets to add to the slide show, including still images and additional audio clips.

Preview the Crew slide show to see how it plays back. Use the Previous Marker and Next Marker buttons on the Control Panel to skip between slides.

FIGURE 12.35

The Slideshow container lists the slides and accompanying audio tracks to be played in the specified order.

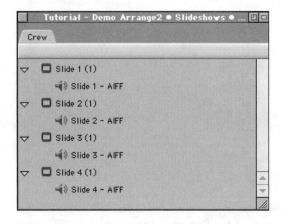

FIGURE 12.36

Use the Slideshow Editor to organize the available image and audio assets into a slide show.

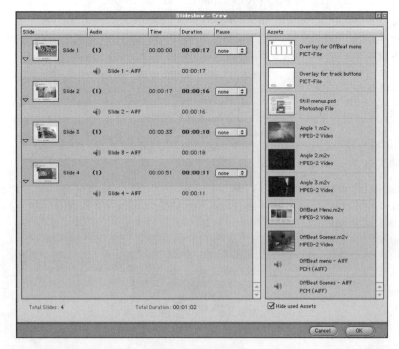

Working with Scripts

DVD Studio Pro supports programming of the behavior of DVD productions using scripts. DVD players, hardware and software, support a simple programming language, including a small number of variables to remember settings. With scripts, a production can remember a user input, change the navigational structure, weave together alternate play orders, and even behave randomly. The scripting language can perform computations, access and set the current settings, such as tracks and audio streams, and test values to perform different actions.

The RandomPlay tile in the Graphical View is a DVD Studio Pro script (see Figure 12.37). The tile shows part of the contents of the script.

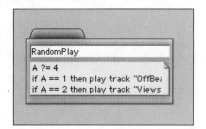

FIGURE 12.37

The RandomPlay script tile defines programmable behavior.

Double-click on the tile to open the Script Editor. The RandomPlay script generates a random number between 1 and 4 in the variable A, and tests the number to randomly play a video track or slide show (see Figure 12.38).

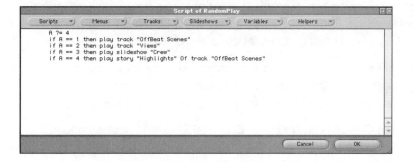

FIGURE 12.38

Use the Script Editor to construct a script—complete with variables, expressions, and logic functions.

You can use the pop-up button menus at the top of the window to explore the available project assets and scripting variables and commands, and then insert them into the script.

The RandomPlay script is linked from the Main menu. Select the Main menu tile, and review its properties. In the Timeout section, the Action after timeout is set to call this script.

Preview the Main menu, and wait for the timeout period to elapse. The Log section in the Debugging area on the right of the Preview screen shows the script being executed and the random value that was computed (see Figure 12.39).

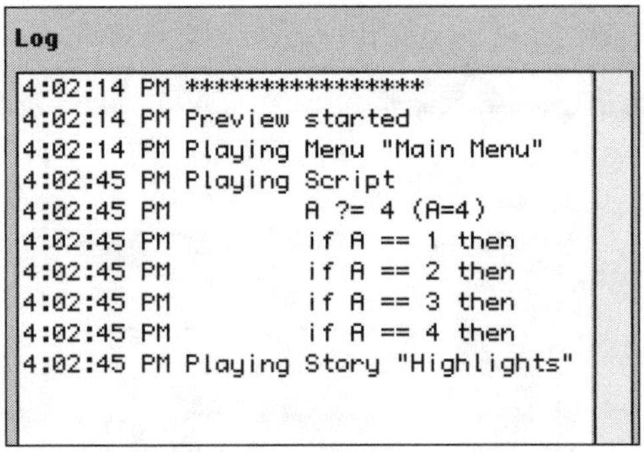

FIGURE 12.39

The Preview Log area shows the script being executed to randomly choose a menu selection.

```
Log
4:02:14 PM ******************
4:02:14 PM Preview started
4:02:14 PM Playing Menu "Main Menu"
4:02:45 PM Playing Script
4:02:45 PM          A ?= 4 (A=4)
4:02:45 PM          if A == 1 then
4:02:45 PM          if A == 2 then
4:02:45 PM          if A == 3 then
4:02:45 PM          if A == 4 then
4:02:45 PM Playing Story "Highlights"
```

Creating Web Links

DVD Studio Pro provides a mechanism for linking from a DVD production to a web site when played on a computer. This uses the Apple DVD@CCESS feature, which requires that the support for these links be built in to the DVD player application, as it is with newer versions of the Apple DVD Player (check the Preferences dialog box to enable this option). This feature is also supported in some Windows DVD player applications. DVD Studio Pro also can add installer programs to your final DVD for Macintosh and Windows computers.

Web links can be attached to a track, menu, or slide show, but not to a button. However, you can link a button to a menu with a web link, as in this example, in which the fourth button on the Main menu links to the Online menu.

Select the Online menu tile in the Graphical View, and double-click on the thumbnail to open the Menu Editor. This menu is used to display a warning that a web link is being accessed (see Figure 12.40).

The @ccess section in the menu properties contains an @ccess URL entry that is set to a URL on the Apple web site (see Figure 12.41).

Preview the Main menu, and use the navigation controls to select the Online button. As the Online menu is displayed, the web link is also opened in a browser.

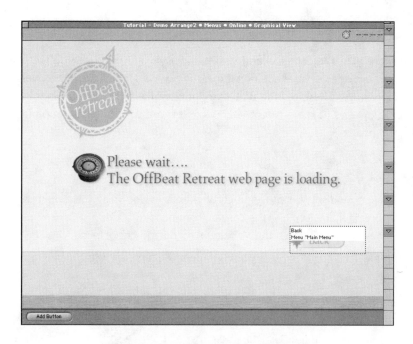

FIGURE 12.40

The Online menu links to an associated web page.

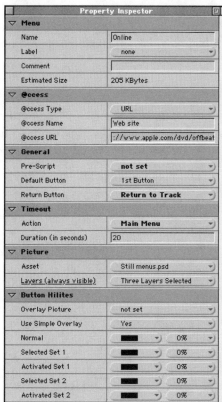

FIGURE 12.41

The Menu properties can contain a web URL to be executed by a DVD player application using the Apple DVD@CCESS feature.

Visualizing a Project

In addition to the Project View and Assets windows and the Assets file list, DVD Studio Pro provides several additional tools for viewing and editing the overall project structure. These include text descriptions of the project contents and Matrix table views to cross-reference how assets are used and navigation flows within the project.

Using the Log Window

The Log window displays status and error messages, including the debugging log from the Preview session, and the results from building a disc. To review the current log messages, pull down the Windows menu and choose Log.

Using Text Descriptions

DVD Studio Pro also can generate text descriptions of individual elements and of the entire disc. Select a specific tile or click on the window background to select the disc, pull down the Item menu, and choose Show Description of the selected element. DVD Studio Pro then displays the Log window with a formatted text list of each container and item (see Figure 12.42) at the end of the log listing. This is useful for checking the structure and contents of your disc.

Using Matrix Views

DVD Studio Pro provides another different view of your project with the Matrix views. The more methodical you are about organizing and naming your project assets and elements, the more useful these views can be to see patterns and inconsistencies in the design.

Pull down the Matrix menu, and choose Assets of Disc to display the Assets Matrix, which shows how the available assets are assigned to different tracks (see Figure 12.43).

Move the cursor over the grid, and click an asset to assign and de-assign assets to the corresponding track.

```
Disc "Tutorial Disc" {
    // Disc
    label                               0
    comment                             " "
    // General
    discCurrentLanguage                 Language "english"
    discMedia                           discMedia_DVD_ROM_12_SL
    discNumberOfSides                   1
    discRegionCode                      1
    discRegionCode                      2
    discRegionCode                      3
    discRegionCode                      4
    discRegionCode                      5
    discRegionCode                      6
    discRegionCode                      8
    discCSS                             off
    discStartJump                       Menu "Main Menu"
    // Disc Menu Settings
    discTVSystem                        NTSC
    discAspectRatio                     aspectRatio_4to3
    // Variable Names
    scriptVariable_1                    "A"
    scriptVariable_2                    "B"
    scriptVariable_3                    "C"
    scriptVariable_4                    "D"
    scriptVariable_5                    "E"
    scriptVariable_6                    "F"
    scriptVariable_7                    "G"
    scriptVariable_8                    "H"
    // Remote-Control
    discRemoteControlButton_Title       Menu "Main Menu"
    discRemoteControlButton_Menu        Menu "Scene menu"
    discRemoteControlButton_Track       notSet
    discRemoteControlButton_Audio       notSet
    discRemoteControlButton_SubTitle    notSet
    discTimeSearchTimePlay              prohibited
    AssetFolder {
        // Asset Container
        label       0
        comment     " "
        PhotoshopAsset "Overlay for OffBeat menu" {
            // Photoshop
            label       0
            comment     " "
            // General
            assetFile   "Macintosh HD:New Apps (Mac OS 9):DVD Studio Pro:DVD
            layer       "Picture"
        }
```

FIGURE 12.42

DVD Studio Pro can display text descriptions of the entire project or individual elements.

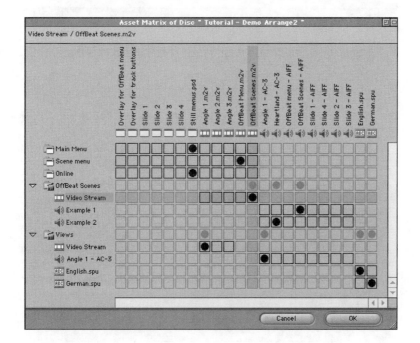

FIGURE 12.43

Use the Assets Matrix to display and assign the available assets to different tracks.

Select Jumps of Menu to display the Jumps Matrix. It shows how jumps and links are assigned to menus and buttons (see Figure 12.44).

This is useful to find where a particular element, such as a story or script, is linked within the project.

Finally, select Layers of Menu to display the Layers Matrix. It shows how layers of Photoshop files are assigned to menus and buttons (see Figure 12.45).

FIGURE 12.44

Use the Jumps Matrix to display and assign jumps and links to menus and buttons.

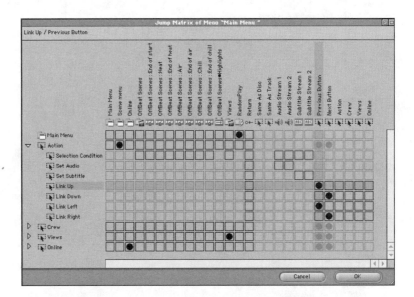

FIGURE 12.45

Use the Layers Matrix to display and assign layers of Photoshop files to menus and buttons.

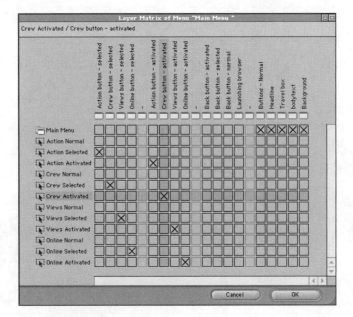

Importing Assets

DVD Studio Pro is designed for assembling preformatted assets into a final DVD production. It does not perform any automatic format conversion. All imported content first must be edited into DVD-ready format, divided into individual clips for each track or menu in which they will be used, and compressed appropriately to confirm to the requirements of DVD playback. See the DVD Studio Pro documentation for complete specifications of the input formats.

DVD Studio Pro supports both standard 4:3 (1.33) aspect ratio and 16:9 (1.78) widescreen anamorphic aspect ratio. If you are creating a 16:9 project, the assets must also be prepared accordingly. See the DVD Studio Pro documentation for more detailed information on supported media formats, resolutions, sample rates, and so on.

The DVD standard imposes maximum bit rate requirements for tracks so that they can be played on inexpensive set-top hardware. When using tracks with multiangle video, the maximum bit rates for each individual video stream are lower, depending on the number of angles.

Importing Graphics Content

DVD Studio Pro imports still images in Photoshop format (.psd) to use for menus, buttons, and slide shows. All the graphics elements for menus, including the background and button states, can be saved as layers in a single file.

Motion menus are actually created from video clips, with the button graphics elements composited on top of the video.

Graphics images used in slide shows must match the resolution of your project.

As you prepare menu graphics, be aware of the difference in aspect ratio between computer displays and television screens. The images you edit on the computer are shown on a computer monitor with square pixels, whereas the final DVD will be slightly squeezed when displayed on a TV set with rectangular pixels. To compensate for this difference for NTSC displays, you can prepare your graphics images at 720×540 resolution and then resize them to 720×480 to be stored on the DVD. Unfortunately, this resizing itself can produce artifacts, particularly in thin lines, so you will need to experiment to achieve a preferred result.

Importing Audio Content

DVD Studio Pro imports audio clips in three formats: PCM (AIFF or WAV), MPEG-1 audio, and Dolby AC-3.

The QuickTime MPEG encoder (provided with DVD Studio Pro) can convert audio files to PCM format.

DVD Studio Pro also includes the Apple A.Pack application for creating multitrack Dolby Digital AC-3 audio streams. The DVD Studio Pro Tutorial files, under the Files to Encode folder, includes a folder of Sample Files for AC-3 Encoding. You can assign these to the Input Channels in the A.Pack window to create a surround-sound audio stream (see Figure 12.46). You can also use A.Pack to process files in batches.

FIGURE 12.46

Use the Apple A.Pack application to create multitrack Dolby Digital AC-3 audio streams.

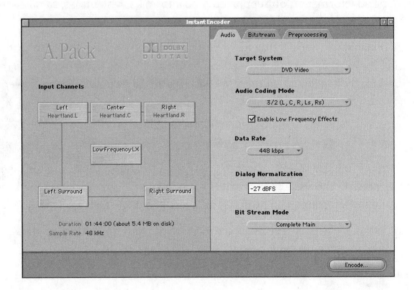

A.Pack also includes the AC-3 Monitor to play back an encoded AC-3 file (see Figure 12.47), either by downmixing to stereo or through special ASIO audio playback hardware. AC-3 Monitor also can decode an AC-3 file into separate PCM audio streams for each channel.

Background audio for menus should be designed for looping. Background audio also needs to be subtle because listening to a clip repeat over and over again can be very irritating.

All audio clips used in a slide show must be in the same format.

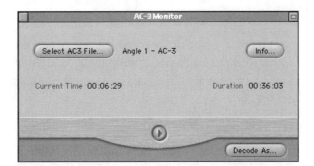

FIGURE 12.47

Use AC-3 Monitor to play back encoded AC-3 audio streams.

Importing Video Content

Video for motion menus should be designed to loop without an obvious jump between the last frame and the start frame (for example, by panning over a repeating texture or rotating an object through one resolution). You can also introduce a transition effect, such as a fade at the loop point.

Video for motion menus and for interactive markers (buttons over video clips) actually have the buttons and other background elements composited over the video material. The button highlight graphics are then provided separately.

All video clips used for multiangle tracks must be in the same format—with matching resolution, frame rate, length, and video-encoding format.

Building the Project

As you develop your DVD project, DVD Studio Pro checks for valid formats as you add assets, and it identifies incomplete streams in italics. It also provides tools, such as the item Descriptions and Matrix views, to check your ongoing design (refer to "Visualizing a Project" earlier in this chapter).

You also can use the Preview mode in DVD Studio Pro to check the look and navigational flow, and use the Debugging log to verify the actions being performed. However, depending on the speed of your processor, the number of angles that can be previewed may be limited.

When you have completed authoring your DVD project, you can build it and burn it to disc. DVD Studio Pro first builds the DVD files on hard disk, and then can output your production in several ways.

Building the Project to Hard Disk

To build your project to hard disk, pull down the File menu, and choose Build Disc. DVD Studio Pro prompts for the destination folder, and begins multiplexing together the menus and streams into the final DVD format. It displays a Progress window that shows the name and bit rate of each track as it is processed (see Figure 12.48).

FIGURE 12.48

The Build Progress window shows each track being multiplexed into the final DVD data, and also shows its associated bit rate.

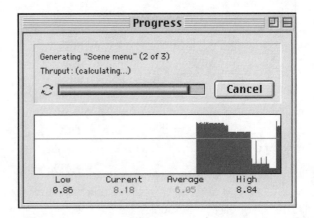

If an error occurs during multiplexing, typically because the bit rate is too high, DVD Studio Pro opens the Log window to display the error messages. Otherwise, when the build is complete, it opens the Log window with a confirmation status message (see Figure 12.49).

FIGURE 12.49

When the build completes, the Log window displays a confirmation status message.

```
                                          Log
11:33:43 AM Starting Up
11:39:17 AM Start Building Disc "Tutorial Disc"
11:39:17 AM Building Track "OffBeat Scenes"
11:39:45 AM Building Track "Views"
11:40:14 AM Generating Language "english"
11:40:14 AM Generating "Main Menu"
11:40:19 AM Generating "Scene menu"
11:40:26 AM Generating "Online"
11:40:27 AM This disc complies to version 1.0 of the DVD-Video Specification
11:40:27 AM Building finished.
```

The result of the build is a folder on hard disk with DVD-format folders and files, under a VIDEO_TS folder (see Figure 12.50).

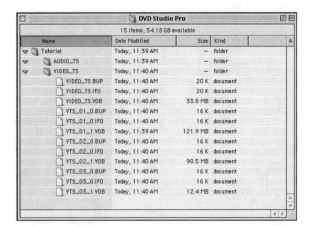

FIGURE 12.50

The build creates the standard DVD-Video format VIDEO_TS folder and data files in the specified folder on hard disk.

You can then play the DVD contents from these files on hard disk. With the Mac OS 9 Apple DVD Player, first enable this in the Preferecnes dialog box. You can then pull down the File menu, and choose Open VIDEO_TS to open and play the DVD directories from hard disk.

Building and Exporting the Project

With DVD Studio Pro, you can burn your project to a DVD disc or export it in several formats to burn copies later.

You can burn the project to a DVD recorder, including the DVD-R SuperDrive or another attached DVD-RAM drive. You can save it as a disc image file (.img), which can then be used to burn multiple copies to DVD with the appropriate tools. You also can record the project to a DVD tape drive, which is to be used to manufacture copies at a disc-replication facility.

To export the project, pull down the File menu, and choose Build & Format Disc. DVD Studio Pro first prompts for the destination folder to build the DVD files to hard disc and then displays the Format Disc dialog box (see Figure 12.51). You can choose to create a disk image file or record to a device, including an available DVD recorder or a DLT tape. If you select a DVD-R recorder, you can choose to simulate the burn process first to check for errors in writing to the device.

DVD Studio Pro multiplexes the project into the final DVD format on hard disk and then outputs it in the specified format.

FIGURE 12.51

*Use the Format Disc
dialog box to save
your project to hard
disk as an image
file, or to record it
to a DVD disc or
DLT tape.*

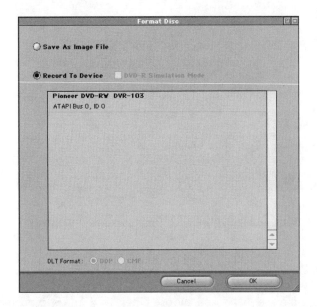

Summary

Personal DVD authoring tools, such as Apple iDVD, are very effective for creating a quick DVD from a collection of video clips that are organized into menus linked to the clips. They provide predesigned graphical themes, automated assistance for laying out menus, and built-in conversion of media assets to DVD formats.

Professional tools, such as DVD Studio Pro, go far beyond these basics to open up almost the full capability of the DVD-Video format, with custom menu selection graphics, alternate streams, subtitles, linked video stories, and scripting. They also provide a more sophisticated interface for viewing the DVD structure and elements, and for accessing individual properties. For professional replication, DVD Studio Pro supports authoring DVD-9 discs and writing to DLT tape.

Chapter 13, "Professional DVD Authoring with Sonic ReelDVD," describes a comparable professional DVD authoring tool for Windows.

Professional DVD Authoring
with Sonic ReelDVD

CHAPTER 11, "PERSONAL DVD AUTHORING WITH SONIC DVDIT!" showed how the DVDit! personal DVD authoring application from Sonic Solutions simplifies DVD authoring by letting you just design your menus while it takes care of the details, such as automatically creating menu buttons with thumbnails for clips, building the menu navigation, and converting clips to DVD format. Although DVDit! provides the capability to customize both the graphical design and menu structure of your DVD productions, by simplifying the authoring process it does limit your ability to take advantage of the capabilities of the DVD format.

This chapter introduces ReelDVD, a professional DVD authoring tool from Sonic Solutions for assembling a DVD production from a collection of prepared media assets. Like Apple's DVD Studio Pro (introduced in Chapter 12, "Professional DVD Authoring with Apple DVD Studio Pro"), professional tools, such as ReelDVD, provide direct control over authoring a DVD production—including multiple audio and subtitle streams, motion menus, menu highlights, and navigational linking.

ReelDVD is a tool for authoring, in the strict sense of combining a collection of assets and linking them together. It is not a graphic design tool or multimedia editor. ReelDVD is the final step in the production pipeline, after you have prepared all your assets and are ready to link them together into an interactive DVD production.

The idea is that you can use the appropriate professional tools for preparing materials. You will need a video editor, such as Adobe Premiere, to prepare your video and audio clips, and a graphics and image editor, such as Adobe Photoshop, to prepare your menus and other graphics. You then can use ReelDVD to organize your assets into tracks, add interactive button highlights (for menus and other navigation), and then link them together.

With this approach, ReelDVD offers immense creative freedom. Because there is no special menu editor, your menu designs are not restricted to a limited set of features. Instead, a menu in ReelDVD is just a track with some visual background and overlaid graphics. As a result, there is no limitation on button designs because you supply the graphics. And "motion menus," with background video and video in button thumbnails, are not any special case, either, because you can use any background content for menus, still or video. Of course, it is still your responsibility to create the appropriate video for these kinds of uses, such as a video background with button thumbnail videos overlaid on it.

This chapter reviews the capabilities of ReelDVD by using the sample ReelDVD Tutorial project provided with version 3.0. It begins by exploring each element of the ReelDVD interface and then provides more details on specific advanced DVD authoring features, including video chapters, slide shows, multiple audio and subtitle streams, menu and button design, and navigational links. The chapter concludes with information on importing assets, and building and exporting a project.

About Sonic ReelDVD

ReelDVD from Sonic Solutions (www.sonic.com) is a professional-level authoring tool designed for corporate video producers, priced at about $1,499. ReelDVD uses a convenient drag-and-drop interface and simple workflow to provide access to a focused set of advanced features designed for its target audience, such as up to eight audio and 32 subtitle streams, without attempting to support the full-feature set of the DVD-Video standard. ReelDVD requires Windows NT 4.0, Windows 2000, or Windows XP systems.

Sonic provides even higher-end tools for professional DVD publishing, DVD Producer and DVD Fusion—on Windows and Macintosh, respectively. For complete control over DVD authoring, Sonic also produces Scenarist and DVD Creator, the standard DVD production systems for commercial "Hollywood" titles on Windows and Macintosh, respectively. (Sonic Scenarist is described in Chapter 14, "Feature Film DVD Authoring with Sonic Scenarist.")

ReelDVD was designed to provide access to the most useful DVD authoring features for independent and corporate video producers, while maintaining a familiar style of user interface and simple workflow. The key DVD features that it offers include multiple audio and subtitle tracks; and explicit control over layered video, images, menu buttons, and subtitles.

ReelDVD version 3.0 was released in May 2002. It extended the support for multiple streams to up to eight audio and 32 subtitle streams. It also updated the support for DVD drives to include rewritable DVD-RW and DVD+RW. The ReelDVD software is copy-protected with a hardware dongle that must be inserted in the parallel port.

Exploring a Project with ReelDVD

This chapter uses the *Facepainting* Tutorial project included with ReelDVD version 3.0, which includes examples of the major features of DVD design. This section introduces the components of the ReelDVD interface by using them to explore the Tutorial project and understand its structure.

Exploring ReelDVD

To start exploring ReelDVD, first launch the application. ReelDVD opens with the default window layout (see Figure 13.1). The ReelDVD interface is built around a graphical view of the navigational flow of your project, with additional windows for laying out multiple streams in a track, and for designing menus and button links.

The main ReelDVD application window is divided into four basic work areas: Storyboard area, Track window, Preview window, and Explorer window. You can reposition, resize, and dock these windows as desired while you are working on your project, or use the View menu or Toolbar buttons to open and close them.

The Explorer window at the top right is used for locating and copying source file assets to your production. It provides folders and files panes like Windows Explorer; as well as options to filter the contents of a folder to display just video, audio, or image files.

The Storyboard area across the top of the application window is the main work area. You can add assets (video, audio, still image, and subpictures) by dragging files from the Explorer window, and you can define navigational links between tracks.

FIGURE 13.1

*The ReelDVD inter-
face includes the
Storyboard area,
Explorer window,
Track window, and
Preview window.*

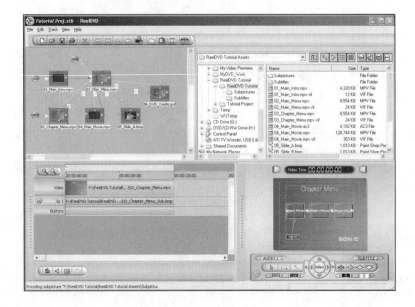

The Track window at the bottom left is used to assemble individual tracks, including trimming video, assembling slide shows, creating chapter points, adding audio
and subpicture streams, and setting language attributes.

The Preview window at the bottom right is used in two modes. In Design mode,
it is used to visually edit the layout of menu buttons and subtitles. In Simulation
mode, it is used to play back the project to preview its current state.

ReelDVD also uses a separate Information window to display status, warning, and
error messages. You can view additional details about the messages, cut and paste
the message text, and save the messages to a log file.

The toolbar at the top of the application window provides access to the most-
often-used functions, including File menu commands (New, Open, Save, Print
project), Edit commands (Clear Selected Objects), options for the Storyboard
display (Show/Hide different types of links, Zoom In/Out), View menu commands
(Show/Hide Explorer, Preview, Track Editor windows), and the Make Disc
command to output your production. The toolbar also can be detached and
freely repositioned.

Using the Explorer Window

The ReelDVD Explorer window in the top right of the application window is used to locate and drag source files into your project, including video and audio clips, menu graphics, and subtitles (see Figure 13.2). If the Explorer window is not currently visible, pull down the View menu and choose Explorer Window, or click on the corresponding button on the toolbar.

To locate source files for your production, use the Folders pane on the left side of the window to browse through the tree view of your discs and folders. Then, use the File pane on the right to scroll through the list of files in the selected folder. You can use the buttons above the File pane to filter the file list and display only files of the corresponding type: Video, Audio, Image, or All files.

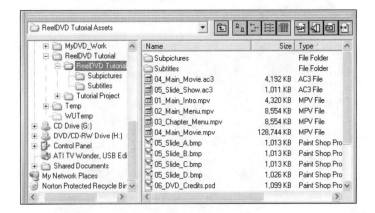

FIGURE 13.2

Use the ReelDVD Explorer window to browse for source file assets of different types to add to your project.

Exploring the Navigation in the Storyboard Window

In ReelDVD, a production consists of a linked collection of menus and tracks. Each track is a piece of content, video or slide show; possibly with additional video, audio, and subtitle streams. Each content track is a linear element that is intended to be played from beginning to end. Menu tracks then define the navigational paths to access the different tracks. In addition, you can define navigational links between the tracks themselves, both for when play reaches the end of the track and in response to user key presses on the DVD Remote Control.

Note that ReelDVD does not have a hard distinction between content and menus. Some video clips and still images may have titles and button graphics designed into them, and are therefore intended for use as menus. Some video content also may have button graphics composited on them, and therefore can have active links even when a video clip is playing. It is up to you to define interactive hot spot regions in a track, presumably corresponding to the button graphics, and then link these to destination tracks.

Similarly, there is no default behavior for navigating through tracks; you link them together as needed. A video menu or a clip may link back to itself to repeat, or can link to another menu or clip when it finishes playing.

You can drag the track icons around to rearrange them to help you visualize the navigational structure of your project, and use the Zoom button on the toolbar to zoom the view in and out (see Figure 13.3).

FIGURE 13.3

Use the Storyboard area to view the navigational design of your project, with tracks and links between them.

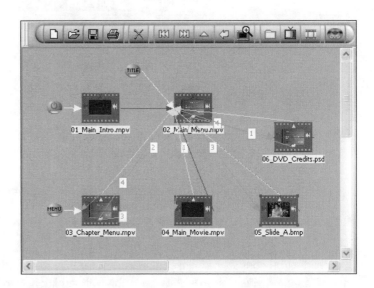

To add a track to your production, simply drag one or more video or still image files from an Explorer window into the Storyboard area. ReelDVD creates a Track icon for each source file, with a thumbnail of the first frame of the video clip. Similarly, you can add audio, subpictures, and subtitles to a track by dragging the corresponding file onto a Track icon in the Storyboard window. For more explicit control of the order of streams in a track, you also can add assets in the Track window.

You can define the links between tracks simply by clicking and dragging from the link point to another track (see the section titled "Creating Navigational Links," later in this chapter). The links between tracks are shown as arrows, color-coded for different kinds of links. These links correspond to key presses on the Remote Control: Next for Skip Forward, Previous for Skip Backward, Return or Up for Return, and Command for menu selections. The Next link also defines the next track to be played when the Player reaches the end of this track.

The Storyboard also contains three special icons corresponding to global DVD settings (yellow arrows). The AutoPlay icon links to the track that will play automatically when the DVD is first inserted into a Player. The other icons link to the tracks that will be played when the viewer presses the Title and Menu keys on the Remote Control.

As shown in the Storyboard area visualization, the structure of the Tutorial project is designed around the Main menu (file 02_Main_Menu.mpv). This contains links to several submenus, as is typically done with DVD productions:

- A chapter index menu (03_Chapter_Menu.mpv)
- The main video clip (04_Main_Movie.mpv)
- A slide show (05_Slide_A.bmp)
- A credits screen (06_DVD_Credits.psd)

The AutoPlay icon links to an initial Introduction screen (01_Main_Intro.mpv) that then links to the main menu. The Title and Menu button icons link to the Main and chapter index menus, respectively.

Note how the use of a consistent and descriptive naming convention helps to organize the source asset files and the DVD design and layout area.

Previewing the Project

Besides viewing the navigational structure of a project in the Storyboard area, you also can explore the design of a project by actually interacting with it using the Preview mode built in to ReelDVD.

The Preview window in the bottom right of the application window is used both for editing the layout of graphical buttons and subtitles, and for simulating the playback of your DVD production. Click on the Simulation On/Off button on the lower left of the Preview window controls to toggle between these two modes. In Design mode, the button is red, and the control panel contains controls for designing menus and subtitles. In Preview mode, the button is green, and the control panel contains controls, just like a DVD remote.

To preview the project as it would play on a DVD, first click on the AutoPlay icon in the Storyboard area to select the starting point for the preview. Click on the Preview window mode button to change it to green, and use the play controls on the right of the panel to start Play and to stop the preview.

The DVD production begins by playing the introductory sequence, which is simply a video clip that fades up to the main menu; including the background motion video and graphics, and the menu buttons composted into the clip (see Figure 13.4).

FIGURE 13.4

Use Preview mode to review your project design and DVD navigation, beginning at the Main menu.

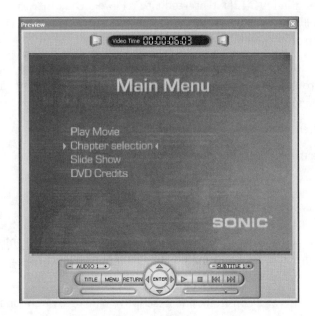

The Main menu is then displayed. This is actually another video clip, which starts with the static menu, fades to a subtle background video sequence, and then fades back to the static map background so that it can repeat. The result is a "motion menu," which has the appearance of a motion video background behind the menu graphics and buttons. Of course, this effect is created by compositing the graphics over the background video in a video editor, adding the fades, and then saving the result as a new source file to import into ReelDVD.

Click the navigation buttons in the center of the control panel (Up, Down, Left, Right) to move between menu buttons, and click on Enter to activate the current button. These button locations and the navigational paths between them were created in ReelDVD using the Design mode in the Preview window. The button highlights, which can be different for each button, were defined as subpicture graphic layers with the track, along with the color schemes for the highlights.

Select the bottom DVD Credits buttons on the Main menu to view the Credits screen. This menu contains a static image with one button to return back to the main menu.

Select the middle Slide Show button on the Main menu to view the slide show of still images. Each image is displayed for 10 seconds and then automatically advances to the next image. A background music audio track also plays with the slide show (see Figure 13.5). When the slide show ends, the DVD playback returns to the Main menu.

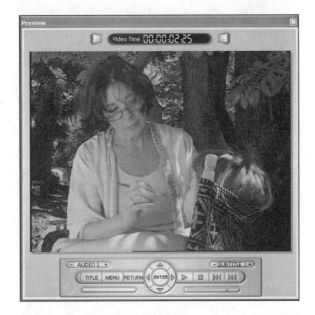

FIGURE 13.5

The Slide Show menu selection displays a timed sequence of still image slides with a background audio clip.

You also can use the menu buttons on the left side of the control panel area to jump to the corresponding disc menus that were defined in the Storyboard area: Title to return to the Main or top menu, Menu to jump to the chapter index menu, and Return to go back the previous menu.

Select the top Play Movie button on the Main menu to play the main video clip in the Tutorial. The video includes a subtitle track (see Figure 13.6).

As you play the clip, use the play controls to Skip Forward and Skip Backward to the adjacent chapter or track. Use the Volume slider underneath to adjust the playback volume level.

The track includes a subtitle stream, with text of the audio commentary timed to the clip.

The audio and subtitle stream indicators at the top corners of the control panel display the currently playing stream. Click the Subtitle button to enable and disable the subtitle display.

Select the second Chapter Selection button on the Main menu to view the Chapter Index menu. This shows the three chapters in the main video clip (see Figure 13.7).

FIGURE 13.6

The Play Video menu selection displays the main video clip with accompanying subtitles.

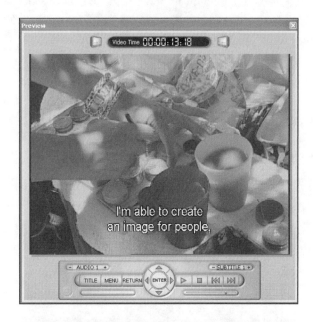

FIGURE 13.7

The Chapter Selection menu item displays the Chapter Index menu with motion video for the clip thumbnail buttons.

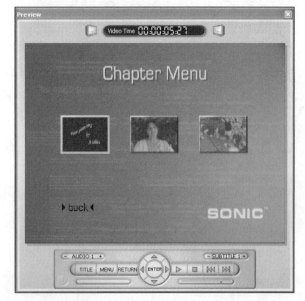

The Chapter menu is a second kind of "motion menu," having the appearance of a still background with motion video in the thumbnail buttons for the clips. Again, to ReelDVD, this is just a track with video and links. The video clip in this track was composited together by combining the background graphic, the menu title text and button graphics, and the miniature video clips of the chapters. The final composited clip was then imported into ReelDVD, along with the button highlight subpictures.

The cursor movement between the buttons also must be explicitly specified in ReelDVD. Clicking the Left or Right buttons steps the current selection between the three chapter buttons. Clicking Up or Down moves the selection between the first clip and the Back button.

When you are finished simulating the project in the Preview window, click the Stop button to stop playback, and then click the Simulation button so that it is red.

Using the Track Window

Each Track icon in your DVD presentation must have one video stream, which can be motion video or a series of still images. Each track also can include multiple audio and subtitle streams that synchronize with the video, as well as button highlights.

The Track window at the bottom left of the ReelDVD application window is used to assign and synchronize the multiple streams in a track. Although the window layout is similar to a timeline used in a nonlinear editor, such as Adobe Premiere, it is not used for editing the streams; it is used just for organizing and positioning them in the playback of the track and for adding chapter points.

When you click on a video clip Track icon in the Storyboard window, ReelDVD displays its streams in the Track window. ReelDVD supports two types of additional streams: audio and subpicture. Subpicture streams are used for all graphics and text overlays, including subtitles and menu button highlights.

Tracks can contain up to eight audio streams for multiple language support, or alternate dialog and music tracks. Tracks can have up to 32 subtitle streams for multiple language support, or other alternate text or even graphical annotation.

Click on the Main_Movie video Track icon (04_Main_Movie.mpv) to display its streams in the Track window (see Figure 13.8). It contains the main video stream (04_Main_Movie.mpv MPEG-2 video), its associated audio stream (04_Main_Movie.ac3 Dolby Digital audio), and a subpicture track with a series of subtitles (Subtitle.01.bmp still image).

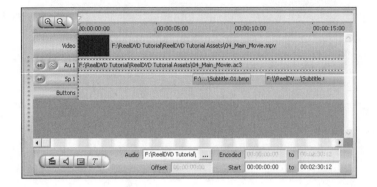

Drag the green Timeline cursor to view the corresponding timecode and video in the Preview window. Click the Zoom In and Zoom Out buttons at the top left of the Track window to view the full tracks. The track also has a series of chapter points defined within it, indicated by yellow triangles above the timeline and vertical dashed lines across the streams.

You can add new streams by dragging and dropping a file from the Explorer window to the Track icon in the Storyboard window or to the Track window. But for more control over the assignment of specific streams to specific tracks, you also can use the buttons at the lower left of the window to add a new audio, subpicture, or subtitle stream (the first button adds a new chapter point).

Each asset in ReelDVD is associated with a file on disk. Click on a stream to display its attributes in the fields below the timeline.

For audio streams, the Audio field shows the source audio filename. The Start field shows the timecode within the main video stream when playback of the audio will begin and end. ReelDVD also can use timecode in Dolby Digital audio files to sync to video timecode.

For subpicture streams, the Subpicture field contains the Start time and a Type field for a Menu or Simple (timed) or Infinite graphic overlay.

When a track contains a subpicture stream, ReelDVD also automatically adds a button stream, which contains the button hot spots and link commands, as defined in the Preview window and Storyboard area, respectively.

Working with Video Tracks and Chapters

The most visible feature of DVD design is the interactivity, with menus and links between video clips. But even a single clip can be quite long (for example, a two-hour movie), so the DVD format provides a second form of interactivity in the form of chapter points for skipping between predefined points within an individual clip.

While you are watching a clip, you can press the Skip Forward and Skip Reverse buttons on the Remote Control to skip to the next or previous chapter point. Chapter points also can be used for scene index menus to provide a visual index of a clip or group of clips.

Click on the Main_Movie video Track icon in the Storyboard area to display its streams in the Track window (see Figure 13.9).

To view the entire track, click on the Zoom Out button at the top left of the Track window to zoom back to see the entire timeline, with its associated audio stream, and a subpicture track with subtitles. To make more room, you also can hide the Preview window by using the View menu or the toolbar.

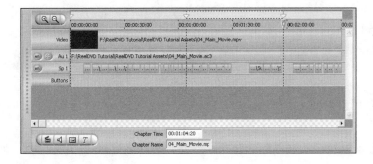

FIGURE 13.9

Zoom out the Track window to view the chapter points.

Creating New Tracks

Each track in ReelDVD contains one main video stream. A video stream can be an MPEG (MPEG-1 or MPEG-2) motion video sequence or a series of still images for a slide show.

To build a new video track like this, you first create the track by dragging and dropping the background video clip file from the Explorer window into the Storyboard area. ReelDVD then creates a new Track icon, labeled with the clip filename.

Then you simply drag and drop the associated audio clip file onto the Track icon. ReelDVD automatically creates an audio stream in the track, and inserts the audio file at the start of the stream.

You can add up to eight audio streams to each track. The viewer can switch between these streams by pressing the Audio button on the Remote Control, or they can be selected automatically by the current language setting in the Player.

You can create an audio stream from one audio file or assemble multiple shorter files into a single stream. The audio stream cannot be longer than the main video stream, and there cannot be any gaps between multiple clips in a single stream. Also, you must pay attention to how you assign audio to the available streams, both within a track and across tracks. You cannot have an empty track above a higher-numbered stream (that is, stream 3 used, but stream 2 or 1 empty). Also, all the streams in a specific stream number must be in the same format across all the tracks (in the same audio format and bit rate).

Creating Chapter Points

The chapter points defined in the track are indicated by yellow triangles above the timeline and by vertical dashed lines across the streams.

To create a new chapter point, first drag the green cursor in the timeline to the approximate position of the new chapter. As you drag the cursor, ReelDVD displays the corresponding video in the Preview window, and updates the timecode above it. You can be more precise in positioning the cursor by zooming in the timeline, and you can adjust the chapter point after it is created.

Then, click on the New Chapter button at the bottom left of the Track window to create a new chapter point at the current cursor position. ReelDVD adds a new yellow triangle chapter marker to the timeline and draws a vertical dashed line down across the streams. Because of the way MPEG video is compressed in groups of frames, the chapter position may need to be adjusted slightly to the nearest group boundary.

To view and adjust a chapter point, click on the gray bar to the right of a chapter marker triangle. ReelDVD displays the Chapter Time and Name at the bottom of the window. To adjust the chapter point, drag the chapter marker or type a new timecode into the Chapter Time field.

Working with Slide Shows

Tracks in ReelDVD can contain a video clip or a single still image (typically for a menu), or a slide show with a series of still images. ReelDVD supports two different forms of still image slide shows: a pretimed slide show and a still show that the viewer manually advances through.

A slide show in ReelDVD is a timed presentation of images, each displayed for a duration set by the DVD author and then automatically advancing to the next image. Slide shows can have one or more audio or subtitle tracks to accompany the slide presentation.

Still shows do not advance automatically; instead, the viewer must press a key on the Remote Control to step through the images. Because still shows do not have a fixed duration, they do not have audio or subtitle streams.

Click on the slide's video Track icon (05_Slide_A.bmp) to display its streams in the Track window (see Figure 13.10). The main video stream contains a series of still images. The audio stream uses the 05_Slide_Show.ac3 background track.

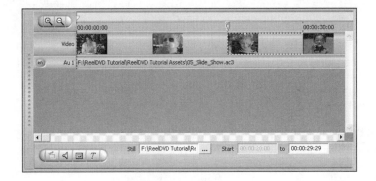

FIGURE 13.10

A slide show contains a sequence of still images, displayed automatically for a specified duration with an accompanying audio stream.

Creating a Slide Show

To create a new slide show or still show, drag and drop the first image file onto the Storyboard area. ReelDVD prompts you to specify the type of track to be created from the image: a Still Menu, a Still Show, or a Slide Show. ReelDVD then creates a new Track icon for the slide show, with one image in the video stream. You can then select the remaining images in the show as a group, and drag and drop them onto the video stream to the right of the first image. ReelDVD will add each image to the stream.

Each image has a default duration of 10 seconds. You can adjust the duration by dragging the edge of the thumbnail in the stream, or by selecting the thumbnail and entering a new duration in the fields at the bottom of the track editor.

Adding Audio

As with a video track, you can add an audio stream to a slide show by dragging and dropping it onto the Track icon. ReelDVD then adds a new audio stream to the track.

If the audio file in the audio stream is shorter than the duration of the slide show in the video stream (typically because it is intended to be used as a repeating background), you can drag multiple copies of the audio file (or different files) to the stream to fill in the duration of the track.

Working with Subtitles and Languages

In addition to multiple audio streams, tracks can contain multiple subtitle streams. Like audio, only one subtitle can be displayed at a time.

Subpicture streams are used to overlay graphics and text over the video or images in a track. Subpictures are created from a limited palette of only four colors (two bits).

For menus, subpictures are used to create the interactive menu button highlights composited over the background static menu image.

For subtitles, multiple subpictures are displayed in a timed sequence over the background video or slide show. Subtitles are displayed only if they have been enabled by the viewer or player.

Menu subpictures and subtitles are simply image files that are overlaid on the main video stream. They can be imported from image files created outside of ReelDVD, or subtitles can be created with the Subtitle Editor built in to ReelDVD.

Click on the Main_Movie video Track icon to display its streams in the Track window with a series of subtitles (refer to Figure 13.8 and 13.9). These subtitles are synchronized to the playback of the video and audio streams. ReelDVD supports two types of subtitles: Simple subtitles with a specified duration, and Infinite subtitles that display until the next subtitle or to the end of the chapter.

Using Subtitles

You can create subtitle images manually as an image file in a graphics editor. ReelDVD also provides a built-in Subtitle Editor. Click on the last button, New Subtitle, on the lower left of the Track window to display the Create Subtitle dialog box. You can then edit the text; adjust its attributes, screen location, color, and contrast; and adjust the start and stop time. You also can edit an existing subtitle at the current position of the green timeline indicator.

The Tutorial includes a series of subtitle images in the Subtitles folder (Subtitle.01.bmp) with the text of the voice-over audio (see Figure 13.11). The text is defined with the face of the characters, plus an inner and outer edge to help the text stand out from the video background.

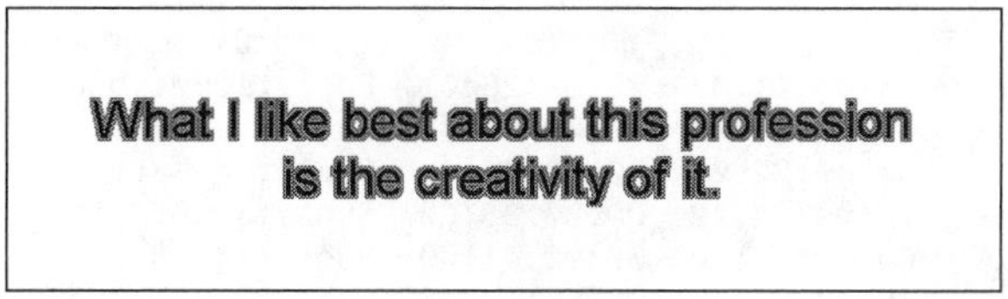

What I like best about this profession is the creativity of it.

FIGURE 13.11

Subtitles are defined as four-color graphics image files.

Subtitle images can be imported into ReelDVD as individual files or in a group using a subtitle script. The tutorial includes a subtitle script file (subtitles.sst) that lists all the individual subtitle image files (see Figure 13.12). The script file contains display information, and it also contains a timed list of the subtitles to be displayed with start and stop times.

Setting Languages

By offering multiple streams of audio and subtitles, a DVD author can make content available in multiple languages. Although the DVD viewer can use the Audio and Subtitle keys on the Remote Control to manually select a desired language on each disc, the DVD specification provides a better way. DVD authors can tag individual streams as containing specific languages. This means that the viewer can select the desired audio and subtitle languages in the Player setup menu, and each disc that they play will then automatically display the associated stream in the desired language.

```
st_format 2
SubTitle        Face_Painting
Display_Star    non_forced
TV_Type         NTSC
Tape_Type       NON_DROP
Pixel_Area (2 479)
Display_Area (0 2 719 479)
Color (3 3 4 4)
Contrast(7 15 15 0)
BG   (255 255 255 = = =)
PA   (0 0 0    = = =)
E1   (255 0 0 = = =)
E2   (0 0 255 = = =)
directory F:\\ReelDVD Tutorial\ReelDVD Tutorial Assets\Subtitles
################################################
SP_NUMBER       START           END         FILE_NAME
1           00:00:07:10    00:00:11:00    Subtitle.01.bmp
2           00:00:12:00    00:00:17:00    Subtitle.02.bmp
3           00:00:17:01    00:00:21:00    Subtitle.03.bmp
4           00:00:21:03    00:00:26:07    Subtitle.04.bmp
5           00:00:26:10    00:00:31:24    Subtitle.05.bmp
6           00:00:32:01    00:00:34:20    Subtitle.06.bmp
7           00:00:34:22    00:00:38:20    Subtitle.07.bmp
8           00:00:39:00    00:00:41:00    Subtitle.08.bmp
9           00:00:41:03    00:00:44:00    Subtitle.09.bmp
10          00:00:44:03    00:00:47:02    Subtitle.10.bmp
11          00:00:47:04    00:00:49:03    Subtitle.11.bmp
12          00:00:50:11    00:00:51:15    Subtitle.12.bmp
13          00:00:52:00    00:00:54:15    Subtitle.13.bmp
14          00:00:54:19    00:00:55:18    Subtitle.14.bmp
15          00:00:56:00    00:00:57:15    Subtitle.15.bmp
```

To assign a language to an individual audio or subtitle stream, click on the Language button on the left of the stream in the Track window, and then select the desired language code from the Select Language dialog box (see Figure 13.13). When you select a language code, it is used as a global setting for the disc, and is applied to the specified stream position (that is, Audio 2) for all tracks in the project.

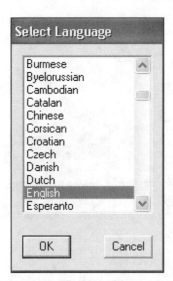

FIGURE 13.13

Use the Select Language dialog box to specify the language code for an individual audio stream.

You also can review and set the language codes for each audio and subtitle stream in the Languages tab of the Project Settings dialog box (pull down the Edit menu and choose Project Settings).

Working with Menus and Buttons

As explained previously, ReelDVD does not treat menus as a special type of object. A menu is simply a track with menu text and button graphics, and their associated button hot spots and links. The menu track can be a still image or a video clip, created in a separate image or video-editing application, and imported into ReelDVD with the menu text and graphics already composited into the image or video file.

Click on the DVD Credits menu track (06_DVD_Credits.psd) to display its streams in the Track window (see Figure 13.14). It contains the main video stream with a still image, no audio stream, a subpicture track with the button highlight graphics, and the corresponding Buttons layer with hot spots and links.

With ReelDVD, the graphics used to highlight buttons are specified in layered Adobe Photoshop files. For still image menus, the highlights can be stored as a separate layer in the same file with the still image. Motion video menus can be stored in a separate image file.

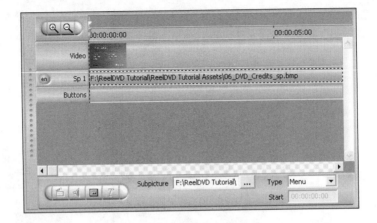

Creating Menu Tracks

To build a menu track, first create the track by dragging the background still image or video clip file from the Explorer window into the Storyboard area. If you are creating the track from a still image, ReelDVD will prompt for the type of track you are creating: Still Menu, Still Show, Slide Show, Still Menu with Subpicture, or Slide Show with Subpicture. The subpicture options appear when the file contains multiple layers.

Menu highlight graphics are imported into ReelDVD as layered Photoshop files, with the highlights for each button in separate layers. This process is much more efficient if you maintain a consistent structure and naming convention for the layers.

When you import an image file for still menus with subpicture layers, ReelDVD also prompts you to select the layers from the file. The Select Layers dialog box displays the layers in the file, and can automatically generate the subpicture stream with the menu button hot spots, and even the standard links between the buttons based on their layout.

ReelDVD then creates a new Track icon, labeled with the clip filename. You can also drag an associated audio file onto the Track icon. ReelDVD automatically creates an audio stream in the track, and inserts the audio file at the start of the stream.

Creating Menu Buttons

The menu background images (or videos) and subpicture overlays that you import into ReelDVD provide the graphical design for the menu screens, buttons, and overlays; but you still need to add the elements that provide the interaction. They define the button hot spot regions, set the colors used for highlights, and define the links between buttons. All of these actions are done in the Preview window.

The Preview window is used for editing the layout of graphical buttons and subtitles, and for simulating the playback of your DVD production. Click on the Simulation button on the left of the Preview window controls to toggle between these two modes. In Preview mode, the button is green, and the panel contains controls like a DVD remote. In Design mode, the button is red, and the panel contains controls for designing menus and subtitles.

The Design mode controls include the audio and subtitle stream indicators at the top corners of the panel, the editing control buttons on the left, the button link tools in the center, and the color mode buttons on the right.

Click on the Main Menu track in the Storyboard area to display its design in the Preview window (see Figure 13.15). The button elements displayed in Design mode include the hot spot rectangles outlined around the buttons, the button highlights graphics and colors, and the link arrows between the buttons.

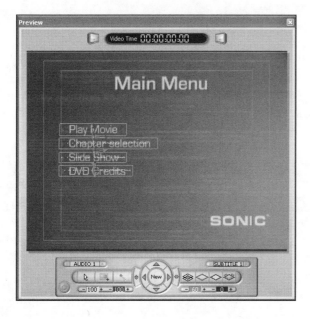

FIGURE 13.15

Use the Design mode of the Preview window to define each button in the Main menu, including the hot spot region, highlight colors, and links for navigating between buttons.

To create menu buttons, click on the Create Menu Buttons tool on the left of the controls (rectangle icon), and drag a rectangular outline over the button graphic in the menu background to outline a hot spot region. This defines an interactive button area in the menu, which is then used to define the button link and as a mask for the highlight subpicture graphic.

Use the Link buttons around the center of the controls to define the paths between the buttons (Up, Down, Left, Right). Use the Link Vertically (Up/Down) and Link Horizontally (Left/Right) to the left and right of the center control to create bidirectional links. These links specify the order in which the Player will highlight the buttons when the viewer presses the Up/Down/Left/Right keys on the DVD Remote Control.

Use the button Color buttons on the right of the controls to select the highlight color schemes for each of the button interaction modes: Original Color, Display Color when not selected, Selection Color when selected, and Action Color when activated by pressing the Enter key. For each mode, use the four colors along the bottom of the controls to select the color and contrast value for the (up to) four different colors used in the highlight subpicture image.

In this way, you can create buttons of arbitrary shapes, create an associated high-light overlay to surround (or even overlay) the button shape, and then specify the colors used to highlight each button as it is selected.

Creating Navigational Links

ReelDVD uses the Storyboard area to define and view links between the tracks in a project (see Figure 13.16). To better visualize the navigational structure of your project, you can enlarge and undock the window, and use the toolbar buttons to zoom in and out and to hide and unhide the different types of link arrows.

FIGURE 13.16

Use the Storyboard area to create links between Track icons by dragging arrows from the appropriate edge of the source tracks.

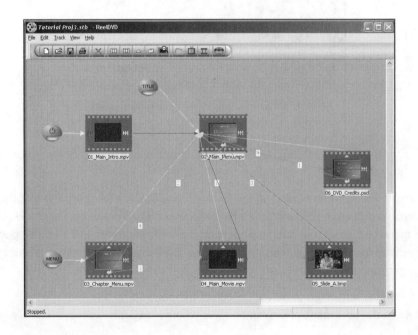

Defining Global Links

The DVD specification includes the capability to designate three tracks that the viewer can access directly at any time by pressing dedicated buttons on the DVD Remote Control. The Storyboard contains three special icons corresponding to these global DVD settings (shown with yellow arrows).

The AutoPlay icon sets the track that will play automatically when the DVD is first inserted into a Player. This can simply be the main menu for the disc, or it can be used for an opening sequence or copyright notice.

The Title icon sets the track that will play when the viewer presses the Title key on the Remote Control. This is intended to access the main menu for the disc.

The Menu icon sets the track that will play when the viewer presses the Menu key on the Remote Control. This is designed to access the Main menu for the current title or section of the disc. In the Tutorial project, it links to the Chapter Index menu.

To create these links, simply click and drag from the lower part of each icon to the Track icon that is to be accessed from the corresponding button. ReelDVD draws a yellow arrow from the icon to the Track icon. By default, ReelDVD designates the first Track icon created as the AutoPlay track, but this can be changed. You should define all three of these actions for your production so that the viewer can take advantage of this DVD navigation convention.

Defining Track Links

The DVD specification also includes three navigation buttons that apply to each individual track: Next, Previous, and Return. The red outer portion of each Track icon contains four different kinds of link arrows to display the navigation through that link. To create these links, drag an arrow from the associated edge of the Track icon to the linked track.

The Next link (from the right edge of a Track icon, with a blue arrow) sets the track that the Player will jump to when the viewer presses the Skip Forward key on the Remote Control. It also is used to indicate the next track to be played when the Player reaches the end of this track.

The Previous link (from the left edge, with a red arrow) sets the track that the Player will jump to when the viewer presses the Skip Backward key. These keys are commonly used to skip through chapters in a longer DVD presentation.

The Return or Up link (from the top edge, with a green arrow) sets the track that the Player will jump to when the viewer presses the Return key. This is typically used to return to the next higher level of a menu hierarchy.

If the destination track for a link is a video track with chapters defined in it, ReelDVD displays a Select Chapter dialog box to select the destination point within the video clip. The dialog box includes a list of the chapter points, with a thumbnail image of the video clip at that point to help select the appropriate chapter.

Again, you should define these actions when they make sense to help the viewer take advantage of DVD conventions to navigate your disc. In particular, you must define the Next link so that the DVD Player knows what to do at the end of a track. A menu track typically jumps back to the beginning of the same track, so that it continues to be displayed until the user makes a selection, and any motion menu elements or an audio track continue to repeat. A video track may jump back to the menu from which it was accessed, or it may jump to another video track in a sequence.

Defining Menu Command Links

Track icons that contain menus with button hot spots also need to have the destination for the button links defined.

When a button is created in a track, the Command link (from the bottom edge) is used to define a button link to another track (magenta arrow) or a chapter within a track (orange arrow).

To create button command links, drag an arrow from the bottom edge of the Track icon to the linked track. ReelDVD displays a Choose Command Button dialog box to select the source button for the link being created.

Creating and Importing Assets

ReelDVD is designed for assembling precreated asset files into a final DVD production and adding the interactive navigation. It does not perform automatic format conversion. All imported content first must be edited into DVD-ready format, divided into individual clips for each track or menu in which they will be used, and compressed appropriately to meet the requirements of DVD playback.

The DVD specification and the ReelDVD authoring layer impose constraints on mixing different types of material in the same project. For example, all video in the project must be compressed in the same MPEG format (either MPEG-1 or MPEG-2) and have the same aspect ratio. ReelDVD supports both the standard 4:3 (1.33) aspect ratio and the 16:9 (1.78) widescreen anamorphic aspect ratio, automatically resizing graphics to letterboxed format when needed.

Similarly, all the clips used in an individual audio stream must have the same format and bit rate, and all streams in the same position in all tracks must also share the same format. There also cannot be any gaps in the audio or subpicture streams within a track.

The global format settings for a project are defined under the Project tab of the Project Settings dialog box (see Figure 13.17). See the ReelDVD documentation for complete specifications of the input formats and requirements.

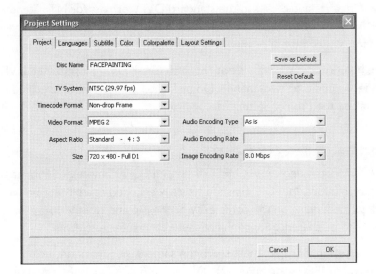

FIGURE 13.17

Global format settings for all assets in the project are defined under the Project tab of the Project Settings dialog box.

Importing Still Image and Subpicture Content

ReelDVD imports still images in a variety of formats to use for menus, buttons, and slide shows. All the graphics elements for menus, including the button highlights, can be saved as layers in a single Photoshop format (.psd) file. ReelDVD supports both NTSC and PAL video resolutions.

Motion menus are actually created from video clips, with motion video buttons and the static menu titles and button graphics elements are composited on top of the video.

Subpicture images must be the same size as the background image or video. Subtitle images can be imported as individual images, or using a subtitle script file (.sst).

As you prepare menu graphics, be aware of the difference in aspect ratio between computer displays and television screens. The images you edit on the computer are shown on a computer monitor with square pixels, whereas the final DVD will be slightly squeezed when displayed on a TV set with rectangular pixels. To compensate for this difference for NTSC displays, you may want to prepare your graphics images at rectangular aspect ratio resolution and then resize them to 720×480 to be stored on the DVD. Unfortunately, this resizing itself can produce artifacts, particularly in thin lines, so you will need to experiment to achieve a preferred result.

Importing Audio Content

ReelDVD imports audio clips in the standard DVD formats for NTSC and PAL: linear PCM (AIFF or WAVE), MPEG-1 audio, and Dolby Digital AC-3. These can be used for mono, stereo, or multichannel sound.

Because MPEG audio support is not required for all DVD Players, ReelDVD can transcode the audio to two-channel Dolby Digital 2.0 format, as specified in the Project tab of the Project Settings dialog box.

Importing Video Content

ReelDVD imports video clips in MPEG-1 and MPEG-2 compressed format at NTSC and PAL resolutions. MPEG-2 clips are typically encoded at a bit rate between 4 and 6Mbps, depending on the complexity of the clip and whether the available bit rate needs to be shared among multiple audio and subtitle streams.

All video assets in a project must share the same basic format, including the compression type (MPEG-1 or MPEG-2), TV system (NTSC or PAL), aspect ratio (4:3 standard or 16:9 widescreen), and frame resolution (that is, NTSC 720×480).

Building the Project

When you have completed authoring your DVD project, you can build it and burn it to disc. With ReelDVD, you first can use the simulation mode in the Preview window to check the design and flow of the project. You then can build your project to hard disk for further testing and to share with others. Finally, you can build a disk image file; and burn your project to DVD or CD disc, or to DLT tape for replication.

Simulating the Project

The Preview window in ReelDVD is used for both designing DVD menus and simulating the DVD playback. To switch between Design and Simulation mode, click on the button at the bottom left of the window. In Simulation mode, the button is green, and the bottom panel contains the standard keys found on a DVD Remote Control (refer to Figure 13.5).

To test the playback of the entire DVD, first click on the AutoPlay icon in the Storyboard area to select it and then press the Play button on the Preview window controls. ReelDVD will begin playing the project, beginning with the AutoPlay track.

As you play though your project, check the design of each menu, the layout of the buttons and positioning of the button hot spots, and the paths and highlighting for selection states. Check both the project flow during playback, and the navigational links between menus and buttons. Also, check the default language and alternate audio and subtitle tracks, if any.

Building the Project to Hard Disk

ReelDVD builds your project by first multiplexing the individual tracks and streams to create a DVD-Video format volume on your hard disk (the VIDEO_TS directory). You can also choose to create a Disc Image file from DVD volume, ready to burn to a DVD or CD disc, or to a DLT tape.

To build your project to hard disk, pull down the File menu and choose Make Disc (or click on the rightmost Make Disc button on the toolbar). ReelDVD displays the Make Disc dialog box (see Figure 13.18). Click to select the Create DVD Video Files option in Step 1, specify the output directory in Step 2, and then click on Start to begin. ReelDVD then displays progress messages in the Information window as it builds your DVD (see Figure 13.19).

After the DVD volume is created, you can use a DVD Player application to play the DVD and to check its design and links again.

Burning the Project to Disc or DLT Tape

To burn the project to disc or copy it to tape, use the Make Disc dialog box to create the DVD volume, and also select Create DVD Image File and Write to Device in Step 1. Then, specify the Target Device DVD burner. You also can select a DLT (Digital Linear Tape) tape drive device to output your project to DLT tape to be manufactured at a DVD replication plant. Also, specify the target directory and DVD or CD device.

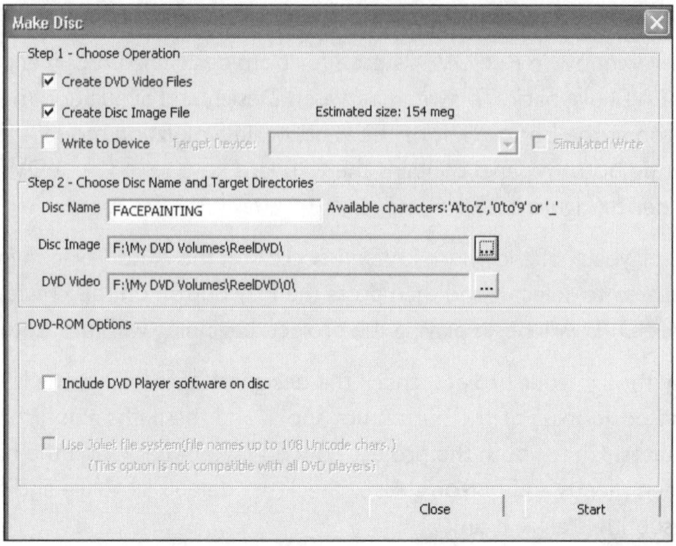

FIGURE 13.18

Use the Make Disc dialog box to create a DVD volume on hard disk, and to burn your project to DVD or CD disc.

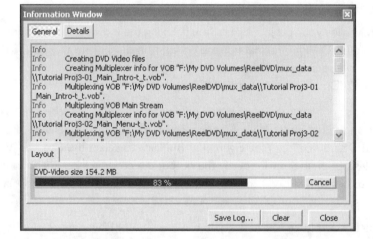

FIGURE 13.19

As it builds your disk, ReelDVD displays status and progress messages in the Information window.

Summary

Personal DVD authoring tools, such as Sonic DVDit! and Apple iDVD, are very effective for creating a quick DVD from a collection of video clips, organized into menus linked to the clips. They provide predesigned graphical themes, automated assistance for laying out menus, and built-in conversions of media assets to DVD formats.

Professional tools, such as Sonic ReelDVD, go beyond these basics to open up more extensive access to the capabilities of the DVD-Video format—with custom menu selection graphics, alternate streams and languages, subtitles, and explicit navigational links. They also provide a more sophisticated interface for viewing the DVD structure and elements, and for editing streams within individual tracks.

With ReelDVD, you can use the Track window to build tracks with multiple audio and subtitle streams. Then you can design the menu button hot spots, graphics, and interaction in the Preview window. Then create the navigational links between tracks by drawing links in the Storyboard area, and simulate the resulting DVD production in the Preview window. ReelDVD provides direct control over DVD features, including menu button highlight graphics, navigational links, and the selection and timing of audio and subtitle streams. Since you explicitly create all menu graphics and video elements, ReelDVD can build motion menus with video backgrounds and clip thumbnails. And you can export to disk or a disc image; burn a DVD directly, or, for professional replication, ReelDVD supports writing to DLT tape.

Chapter 14, "Feature Film DVD Authoring with Sonic Scenarist," describes the next step in authoring tools. Sonic Scenarist removes any user interface abstraction layer for DVD design to provide direct access to the underlying data structures and functions of the DVD-Video specification.

Feature Film DVD Authoring with Sonic Scenarist

CHAPTER 13, "PROFESSIONAL DVD AUTHORING WITH SONIC REELDVD," introduced ReelDVD—a professional DVD authoring tool that goes beyond the capabilities of consumer tools to provide more advanced DVD features. Some of its features are multiple audio and subtitle streams, motion menus, menu highlights, and navigational linking.

Professional tools, such as ReelDVD, are designed to provide the most useful DVD-authoring features for a target audience of independent and corporate video producers, while still maintaining a familiar style of user interface and simple workflow. However, this layer of user interface abstraction prevents access to the full capabilities of the DVD-Video specification. Sonic also offers higher-end professional tools, such as DVD Producer and DVD Fusion. For complete control over DVD authoring Sonic produces Scenarist and DVD Creator—the standard DVD production systems for commercial "Hollywood" titles on Windows and Macintosh.

Sonic describes Scenarist as the world's most comprehensive DVD authoring system—providing the broadest support of the DVD specification. It is used by Hollywood post-production facilities to produce the majority of commercial DVD titles in release today. Some of the more advanced DVD features provided by Scenarist include non-seamless and seamless multiangle switching, karaoke support, and active subpictures.

Whereas professional tools, such as ReelDVD, package up the DVD specification to provide access to higher-level objects (such as tracks, streams, and chapters) Scenarist is more like a microscope—drilling down to the intimate details of the DVD data structures.

Although Scenarist is much too complex to describe in detail in this single chapter, it provides a useful vehicle for exploring and understanding the low-level details of the DVD specification. This chapter provides an overview of the main elements of the Scenarist interface, and uses them to demonstrate the data elements used to construct a DVD production.

About Sonic Scenarist

Scenarist from Sonic Solutions (www.sonic.com) is a comprehensive DVD authoring system, which is used to produce Hollywood DVD titles for commercial release. Sonic acquired the Scenarist product from Daikin Industries in February 2001, and introduced a Sonic-branded Scenarist version in April 2001. This version added the Sonic DVD and CD disc-imaging engine and supported the Sonic SD-series of hardware MPEG encoders. Scenarist 2.6 was released in early 2002, and added support for Pioneer DVD-R for general drives and DTS files created using the Surcode Surround Sound Software Encoder. The Scenarist software runs on Windows and is copy protected with a hardware dongle.

Sonic also bundles Scenarist as a workstation product, and supports the use of the Sonic SD-1000 MPEG-2 encoding hardware for professional cinematic-quality video compression.

Creating a Scenario Project

The first step in creating a new project or scenario in Scenarist is to define the global project settings. Scenarist provides a Project Wizard to step you through this process.

The Wizard is used to define default settings for a project, although these can be changed or refined during authoring, or for different elements in the project (see Figure 14.1).

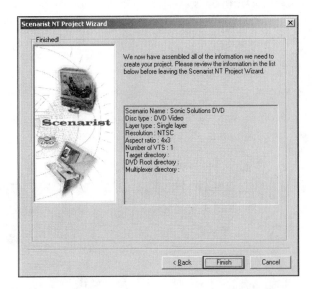

FIGURE 14.1

The final screen of the Scenarist Project Wizard summarizes the global project settings.

Exploring the Scenarist Interface

Scenarist uses a tabbed interface to provide access to the multiple views and associated editors for building and managing a DVD scenario (see Figure 14.2).

The main Scenarist window has a large editor area at the top, and smaller information and browser windows at the bottom. There is also a row of toolbar buttons at the top of the window to provide access to commonly used commands.

The main editor area is divided into two panes, with the left providing a hierarchical directory view of your assets, and the right providing a work area with detailed views of the objects being edited. Scenarist provides access to the four main editors or views in this area. Click on the tabs above the work area to switch between the selections:

- The **Data Editor** is used to register and manage the assets in the project. Scenarist maintains a database of links to all the assets files registered in the project, including video and audio clips.

- The **Track Editor** is used to combine assets into tracks, synchronize multiple streams, set languages, and create menus.

- The **Scenario Editor** is used to organize tracks into programs and titles, and create navigational links between them.

- Finally, the **Layout Editor** is used to lay out the project into a DVD volume, format it into a DVD image, and premaster the disc to a DVD disc or DLT tape.

Scenarist also provides several other windows for specific editing tasks, including the Simulation window to edit menu buttons and subpictures, and the Subtitle Editor.

The area at the bottom of the main Scenarist window includes several tabbed informational windows, including status information, and a Property Browser to view and set attributes for the currently selected asset.

FIGURE 14.2

The Scenarist interface provides tabbed access to Data, Track, Scenario, and Layout Editors for managing different views of your project.

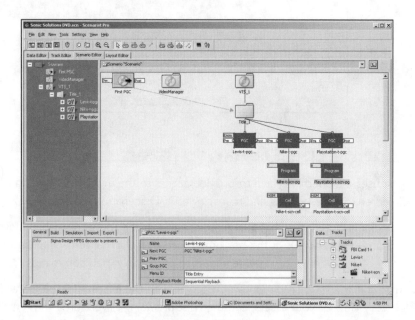

Exploring a Scenario

Scenarist refers to a disc design as a *scenario*, and provides the Scenario Editor tool to create and manage the components of your disc. This includes the actual media streams (video, audio, and images), the menus and navigation linking them, and the logical grouping of this material into different sets. The disc organization is represented graphically in the Scenario Editor, with different icons for each type of component—folders and data (see Figure 14.3).

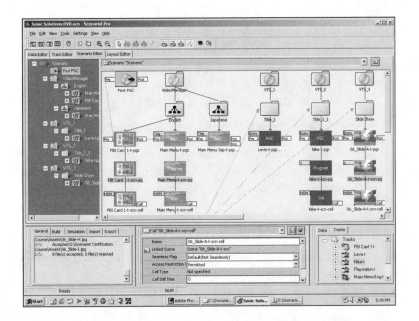

FIGURE 14.3

*The Scenario Editor
is used to browse
and modify the
organization of the
disc into title sets
and program chains.*

The two main organizational elements of a DVD are the Video Manager (VMG), which contains the global system parameters, introductory sequences and typically the main menu; and one or more Video Title Sets (VTS), which contain a set of DVD content in common formats and are organized with a common menu structure. The VMG and each VTS also can contain multiple language domains, to organize the presentation for different languages.

The general organization of a disc within the Scenario Editor is as follows:

> Video Manager (VMG)
>> Language folder(s)
>>> Title menu
>>> Assets (content)
>>>
>>>   . . .
>
> Video Title Sets (VTS)
>> Language and Title folder(s)
>>> Root menu
>>> Assets (content)
>>>> Program chains (PGC)
>>>> Program (PG) (for example, video chapter)
>>>> Cell (smallest general navigation unit)

The Video Manager (VMG)

The Video Manager (VMG) contains the global information and directory for the disc, including domains for multiple languages and regional and parental control settings. The VMG also typically contains the main title menu for navigating the entire disc and any introductory video clips, such as copyright notices.

There is only one VMG, and Video Manager icon, in a project.

The first PGC icon links to the program chain that has been designated to be played when the disc is first inserted in a DVD player. This is typically used to play an introductory sequence and then display the main menu.

The Video Title Set (VTS) and Languages

The Video Title Set (VTS) is a method of grouping content defined in the DVD-Video format. Typically, it is not made available in lower-end tools. The VTS grouping provides two important benefits for organizing your disc.

First, you can organize your material into logical groups with their own distinct menu hierarchy. This is actually the reason for having the separate Title and Menu keys on the DVD remote control. The Title key jumps back to the main or top menu for the entire disc. The Menu key is typically used to jump back to the top menu for the current logical section of the disc—as organized into the current VTS.

Secondly, many of the rules requiring that all source material be formatted, encoded, and organized in streams in compatible formats apply only within a VTS—not across an entire disc.

For both of these reasons, commercial movies on DVD often organize the movie into one VTS in widescreen video format and with multiple language and subtitle tracks. Then ancillary material, such as "the making of" documentaries shot in standard video format, is placed into a separate VTS.

A project can contain multiple VTS folders. Video Title Sets and the Video Manager then can include multiple Language folders to support multi-language discs, with multiple audio streams, subpicture streams for subtitles, and even menu hierarchies for different languages.

Titles and Program Chains (PGC)

Each VTS can contain many menus and titles. Scenarist uses Title folders to organize different collections of content.

A Title is a logical group of material within a VTS; typically a specific piece of material, such as a video clip or slide show.

The material in a Title is then divided into program chains (PGCs). PGCs are the basic unit of playback for a DVD, and contain both playback and navigation information. The basic navigation of a DVD consists of playing each program chain (for example, a video clip), and specifying pre- and post-commands to control the navigation between each such unit.

However, a program chain can be much more sophisticated, and can actually define a list of materials to be played in a specified order. In this way, you can create multi-story discs, with user- and program-controlled branching to present alternate versions of the same program material.

The Program Chain icon then contains a vertical string of icons for its contents, programs, and cells. A *program* is typically a sequential piece of material, such as a video chapter. A *cell* is the smallest general navigation unit for defining jump points in your material, with the video and audio content. A menu PGC also contains a Buttons (menu) icon.

To simplify the Scenario Editor display, you can collapse the elements of the PGC to just show the main icon.

Basic link navigation in defined in Scenarist by drawing link arrows between the program chains. Scenarist also supports the more sophisticated capabilities of the DVD-Video specification for conditional branching and executing navigational commands.

Using the Template Wizard

To simplify the effort of creating scenarios from scratch, Scenarist includes a Template Wizard to create two common project organizations.

The Loop Wizard is used to play a list of clips. It creates a sequential list of PGCs that link from one to the next, and then loops back to the beginning. You can also specify an introductory clip that plays once.

The Branch Wizard creates a menu structure that can be used to select one clip from a list, and then branches back to the menu.

Editing Tracks

The Scenarist Track Editor is used to organize tracks from multiple streams (see Figure 14.4). The left pane of the window shows a directory view of tracks and their contents as folders. The right pane displays a work area view with track asset icons, and a Timeline view of the streams in a track.

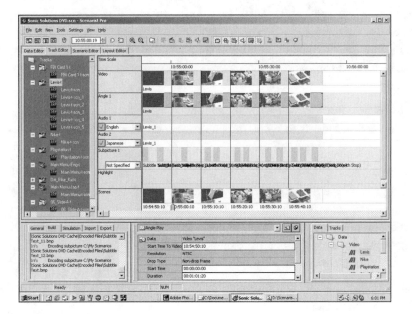

You can drag-and-drop assets into a track folder in the Scenario Editor or into the Track Editor. As you add assets, they are automatically registered in the Data view, and are also added as new streams in the Timeline.

Using the Timeline View

The Timeline view in the right pane shows the streams in a track, including Video, Audio, Still, Subpicture, and Highlight. These are synchronized to the top Time Scale stream.

Scenarist supports multiangle tracks, with multiple video streams. Multiangle tracks can be seamless if they share the same audio streams, so the viewer can switch between different views of a music concert without any glitches or breaks in the playback. Multiangle tracks also can have a different audio stream for each video stream. In this case, the playback is non-seamless, because there can be a brief interruption when switching between streams.

A track also can contain a series of still images to use as a slide show or a still show. Slide shows are designed to automatically advance after a specified duration, and can have an accompanying audio track. Still shows are designed to be manually advanced by the viewer by pressing a key on the remote control—and still shows do not have any audio.

Scenarist provides several powerful editing tools for working with tracks. You can change settings for multiple streams with a single command, for example, to set the language code. You also can combine multiple video files into a single track so that they will be concatenated into a single video stream on the disc. The Timeline view also is used to define chapter points within the track.

Using the Subtitle Editor

Scenarist also includes a Subtitle Editor to create text subtitles to overlay on video tracks. The Subtitle Editor is used to edit and format text strings. Subtitles are actually created as subpicture graphic objects, which can be synchronized with the video playback.

Creating Menus

You can create a menu in Scenarist as a still or a video track, with a subpicture layer to define the button highlights. As described in the previous two chapters, the background picture has the menu button graphics composited into the image, and the subpicture layer defines the highlight graphics effects. You then edit the interactivity for buttons on the menu in the Simulation window (see Figure 14.5).

Creating Buttons

You begin creating buttons in the Simulation window by drawing the highlight regions around the button graphics. Scenarist provides additional tools to help make the button layout consistent by aligning groups of buttons and unifying their height and width.

You then need to create the path links between the buttons to respond to the Up, Down, Left, and Right cursor buttons on the DVD remote control. Scenarist also provides an Auto Route command to create these paths automatically based on the button layout.

FIGURE 14.5

*The Simulation
window is used to
design the interactivity
for menu buttons
and subpictures.*

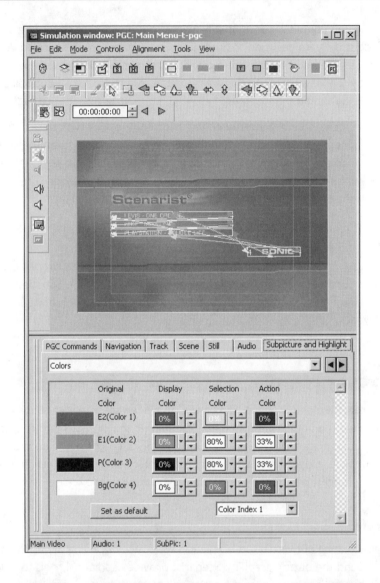

Even better, you can design Auto Action buttons to automatically activate a link. For example, when stepping through a series of linked menus with the chapters in a clip, you can create an Auto Action button so that when the viewer repeatedly presses the next key on the remote control, the menu steps through each chapter, and then automatically jumps to the next chapter, without the viewer needing to explicitly press the Select key to activate a Next button.

Editing Colors

In the DVD-Video specification, subpictures, and therefore subtitles, can only have four colors. These are defined in a palette of 16 available colors, which can be different in each program chain.

The graphics images that you import for menu highlights and subtitles should be defined with four colors, but the colors can be redefined when the subpicture is displayed. In Scenarist, you can define the mapping of input to logical colors. You can even select a range of colors in the input image.

The four colors used for menu button highlights and subtitle text are defined as:

- **E1**. Inner edge, Emphasis 1
- **E2**. Outer edge, Emphasis 2
- **P**. Face/Pattern
- **Bg**. Background

For each of the areas defined by colors in the imported subpicture graphic, you can define the color and contrast (transparency) to be used for the displayed subpicture. For menu highlights, colors are defined for the three button states: Display, Selection, and Action.

Scenarist also supports subpicture effects, animating subpicture attributes, such as location and contrast—along with fade, scroll, and wipe motion effects. You can fade a subpicture for a specified duration between different contrast levels. You can scroll a subpicture up or down across the frame, and optionally out of the frame. You can also wipe a subpicture left or right, changing the color and contrast as it moves. For each of these effects, you can specify the start time and duration of the effect in the Timeline.

Defining Navigation

Scenarist supports three types of navigational flow: links between program chains or tracks, chapter points within a single program or clip, and navigation commands. Navigation commands use the built-in programmability of DVD players to change the flow of DVD playback based on conditional tests of the current DVD settings and saved values.

Program Chain Links

The main form of navigation in Scenarist is between program chains (PGCs). In the Scenario Editor, the PGC icon contains Pre and Post tabs to define links between PGCs (see Figure 14.6). You can click and drag between elements in the Scenario Editor to add one or more commands to the Pre and Post area.

FIGURE 14.6

The Scenario Editor shows navigational links as arrows linking program chains (PGCs).

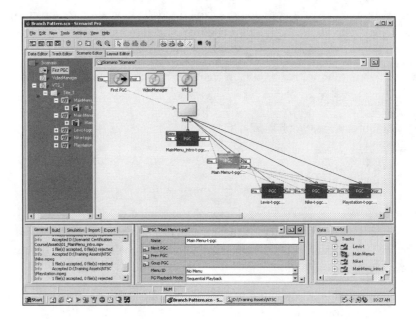

Chapter Links

DVD discs have a second form of navigation when playing a clip—the Previous and Next Chapter keys on the remote. These are defined in the DVD-Video specification as Parts-of-Titles (PTTs), and typically referred to as chapters. Scenarist indicates the chapter-play sequence using numbered flags on the Program (PG) icons. It also provides a Chapters Editor to explicitly add, delete, and rearrange the order of chapters within a VTS.

Navigation Commands

But besides jumps to fixed links, the DVD-Video specification defines a set of commands to control the playback flow of a DVD, including the capability to control the playback program and streams and to perform conditional tests to control the linking.

DVD players include both System and General (user) Parameter registers that can be used to examine and save current playback status.

The 24 built-in System Parameter (SPRM) registers contain the current player settings, including values defined by the viewer as part of the set-up (in otherwords, menu language and parental level), set by the playback navigation (in otherwords, current title), and set by viewer actions or DVD commands (in otherwords, current audio and subpicture streams).

The 16 General Parameter (GPRM) registers are used to store values for use with the navigational commands—for example, to remember when the user uses a menu to choose to play an alternate path story through the DVD content.

The six groups of navigation commands, which either jump to change the navigational flow, or compare and set navigational parameters, are

Link or Jump. Typically plays a video clip, but also can link to a menu or to another set of commands.

Goto. Continue playback at another location on the disc. Used to allow conditional tests based on playback state or user input.

Compare. Compares current register values.

SetSystem. Sets navigation parameters.

Set. Calculates General Parameter values.

In Scenarist, you can place these commands in four areas within a program chain:

- A PGC pre-command to be executed before the PGC plays.

- A PGC post-command to be executed after the PGC plays.

- A cell command to be executed after the cell plays.

- A Btns (Button) command in a menu to link from a menu highlight button.

You can create simple actions by combining these commands, or use the Commands tab in the Simulation Window to create an entire command script.

Although you do not have complete freedom to jump from any part of a Video Title Set into another VTS, you can achieve this effect by creating a dummy PGC in the Video Manager and linking from there to your desired destination in the Scenario.

Building the Project

Scenarist includes the Layout Editor to provide complete control over building your project to hard disk for further testing, creating a disc image file, and burning the result to DVD disc or to DLT tape for replication. The options and working directories for this process are defined in the Layout Editor (see Figure 14.7).

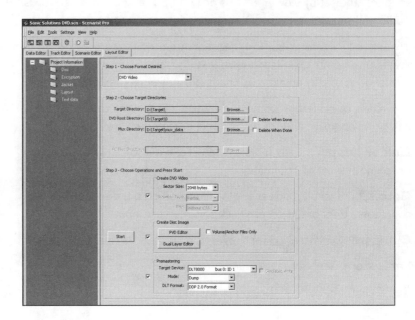

The terminology used for these steps varies, but can be described as follows:

1. **Layout**. Combine the DVD and navigational data into a DVD volume on hard disk. Multiplex the video, audio, image, and subpicture streams, along with navigational information to create the DVD-format video objects. The result is a DVD volume on hard disk with the same DVD directories and files (under VIDEO_TS) that will be burned to disc. The DVD project then can be played and tested from hard disc with DVD Player software application.

2. **Formatting**. Package the DVD volume from the layout into a disc image. The result is a single disc image file that is exactly the format and data to be burned to a DVD disc.

3. **Premaster**. Write a disc image file to DVD disc or DLT tape. The disc image can be burned directly to DVD to create the proper data structures and DVD volume directories. It also can be transferred to DLT tape to be used at a replication facility to manufacture multiple copies of the disc.

Copy Protection

Scenarist supports three DVD copy protection schemes, selected by parameters in the Layout Editor. Some of these can be applied to individual Video Title Sets.

- **Macrovision APS (Analog Protection System)** prevents copying to an analog videotape.

- **CGMS (Copy Generation Management System)** defines the number of copies permitted of the DVD material. This can be set to none, one, or any number of copies. CGMS is defined by a flag in every data sector of a DVD disc.

- **CSS (Content Scrambling System)** encrypts the DVD digital data to prevent it from being read without the proper decryption key.

You also can set the Region Management options to specify that the disc can only be played in certain geographical regions of the world. This is intended to inhibit piracy by creating discs that will only play back on players in a specific region.

Creating the Layout

The Layout Editor contains a directory area and a work area, with the layout process organized into three steps.

Scenarist can create three types of DVD discs: DVD-Video, DVD-ROM (computer only), or Enhanced DVD (DVD-Video plus DVD-ROM data).

The Layout Editor provides explicit control over the working directories used to assemble, layout, and format the disc volume and image. You can assign these directories to different discs, and also specify whether the intermediate directories are deleted to save space:

DVD Root	Copies DVD-Video files.
DVD Mux	Creates the multiplexed video object files.
PC Data	PC files used in DVD-ROM or Enhanced DVD.
Target directory	Disk image file.

Authoring a disc requires at least three times the disk space of the original assets—to store the original assets, the multiplexed video objects, and for transfer space. For a 4.7GB single-sided, single-layer disc, this requires more then 14GB—or over 18GB if the Root and Mux intermediate directories are not deleted. For an 8.5GB dual-layer disc, the minimum disk space is almost 26GB.

When creating a disc image, Scenarist provides the capability to define Primary Volume Descriptor (PVD) project information. The PVD contains project description information, such as volume name, publisher, preparer, copyright, abstract, and creation date.

Scenarist also can be used to create dual-layer DVD discs. You can explicitly specify the point in a dual-layer disc where the data splits between the two layers. Because the layer transition causes a visible interruption during playback, it is a good idea to plan the breakpoint accordingly. The Scenarist Dual Layer Editor permits you to explicitly arrange the order of files in the disc image, and set the breakpoint between the two layers. You can also control the direction of the spiral paths of the two layers on the disc, both spiraling in the same direction (parallel), or outward and then in (opposite). This determines the length of the break when transitioning between layers, and the amount of data that can be placed on the second layer.

Scenarist supports several DVD features that were intended to provide additional information when playing a disc, but which are not actually used much in consumer products. These include the Text Data extension to provide text information about the disc, such as the disc and track titles, and Jacket Picture information to display a still image picture.

Summary

As you have seen, Sonic Scenarist drills down to the level of the DVD-Video data structures to provide complete control over the DVD design. This lets you author a disc that takes full advantage of the DVD format, including multi-story discs, multiple Video Title Sets with different video formats, multiangle video streams, program chains, and menus with navigational commands accessing the parameter registers, direct control over subpicture palettes and color matching, and even subpicture effects.

These more professional tools, including Apple DVD Studio Pro and Sonic ReelDVD, not only provide access to more DVD features, but also more creative control over the design of menus and button highlights. They also explicitly require that you prepare and encode your video and audio clips before importing them into the authoring tool, which also gives you more control over trading off video and audio quality versus file sizes and bandwidth.

The simpler DVD authoring tools clearly are much more efficient for quickly converting a collection of clips, or a videotape, into DVD format. But it is useful to also be able to roll out the more professional tools for a more customized project. And, even though you might not need the full microscopic detail of Scenarist for your productions, it is very helpful to understand the details of the DVD-Video format so that you can see how the other tools package up the raw DVD functionality to provide simpler, more abstract, interfaces.

Part **VI**

Appendixes

DVD Technical Summary

As YOU HAVE SEEN THROUGHOUT THIS BOOK, DVD is much more than just a better way to watch movies; it is a whole family of formats for different purposes. As discussed in Chapter 1, "Making Sense of DVD," DVD is for video, audio, and data. DVD discs can be manufactured as read-only media, or they can be recorded on the set-top or desktop. A surprisingly large number of variations exist for each version.

This appendix provides a technical summary of the different kinds of DVD formats. For consumers trying to understand the logos on a DVD product, the first section provides a visual index of all the different DVD and CD logos. To help you understand the differences between the physical and logical DVD formats, the second section steps you through the elements of a DVD disc—from physical structure, to file system, to data contents.

Appendix B, "DVD References," provides links to more technical details—from laser wavelengths to the construction of pits on the disc surface. This appendix is intended to help you understand the practical differences between the different types of formats for use on the set-top and the desktop.

DVD Formats and Logos Overview

DVD and CD disks, drives, and players come in a sometimes-bewildering range of formats. This technical summary provides a visual summary of the formats and their purposes. Various industry consortiums have developed trademarked logos that provide end users with a quick indication of the capability of a particular player, drive, or disc media. It still remains your responsibility to understand the specifications of the player, drive, media, and software that you purchase to ensure that the formats that you need are supported.

CD Formats and Logos

Although this book is about DVD, many DVD set-top players, computer drives, and software player applications also support various compact disc (CD) formats.

For checking the types of CD formats that a CD music player, or even set-top DVD player can read and play, Table A.1 lists the logos used to identify the various logical CD formats.

Although a set-top player with these logos can play a manufactured CD in the associated formats, it may or may not be able to read different kinds of recordable discs that contain the same data (as listed in the next table). These days, most CD music players and CD-ROM drives that can play manufactured CD-Audio discs also can play music recorded in CD-Audio format on both CD-R and CD-RW discs.

TABLE A.1   Compact Disc (CD) Logical Formats and Logos

Format	Logo	Supports
CD-ROM	COMPACT disc	*Compact Disc Read Only Memory:* Reads manufactured read-only CD discs. Typically used for computer CD drives that can read manufactured data CDs and audio CDs. Most drives also read recordable (CD-R) and rewritable (CD-RW) recorded formats.
CD-Audio	COMPACT disc DIGITAL AUDIO	*Compact Disc Digital Audio (CDDA, Audio CD):* Plays music CDs, with up to 74 to 80 minutes of digital audio.

Format	Logo	Supports
Video-CD (VCD)	COMPACT disc DIGITAL VIDEO	*Compact Disc Digital Video:* Plays video CDs, with up to 74 minutes of VHS-quality video and audio.
Super Video CD (SVCD)	COMPACT disc SUPER VIDEO	*Compact Disc Digital Super Video (Super VCD):* Plays higher-quality super video CDs, with around 35 minutes of near-DVD quality video and audio, and interactivity.

Logos used with the permission of Philips Electronics.

When recording your own discs, either with a computer CD burner or separate audio recorder product, Table A.2 lists the logos used to identify the physical recordable CD disc media formats that a specific piece of equipment can read and play (if a player) or write (if a recorder or burner).

TABLE A.2   Compact Disc (CD) Recordable Formats and Logos

Format	Logo	Supports
CD-R	COMPACT disc Recordable	*Compact Disc Recordable:* Records to write-once CD discs.
CD-RW	COMPACT disc ReWritable	*Compact Disc ReWritable:* Records to re-recordable CD discs.

Logos used with the permission of Philips Electronics.

DVD Formats and Logos

As with the CD formats, DVD format logos have been developed to identify both the types of logical formats that a product can play, and the physical recordable formats that a player can read or a recorder can write to. It also shows the associated blank DVD media that can be used for recording.

For DVD set-top players and computer drives, Table A.3 lists the logos used to identify the logical DVD video and audio formats that a particular product can read and play. These are the base, prerecorded formats defined by the DVD Forum.

Although a set-top player with these logos can play a manufactured disc in the associated format, it may or may not be able to read different kinds of recordable discs that contain the same data (as listed in the next table). These days, many DVD players and DVD-ROM drives that can play movies on manufactured DVD-Video discs, also can play video recorded in DVD-Video format on recordable (DVD-R) and sometimes ReWritable (DVD-RW) discs.

TABLE A.3 DVD Video and Audio Logical Formats and Logos

Format	Logo	Supports
DVD-ROM	**DVD** **R O M** ™	*DVD Read Only Memory:* Reads manufactured read-only DVD discs. Typically used for computer DVD drives that can read manufactured data DVDs and DVD-Video discs. Recent drives also read recordable (DVD-R) and often rewritable (DVD-RW) recorded formats. Often also reads CD-ROM, CD-R, and CD-RW formats.
DVD-Video	**DVD** **V I D E O** ™	*Video DVD:* Plays movies on DVD, for two hours or more, with interactive menus.
DVD-VR	No formal logo	*Video Recording:* New enhanced DVD-Video format with non-linear editing capability. Plays discs from set-top DVD recorders that use VR format to provide real-time recording and updating of discs.

Format	Logo	Supports
DVD-Audio	**DVD** AUDIO™	*Audio DVD:* Plays high-fidelity audio DVDs, with graphics and interactivity.

Logos used with the permission of the DVD Format/Logo Licensing Corporation.

The Super Audio CD (SACD) format shown in Table A.4 is an alternate high-fidelity audiophile format promoted by Sony and Philips, among others.

TABLE A.4   Super Audio CD (SACD) Format and Logo

Format	Logo	Supports
Super Audio CD (SACD)	*SUPER AUDIO CD*	*Super Audio CD:* Plays high-fidelity SACD discs, with both SACD and CD layers. Super Audio CD is a registered trademark.

Logo used with the permission of Philips Electronics.

Table A.5 lists the logos used to identify the physical recordable DVD disc media formats that a specific piece of equipment can read and play (if a player) or write (if a recorder or burner).

These are the base prerecorded formats defined by the DVD Forum. The *Multi* designation is used to identify products that support all three recordable formats.

TABLE A.5   DVD Forum Recordable Formats and Logos

Format	Logo	Supports
DVD-R	**DVD** R™	*DVD Recordable:* Records to write-once DVD discs. Includes DVD-R for General consumer recording, and DVD-R for Authoring professional recording with copy protection.

continues

TABLE A.5 Continued

Format	Logo	Supports
DVD-RW	*DVD* RW	*DVD ReWritable:* Records to rerecordable DVD discs.
DVD-RAM	*DVD* RAM	*DVD Random Access Memory:* Records to rerecordable DVD discs with access much like a magnetic disk.
DVD-Multi Player	*DVD* MULTI PLAYER	*DVD Multi Drive Read-Only:* Player that reads DVD-ROM, DVD-R, DVD-RW, and DVD-RAM physical disc formats. Often also reads CD-ROM, CD-R, and CD-RW formats.
DVD-Multi Recorder	*DVD* MULTI RECORDER	*DVD Multi Drive Writable:* Recorder that both reads the Multi formats, and records to DVD-R, DVD-RW, and DVD-RAM physical disc formats. Often also writes to CD-R and CD-RW formats.

Logos used with the permission of the DVD Format/Logo Licensing Corporation.

The DVD+RW formats shown in Table A.6 are alternate recordable formats supported by the DVD+RW Alliance. These are designed to record discs that are compatible with existing DVD players and drives.

However, each format requires the associated media for recording—"plus" set-top recorders and computer burners do not record on "dash" media, and vice versa.

TABLE A.6   DVD+RW Alliance Recordable Formats and Logos

Format	Logo	Supports
DVD+R	DVD+R	*DVD Recordable:* Records to write-once DVD discs.
DVD+RW	DVD+ReWritable	*DVD ReWritable:* Records to re-recordable DVD discs.

Logos used with the permission of Philips Electronics.

DVD Formats: from Discs to Data

The most important concept to grasp in understanding DVD formats is that a DVD is just a system for digital data storage. The data can represent bits and bytes of data documents, such as memos, presentations, spreadsheets, digitized audio, digitized video stream, or a mixture. However, at a low level, a DVD disc just contains a stream of data—binary ones and zeroes.

Before discussing the technical details of how DVD stores those zeroes and ones (and how it enables the stream to be retrieved as a document, a favorite song, or a classic movie) first consider the characteristics of data storage media, files, and file systems. For example, many of us are more familiar with the context of the disks and file systems of your personal computer.

We can think about the protocols and standards of computer file systems as a series of layers, with the upper layers depending upon the lower layers to provide the necessary support. Table A.7 shows a simplified model of how data is organized on a storage device, from the physical medium to data files. Or, in the case of DVD, from the pits on the surface of a DVD disc representing zeros and ones to the VIDEO_TS directory and .VOB files used to store the contents of a DVD-Video disc.

TABLE A.7 Simplified Model of File System Architecture

Layer	Name	What It Defines	Examples
0	Physical Medium	Materials, geometry, size, recording, and playback mechanisms	Floppy disk, CD, DVD, removable disk, hard disk
1	Partition	Layout of data on the disk in blocks	FAT, FAT32, NTFS, MHFS
2	File System	Files that hold information about the file system: which blocks are in use; which blocks are assigned to which files	FAT, FAT32, NTFS, MHFS
3	Operating System	Programming interface to the file system	DOS, Windows, Macintosh OS
4	Application File Format	Detailed layout of data within your files	Word processing and spreadsheet document files, DVD-Audio, and DVD-Video
5	Application	Creates and modifies documents	Word processing and spreadsheet applications, DVD players

The lowest level is the Physical Medium layer, on which the data is stored. Specification of a physical medium must include information about the materials that are used for data storage and the details of the read/write mechanisms. In the case of removable media, the specification needs to include geometry and size information about the media and the cartridge (if any) in which the media reside so that the media can be easily exchanged between drives. Examples of physical media include floppy disks, removable magnetic disks, hard disks, and optical discs, such as CD and DVD.

The next level is the Partition layer, which defines the layout of data on the physical media. The data is laid out in numbered blocks. This layer defines how big the blocks of data will be, where they will be, how they will be numbered, and where the file system will store its private data. The FDISK command on PC platforms is used to create and edit partitions. Examples include FAT for DOS and early versions of Windows, and the Macintosh Hierarchical File System (MHFS). A physical medium can be broken up into multiple logical partitions of different types, each of which can support a file system.

The File System layer is intimately connected to the partition, and frequently has the same name as the partition type. On PC platforms, the file system is created within a partition by the FORMAT command. This command clears the list of file-names, and clears the list of used data blocks.

The Operating System layer provides a programming interface to the file system that application developers use when they code programs.

Finally, application programs sit atop the operating system and store their data in files whose detailed layout depends on the program. The Application File Format layer defines the format of the data stored in files by the various applications that you use on your system. Some applications, such as word processing programs, use very different application file formats that must be converted to share between applications. Other file formats, such as HTML for web documents and DVD-Video, have been standardized for sharing among a wide variety of applications.

DVD File Systems

An important consequence of defining standards using a model like this is that it is possible to change a low-level layer of the system without disturbing the higher levels. An application can handle files on floppy disks, CDs, DVDs, and hard disks because the Application File Format layer talks only to the Operating System layer; it does not see the Physical Medium layer.

However, if you have a disk that has been set up for a specific file system, such as NTFS, it will not work on a computer system that only understands FAT.

When CD-Audio discs were developed, the standards for the discs did not envision their use as data storage devices for computers. Hence, various vendors developed their own proprietary versions of file systems for CDs used as read-only memory—CD-ROM. Some of these file systems were as incompatible as NTFS and FAT—CD-ROMS prepared with the different file systems could not be easily read in the same computer. Soon the vendors developed a standard file system for CD-ROM. The result was the High Sierra format that became standardized as ISO 9660. ISO 9660 was designed to support the then popular DOS operating system, so it lacked support for important features of modern operating systems, such as long filenames.

The developers of DVD learned from the CD-ROM difficulties, and tried to define a file system that would be uniform across all DVDs, and be flexible enough to support all contemplated uses of DVD. The result was the Universal Disk Format (UDF). The UDF, along with some additional standards for the programming interface to the file system, takes care of layers 1 through 4 of the file system architecture and therefore enables the manufacture of DVD players that can process audio, video, and data.

Because all DVD systems use the UDF, ordinary users do not need to concern themselves with the details—any more than they need to understand the nitty-gritty details of FAT or NTFS to make good use of their PC computers.

DVD Physical Media

Two areas left undefined by UDF and its associated file standards are the physical media and the applications.

Physical media for CD and DVD fall into three broad categories:

- Read-only

- Write-once

- Rewritable

Read only means that the information (audio, video, or data) was pressed into the disk at the time of manufacture; the information cannot be subsequently changed and can be read using a read-only drive (for example, CD-ROM).

Write-once media can be written to by the end user by using a write-once drive (for example, CD-R), but once written to, it cannot be changed.

Rewritable media can be written repeatedly on a rewritable drive (for example, CD-RW), though there are limits to the number of rewrite cycles that the media will support.

To understand the differences between the three media and the need for different types of drives to handle the different physical media, consider how a CD or DVD drive reads a disk. The drive focuses a laser beam to a small spot, and scans the spot across the disk. The disk has a layer that reflects the laser light to a detector. The information in the disk is encoded in variations in the reflected light.

There are many physical mechanisms that can be used to vary the reflection. The method used for read-only discs is to vary the physical distance from the reflective layer to the laser, as illustrated in Figure A.1. The reflection from a pit is different from a land because the distance difference causes the laser to focus differently on a pit than a land—pits reflect less light than the lands do.

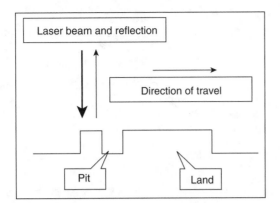

FIGURE A.1

How a laser reads an optical disc.

The method used for write-once disks is based on organic dyes. The reflective layer of the disk has a constant depth groove that is created during manufacture; the reflective layer is coated with a dye layer. During recording and playback, the groove is used to guide the laser. During the recording process, the laser is turned up to relatively high power that can heat the dye layer. The heating causes the dye to become darker and less transparent. When the same laser is used to read out the disk, it is run at lower power. Because the change in the dye is not reversible, the laser can write to a particular part of the disk only one time.

The method used for rewritable disks is based on phase-change media. The active layer of the disk is a sandwich of dielectric, reflective, and recording films. The recording film is a metallic alloy that has relatively high reflectivity when recrystalized by heating, and has relatively low reflectivity when converted to an amorphous state by heating to a melting point, followed by rapid cooling. Pulsing the recording laser to a high power level gives a low reflectivity "pit," and pulsing the recording laser to the lower power level erases it back to the high reflectivity crystalline state. As with the write-once disks, rewritable disks have a constant depth groove that is created during manufacture and used to guide the laser.

Table A.8 shows some selected physical parameters of DVD media. If you combine the various choices for diameter, number of sides, number of layers per side, and laser wavelength; and the choices of read-only, write-once, and rewritable, there are a stunning number of variations at the physical media level using these parameters alone.

TABLE A.8 Selected DVD Physical Parameters

Physical Parameter	Value(s)
*	120mm or 80mm
Disc thickness	1.2mm (two laminated 0.6mm substrates)
Number of sides	1 or 2
Number of layers per side	1 or 2
Laser wavelength	650nm or 630nm

All these variations can be confusing, especially to a typical end user who simply wants to be sure that the hardware, software, and media that they buy will work together. This leads to the notion of formats.

The word *format* has multiple meanings. In the context of DVD, format encompasses parts of all three of these definitions. A DVD format is the result of making choices for the options available in layers 0 to 4 of the simplified model in Table A.7.

For example, DVD-RW is a rewritable version of the DVD-R format, though it differs in several technical details. RW uses constant linear velocity (CLV) rather than constant angular velocity (CAV) for rotation control. This makes it more suitable for sequential access—movies—than for computer data.

DVD-RAM is a rewritable version of DVD-ROM. DVD-RAM uses zoned CLV—sort of midway between CLV and CAV. This provides a balance between the better storage capacity of CLV and the better access time of CAV. This balance makes it a suitable choice for both computer data and movies. DVD-RAM disks usually come in cartridges that are designed to protect the disk. After the disk is written, it can be removed from the cartridge for playback. DVD+RW supports both CAV and CLV, although DVD-RW uses CLV, and DVD-RAM uses zoned CLV. DVD+RW uses a different method for addressing sectors from those the other two media use. Proponents of DVD+RW argue that the differences provide better compatibility with DVD-ROM and DVD-Video with less effort on the part of the user, and also provide better editing capability for disks that have already been written to.

DVD Video Recording is a newer format that is designed for recording in real time to any of the writable DVD media. This format was developed because the formats for prerecorded disks assume that you know the size and running time of the movie or audio track when you start recording—when you actually don't know until you are finished recording. Unfortunately, these formats are not compatible with current DVD Video players. Hence, DVD recording products provide the option to "finalize" or "close" the disc after recording for better compatibility after the size and running time are known.

DVD References

THIS APPENDIX PROVIDES A SHORT LIST of references and web links for DVD-related information and products, with the emphasis on material discussed in the book. The links are organized similarly to the book, with general information, consumer and computer hardware products, and authoring-related software.

See Appendix D, "DVD Authoring Software Gallery," for information and links on authoring tools and related video-editing software.

See the Manifest Technology site for updates to this list: www.manifest-tech.com.

DVD Information Resources

This section includes the primary resources for information on DVD technology, production, and products. (See the DVD FAQ for more links.)

DVD Publications

Taylor, Jim. 2000. *DVD Demystified,* 2nd Edition. McGraw-Hill.

LaBarge, Ralph. 2001. *DVD Authoring and Production*. CMP Books.

De Lancie, Philip, and Mark Ely. 2001. *DVD Production*. Focal Press.

Camcorder & Computer Video Magazine (www.candcv.com)

DV Magazine (www.dv.com)

EMedia Magazine (www.emedialive.com)

Online DVD Resources

DVD FAQ—Jim Taylor

www.dvddemystified.com/dvdfaq.html

Recipe 4 DVD—Bruce Nazarian

www.recipe4dvd.com

Video CD Help

www.vcdhelp.com

Industry Organizations

DVDA—DVD Association

www.dvda.org

DVD Forum

www.dvdforum.com

Recordable DVD Council

www.rdvdm.org

DVD+RW Group

www.dvdrw.org

DVD+RW Resources

www.dvdplusrw.org

DVD Hardware Products

Representative DVD hardware products, including consumer set-top products, computer DVD recorders, and DVD disc media.

DVD Consumer Products/Drives

Pioneer—DVD-R/RW

www.pioneerelectronics.com

Panasonic—DVD-RAM

www.panasonic.com

Philips Consumer Electronics—DVD+RW

www.dvdrecorder.philips.com

Other Computer DVD Drives

LaCie—DVD Drives

www.lacie.com

QPS Inc.—QPS Que! Drives

www.qps-inc.com

Other DVD Media

Maxell

www.maxell-data.com

Verbatim

www.verbatimcorp.com

Vivastar

www.vivastar.com

Integrated DVD Computer Systems

Early computer systems with integrated DVD recorders and authoring software.

Mac OS Systems

Apple Computer—Power Mac, iMac, SuperDrive

www.apple.com

Windows Systems

Compaq—Presario, MyMovieSTUDIO

www.compaq.com

Hewlett-Packard—DVD+RW

www.hp.com

Sony—VAIO Digital Studio PC

www.sony.com/vaio

DVD-Related Software

Software support references for DVD burning and video compression. (See Appendix D for DVD authoring tools and video editors.)

Microsoft Windows Updates

Microsoft—DirectX Download

www.microsoft.com/directx/homeuser/downloads/default.asp

Microsoft—Windows Media Download

www.microsoft.com/windows/windowsmedia/en/download/default.asp

DVD Recording Software

Prassi/VERITAS—PrimoDVD

www.prassieurope.com

Roxio Easy CD Creator and Direct CD (formerly Adaptec)

www.roxio.com

VOB Information Systems—InstantCD/DVD

www.vobinc.com

Video Compression and Conversion Software

Canopus Corp.—ProCoder

www.canopuscorp.com

Discreet—Cleaner

www.discreet.com/products/cleaner

1.33 Standard aspect ratio used for television; one third wider than it is high (4:3). See also *aspect ratio*.

1.78 Widescreen aspect ratio used for film; almost twice as wide as it is high (16:9). See also *aspect ratio*.

1394 See *FireWire*.

16:9 Widescreen aspect ratio used for film; almost twice as wide as it is high (1.78:1). See also *aspect ratio*.

2-3/3-2 pulldown Process used to convert material from film to interlaced NTSC display rates, from 24 to 30 frames per second. This is done by duplicating fields, 2 from one frame and then 3 from the next frame (or 3 and then 2). Both terms are often used interchangeably to describe the effect. See also *inverse telecine*.

4:3 Standard aspect ratio used for television; one third wider than it is high (1.33:1). See also *aspect ratio*.

5.1 Surround-sound audio. See also *Dolby Digital*.

AC-3 See *Dolby Digital*.

AIFF Acronym for Audio Interchange File Format; Macintosh audio file format. Can be used for uncompressed and compressed data. See also *WAV*.

alpha channel Extra information stored with an image to define transparent areas used for keying and superimpositions. Also called an alpha mask. Sometimes present in files prepared using a tool such as Adobe Photoshop or Illustrator.

amplify   Increase the audio volume.

analog media   Audio sources, such as audio cassettes and microphones, and video sources—such as VHS and 8mm VCRs and camcorders—that must be digitized and converted into digital format for processing by a computer. Newer digital formats, such as DV and DVD, have higher resolution and quality than older consumer formats, such as VHS, and also do not degrade in quality when they are copied from one generation to the next. See also *component video, composite video, digital media*.

anamorphic   A method of storing widescreen video on DVDs. The original 16:9 widescreen image is squeezed horizontally and stored on disc in the standard 4:3 video resolution or typically letterboxed on a standard television monitor. The DVD player then stretches it back out to the original aspect ratio for display, either to a widescreen monitor or typically letterboxed on a standard television monitor. See also *aspect ratio*.

animate   To move and manipulate an object over time, such as a title, a superimposed logo, or a transition between frames.

antialias   To smooth out a jagged or stair-step appearance or motion between adjacent points so that it appears continuous.

aspect ratio   The shape of an image or frame, expressed as the width-to-height ratio. Widescreen film uses a 16:9 aspect ratio (1.78:1), whereas standard television uses 4:3 aspect ratio (1.33:1). A DVD disc can store video in either standard or widescreen format. DVD players can automatically format widescreen video for display on standard televisions letterboxing or pan and scan. See also *anamorphic, letterbox, pan and scan*.

asset   Individual element imported into a DVD project, typically from an associated file on hard disk. Assets include video and audio clips, still images, subtitles, and menu and button graphics.

audio stream   Each DVD track can have accompanying audio tracks that play along with the track. The DVD-Video format supports up to eight audio streams per track. See also *video stream*.

AUDIO_TS   The root directory of a DVD-Audio production as stored on a DVD disc. See also *DVD Volume, VIDEO_TS*.

AVI   Acronym for Audio Video Interleave. The old multimedia file format used under Windows for interleaved video and audio streams. See also *Video for Windows,*

Windows Media.

bandwidth   The amount and rate of data that can be processed or transmitted by a given device. An analog modem has very little bandwidth compared to a high-speed cable modem, for instance, so the former cannot download video from the Internet nearly as quickly as the latter. See also *data rate*.

baseband video   See *composite video*.

bit   A binary digit. The fundamental element of computer logic and numbers. Represents one of two values: zero or one, off or on, false or true. See also *byte*.

bit rate   See *data rate*.

bitstream   A collection of data, as in video or audio data compressed to a file or transmitted between devices.

BMP   The standard Windows bitmap still image file format. Bitmap files are not compressed, and are therefore significantly larger than the same image stored in formats such as GIF and JPEG.

BNC connector   A twist-on connector commonly used for higher-end video systems. Used for both analog and digital signals. See also *F connector*, *FireWire connector*, *RCA connector*, *S-Video connector*.

BUP file   Backup file in the DVD-Video disc format for the IFO navigation file of a title set. See also *DVD Volume*.

burn   To record data to a removable disc. Typically used to record a music playlist to a recordable CD or a video production to a recordable CD or DVD.

button   A selectable option on a DVD menu. Buttons can be graphics, text, thumbnail images, or motion video; with graphical highlighting to indicate the current selection state. See also *menu*, *subpicture stream*.

byte   A data element containing eight bits, or 256 distinct values. Commonly used to store a single text character. Computer data transfer rates are traditionally measured in bits, as in Mb for Megabits (millions of bits, with a lowercase "b"); whereas computer data storage is traditionally measured in bytes, as in MB, for megabytes (millions of bytes, with an uppercase "B"). See also *bit*, *GB*, *MB*.

caddy   A case to store and protect a disc when not in use. Many DVD-RAMs use a caddy to hold the disc.

caption   Title text that labels a scene or identifies a location or person onscreen.

capture   To digitize, or import and convert, video and audio into digital format on your computer from external devices, such as a camcorder or VCR. You typically use a special video capture card to input analog video into your computer, and then convert and save it into digital files on your disk. With DV camcorders, you transfer digital data directly into your computer over a FireWire/1394 interface. See also *import*.

CBR   Acronym for Constant Bit Rate. A compression scheme in which each unit of input material is always compressed to the same output size. For MPEG-2 video, for example, this means that the compressed data always has the same data rate (that is, bytes per second), even when the input material is very easy to encode. See also *VBR*.

CD   See *compact disc*.

CD-Audio   A consumer electronics format for prerecorded music on compact disc. CD-Audio discs include only the audio data for each track. Other ancillary information, such as song titles or album and artist information can be accessed from online databases. See also *Video CD*.

CD-R   Compact Disc—Recordable. A write-once compact disc format. Although the disc can be written in multiple sessions by appending more data, the data on each area of the disc can only be written one time. Because the data cannot be erased, the CD-R is useful for making permanent backups. See also *CD-RW*.

CD-ROM   Compact Disc—Read-Only Memory. The read-only compact disc format, used for prerecorded audio and data. See also *CD-R*.

CD-RW   Compact Disc—ReWritable. A re-recordable compact disc format. Contents of the disc can be recorded over, and the entire disc can be bulk erased and reused. See also *CD-R*.

cell   The DVD-Video data element within a program that is the smallest general navigation unit for defining jump points in the video and audio content.

CGMS   Acronym for Copy Generation Management System. The DVD-Video copy management mechanism that defines the number of copies permitted of the DVD material. This can be set to none, one, or any number of copies. See also *content protection*.

channel   The subcomponents of a clip. For images, an alpha channel can contain a matte or mask image to key certain regions of the image to be transparent. For audio, the separate left and right channels of a stereo clip.

chrominance   The color of a video signal. Video signals are split into separate luma and chroma (color) components for higher-quality and more efficient transmission and encoding. The chroma signal is typically split into two components or color difference signals, such as YUV format. See also *luminance*.

clip   A short piece of video or audio, often containing an individual *scene*. You can import clips into a DVD project, or use a video editor to first edit a collection of clips together to create a full production, with transitions between clips, titles, and other added effects.

closed-caption   Text characters invisibly buried within a video signal, which can be decoded and displayed as subtitles by the television set. Independent of any subtitle streams included in a DVD-Video track.

codec   A video or audio compression component that can both compress and decompress (encode and decode) files. Media formats and players, such as Windows Media, RealMedia, and QuickTime have a selection of codecs built in, and can add additional codecs to support new file formats. See also *compress*.

compact disc (CD)   An optical digital disc format used for prerecorded music and computer data storage. The full-size 120mm (12cm) diameter disc originally stored 650MB, or 60 minutes of CD-Audio, now also available in 700MB/80-minute capacity. Also available in smaller sizes and specialty shapes (business cards, for example). See also *CD-R, CD-ROM, CD-RW, DVD, Video CD*.

component video   A video signal that separates the video signal into three separate signals (and three separate wires) to avoid any quality loss from mixing signals. The components can be RGB (red, green, and blue); luma (Y) and two chroma signals, such as Y, Y-R, Y-B; or other formats including YUV, YCbCr, or Y Pr Pb. Requires a separate audio signal and connector. See also *composite video, DV, RF video, S-Video*.

composite   See *superimpose*.

composite video   A video signal that combines the brightness (luminance or luma) and the color (chrominance or chroma) video information into one signal. Because the signal is not modulated, composite video provides higher quality than RF video. Requires a separate audio signal and connector. Also called baseband video. See also *component video, DV, RF video, S-Video*.

compress   To reduce the size of audio or video data through the use of a compression scheme. Also called encode. See also *decompress, lossless, and lossy*.

compressor Program by which files are *compressed*. A compressor which also *decompresses* files (returns them to their original state) is called a *codec*. See also *compress*.

content protection A variety of mechanisms designed to protect DVD content by controlling its use. These include copy protection techniques to prevent the disc from being copied, the Content Scrambling System (CSS) to encrypt the disc contents even if it is copied, and regional management to specify the geographical regions in which a disc can be played.

Content Scrambling System See *CSS*.

Copy Generation Management System See *CGMS*.

copy management Mechanisms designed to control the capability to copy DVD content from a disc. See also *CGMS*.

copy protection Mechanisms designed to protect DVD content from being copied. These include the Macrovision APS to prevent copying the analog video signal and the Copy Generation Management System (CGMS) to specify how many copies may be made of the disc.

crop To make an image physically smaller by trimming away one or more edges. This reduces the dimensions of the image, and reduces the size of the computer file.

cross-fade See *fade*.

CSS Acronym for Content Scrambling System. The DVD-Video copy-protection mechanism that encrypts the DVD digital data to prevent it from being read without the proper decryption key. See also *content protection*.

cut To switch instantly from one clip to another. A video cut appears suddenly onscreen without any other kind of transition effect. The cut is the most basic kind of transition for changing scenes and dropping titles onto the screen. See also *fade, transition*.

DAT The file type used for video data on a Video-CD disc. Contains MPEG-1 video.

data rate The speed at which data is transferred, as in bytes per second. Also called bit rate. For example, the speed to download or stream a video file over the Internet, or the speed at which the file must play from a hard disk. When you create a video or audio file, you can specify the target bit rate at which the file will be played. Also called bit rate. See also *bandwidth*.

decode See *decompress*.

decompress To process a compressed bitstream and recover the original data (if lossless compression), or an approximation of the original (if lossy compression). Also called decode. See also *compress*.

deinterlace To process *interlaced* television video, in which each frame contains alternating pairs of lines from two separate fields captured at slightly different times. The motion between fields can cause visible tearing when displayed on a computer monitor. Deinterlacing uses every other line from one field and interpolates new in-between lines without tearing. See also *interlaced video, NTSC*.

digital media Audio and video sources, such as audio CD, DV, miniDV, Digital8 camcorders, and DVD, that store the audio and video in digital format. As a result, the data can be imported and processed directly by a computer, and copied without any loss from one generation to the next. See also *analog media, DV*.

Digital Theater System See *DTS*.

disc Term commonly used to refer to optical storage devices, such as DVD and CD. See also *disk*.

disc image A single file that contains the data for a complete DVD production. A disc image can be burned very efficiently to a DVD disc because it is in exactly the format that the data will be stored on a DVD. The disc image can be recorded directly to DVD to create the proper data structures and DVD volume directories. It also can be transferred to DLT tape to be used at a replication facility to manufacture multiple copies of the disc. See also *format*.

disk Term commonly used to refer to magnetic storage devices, such as hard disks. See also *disc*.

dissolve A video transition in which one video clip fades into the next. See also *fade, transition*.

DLT Acronym for Digital Linear Tape. A half-inch magnetic tape format used extensively for computer file backup and retrieval. Commonly used for transferring premastered DVD productions to a replication facility for manufacturing.

Dolby Digital   Also called AC-3. Multichannel surround-sound audio encoding, used for cinemas and the home. Supports one to five full-range channels, plus a Low-Frequency Effects (LFE) channel for carrying low bass sounds. The five channels are Front Left, Front Center, Front Right, Left Surround, and Right Surround. Full surround-sound Dolby Digital is referred to as "5.1," for these five channels plus ".1" for the low-frequency channel. DVD-Video discs for NTSC are required to provide at least one Dolby Digital or PCM audio track. PAL/SECAM discs are required to provide at least one Dolby Digital, PCM, or MPEG-2 audio track. Discs may also have a separate stereo track, or DVD players can downmix a surround-sound signal to stereo. See also *Dolby Headphone, Dolby Surround, DTS, SDDS, virtual surround sound.*

Dolby Headphone   Audio signal processing that allows conventional stereo headphones to create a surround-sound effect. See also *Dolby Digital, virtual surround sound.*

Dolby Surround   A method of processing audio to achieve four-channel surround sound with conventional analog audio signals. The signal sounds like normal stereo, with left and right channels when played back through a conventional stereo system. When played through an audio system equipped with a Dolby Surround Pro Logic decoder, it extracts the two additional channels, center and surround. See also *Dolby Digital, virtual surround sound.*

Dolby Surround Pro Logic   The technology that decodes program material encoded in Dolby Surround format.

double-sided disc   A DVD disc with both sides used for data storage (unlike a manufactured DVD-Video or CD-Audio disc with one side used for the label). Often used to distribute two versions of a commercial movie, with a widescreen version on one side and a standard 4:3 aspect ratio on the other. With both sides, the storage capacity doubles from 4.7 to 9.4GB (actually billion bytes). Also called DVD-10. See also *dual-layer disc.*

downmix   To convert from a multichannel audio program to fewer channels. For viewers who do not have a surround-sound audio system, DVD players can downmix the DVD soundtrack to two-channel analog stereo, so the DVD can be played on a television or stereo system.

DTS   Acronym for Digital Theater Systems. A surround-sound audio system used in many movie theaters. An optional format for DVD-Video that requires a separate decoder. See also *Dolby Digital, PCM.*

dual-layer disc   A DVD disc with two layers of data on a side, accessed by refocusing the laser beam through the top layer to read the second layer. Often used to distribute a commercial title that is too long for a single-sided DVD while avoiding the need to continue the movie on a second disc. With the second layer, the storage capacity almost doubles from 4.7 to 8.5GB (actually billion bytes). Also called DVD-9. See also *double-sided disc*.

duplication   To record a small quantity of DVD (and CD) discs using a dedicated recorder. See also *replication*.

duration   A length of time. For a clip, the length of time that it will play, determined by its overall length. Or if the clip has been trimmed, the difference in time between its In point and Out point. See also *timecode*.

DV   A Digital Video tape and compression format for consumer and professional video equipment. The DV compression format is used for DV and Digital-8 camcorders. DV format video and audio can be captured using a FireWire/IEEE 1394 interface. The consumer tape format is more accurately called mini-DV. See also *analog media*.

DVD   Originally an acronym for Digital Versatile Disc (or Digital Video Disc). A family of optical disc formats used both for prerecorded content, especially movies, and as recordable media for consumer devices and computers (that is, DVD-ROM, DVD-R, DVD-RW, DVD-RAM). A family of data format standards for video, audio, and data storage (that is, DVD-Video and DVD-Audio) for consumer electronics products and computers. DVD discs are the same diameter as CD discs (120mm or 12 cm, in diameter), and most formats hold 4.7GB (actually billion bytes) of data on a side. A smaller size mini-DVD disc is also used, especially in camcorders.

DVD-5   Single-sized DVD disc format, with a storage capacity of 4.7GB (actually billion bytes).

DVD-9   Dual-layer DVD disc format, with a storage capacity of 8.5GB (actually billion bytes).

DVD-10   Double-sided DVD disc format, with a storage capacity of 9.4GB (actually billion bytes).

DVD-Audio   A DVD Forum-defined format for high-quality surround-sound audio. Also supports optional text, images, video, and menus. Manufactured or packaged with a version of the album in DVD-Video format. Currently designed for audiophiles, and not supported in many DVD players. See also *DVD-Video, SACD*.

DVD@ACCESS Mechanism for linking from a DVD production to a web site. Developed by Apple and supported in DVD Studio Pro. See also *enhanced DVD, Web DVD*.

DVD Authoring The process of creating a DVD production. This involves designing the overall navigational structure; preparing the multimedia assets (video, audio, images); designing the graphical look; laying out the assets into tracks, streams, and chapters; designing interactive menus; linking the elements into the navigational structure; and building the final production to write to DVD, CD, hard disk, or tape. Consumer DVD Authoring software applications automate much of this process, including compressing the input files into DVD formats and laying out menus with buttons linking to the assets. More professional DVD Authoring tools separate the asset encoding and premastering steps, and provide more control over the DVD design—including button highlights and programmable scripts with navigation commands.

DVD on CD A CD disc containing a DVD-format directory (VIDEO_TS) and files. Storing the contents of a DVD disc on a CD provides a convenient and less-expensive way to share a short DVD production (about 18 minutes at reasonable quality). DVD on CD discs can be played on a computer with DVD player software, but typically do not play on set-top DVD players. To make these discs more universally playable on any computer, some DVD authoring tools provide the option to include a DVD player software application on the CD disc. See also *Video CD*.

DVD Forum An industry consortium of international hardware manufacturers, software firms, and other DVD-related companies that developed the initial standards for the DVD physical disc and logical data formats.

DVD-Multi An umbrella DVD Forum-sponsored logo to identify DVD products, players and recorders, that support DVD-R, DVD-RW, and DVD-RAM formats.

DVD player Either a consumer electronics hardware product designed to connect to a television set to play back DVD movies (a set-top DVD player) or a computer software application that plays DVD movies from a computer DVD drive (a DVD player application). See also *DVD recorder*.

DVD player application A computer software application that plays DVD movies from a computer DVD drive. See also *set-top DVD player*.

DVD-R   DVD Recordable. The DVD Forum-defined write-once DVD format. Because the data cannot be erased, the DVD-R is useful for making permanent backups. Recordable discs are more compatible with set-top DVD players than rewritable discs. See also *DVD-R for Authoring, DVD-R for General, DVD+R, DVD-RW.*

DVD-R for Authoring   Recordable DVD format for professional authoring use. Higher-cost discs that support the professional content-protection features. See also *DVD-R for General.*

DVD-R for General   Recordable DVD format for general consumer use. Lower-cost discs that do not support the professional content-protection features. See also *DVD-R for Authoring.*

DVD+R   Alternate DVD Recordable write-once format developed by the DVD+RW Alliance. See also *DVD-R, DVD+RW.*

DVD-RAM   DVD Random-Access Memory. The DVD Forum-defined, random-access DVD data format. Designed for data storage applications, with the capability to be accessed like a hard disk by reading and writing randomly, and with built-in error correction and defect management. Whereas DVD-RW discs can be over-written 1000 times, DVD-RAM is designed to be written more than 100,000 times. See also *DVD-R, DVD-RW.*

DVD recorder   A consumer electronics hardware product that acts like a digital VCR. Records television programming and input video (such as from a camcorder) to DVD disc. Some DVD Authoring computer software applications also can record directly from video input to a DVD drive. See also *set-top DVD player.*

DVD-ROM   DVD Read-Only Memory. The DVD Forum-defined, read-only DVD format. Used for prerecorded audio and data. Also the computer-readable content on a DVD-Video disc. See also *DVD-R.*

DVD-RW   DVD ReWritable. The DVD Forum-defined, re-recordable DVD format. Like CD-RW, rewritable discs can be reused, but are more expensive than recordable, and are less compatible with set-top players. See also *DVD-R, DVD+RW, DVD-RAM.*

DVD+RW   Alternate DVD ReWritable format developed by the DVD+RW Alliance. Intended to replace the capabilities of DVD-RW and DVD-RAM and also provide higher compatibility with set-top players. See also *DVD+R, DVD-RW.*

DVD+RW Alliance   An industry consortium developed the alternate recordable DVD formats, DVD+R and DVD+RW ("DVD plus"). See also *DVD Forum.*

DVD-Video   A DVD Forum-defined format for movies on DVD, including high-quality video and surround-sound audio; interactive navigation with menus and programmable control; and multilanguage and alternate viewing support with multiple video, audio, and subtitle streams. See also *DVD-Audio, DVD-ROM*.

DVD Volume   The DVD disc directory structure and files. You can create a DVD Volume on hard disk to play and test a project with a DVD player software application or burn the same files to a DVD disc. The DVD Volume is stored under a VIDEO_TS directory for the DVD-Video format. It includes Video Object (VOB) files with the actual multimedia data, video and audio; plus associated navigation information (IFO) and backup (BUP) files that describe their contents. These files are created for each Video Title Set (VTS), with the data split into multiple VOB files so that each file is no larger than 1GB. See also *layout*.

DVD-VR   DVD Video Recording. A modified form of the DVD format used to provide enhanced recording capabilities on some video recorders. Not as compatible with all DVD-Video players.

dynamic range   The difference between the softest and loudest sounds. Decrease to compress the range and reduce noise, or expand to emphasize volume differences.

effect   The result of processing audio and video clips to enhance, improve, or distort them. See also *filter*.

encode   See *compress*.

enhanced DVD   A general term for a DVD-Video disc that also contains computer-readable material. The disc includes both the DVD-Video portion and a DVD-ROM data portion that is ignored by set-top DVD players. The enhanced features may include computer applications (PC- and/or Macintosh-specific, web pages, or dynamic links) from the DVD playback to online web content. Also called hybrid DVD. See also *Web DVD*.

export   To save your production to a file or to an external device. See *import*.

F connector   A video connector with a thin center wire typically used for antenna connections and RF signals. See also *BNC connector, Firewire connector, RCA connector, RF video, S-Video connector*.

fade   A gradual transition from one clip to another. With video, the clip changes from transparent to fully opaque (or vice versa) to fade in or out. With audio, the gain changes between silence and full volume.

field   For interlaced video sources, a full frame is constructed from alternating odd and even lines from two video fields captured at slightly different times. See also *interlaced video*.

filter   A transformation applied to a video or audio clip to enhance it or create a visual or auditory effect. See also *effect*.

FireWire   A digital data interface standard that provides a high-speed Plug-and-Play interface for personal computers. Used for connecting DV camcorders to computers, as well as to hard disk drives and DVD drives. Supports up to 480Mbps data rate. Also known as IEEE 1394 and Sony iLink. See also *USB*.

FireWire connector   A roughly rectangular, hot-pluggable connector used for FireWire/IEEE 1394 digital connections, especially digital video signals, such as from DV camcorders. The connectors can vary in size: full-size (6-pin) for connecting to a computer or hub, and smaller (4-pin) for connecting to equipment, such as DV camcorders. See also *BNC connector*, *DV*, *F connector*, *RCA connector*, *S-Video connector*.

First Play   Identifies the first element to be played when a DVD is first inserted in a player. Typically, an introductory sequence, such as a copyright notice or the main disc Title menu. See also *Title menu*.

format   To prepare storage media, such as CD or DVD discs for writing. Also, in DVD authoring, often used to describe packaging the DVD Volume directories and files from a layout into a single disc image file, ready to burn to a DVD disc. See also *disc image*, *premaster*.

fps   Frames per second. See also *frame rate*.

frame rate   Playback speed as determined in frames per second.

frames   The individual video images that make up a moving sequence. Video formats and individual clips are typically described in terms of the resolution of the individual frames, and the frame rate at which they are played. See also *frame rate*, *field*.

gain   Overall audio output volume. Increase gain to *amplify* a clip, or decrease gain to *attenuate* a clip, making it quieter.

gamma   A display setting related to the brightness of the middle tones of an image. You can adjust the gamma of an image to lighten or darken the midtones (the middle-gray levels), without significantly changing the dark and light areas (the shadows and highlights).

GB Gigabytes (billions of bytes). In computer use, a gigabyte actually represents the closest binary power of 2 to a billion, or 1024 cubed. In general use in advertising DVD disc capacity, however, the number of "GB" is actually used to specify a different value, a billion decimal. See also *byte, MB*.

General Parameter (GPRM) Registers Sixteen general variables in DVD players that can be used to store values for use with scripts and navigational commands to program interactive behavior. See also *System Parameter (SPRM) Registers*.

GIF Acronym for Graphics Interchange Format. A still image file format commonly used on web pages for simple illustrations and animations. Use the JPEG format for photographic images.

GOP Acronym for Group of Pictures. In MPEG-2 video compression, a short sequence of interrelated frames.

hybrid DVD A general term for a DVD-Video disc that contains both video and computer content. See also *enhanced DVD*.

Hz Hertz. A measurement used for audio sampling rate, as in the number of audio samples per second. See also *sample rate*.

IEEE 1394 See *FireWire*.

IFO file Navigation information file for a title set in the DVD-Video disc format. See also *DVD Volume*.

iLink See *FireWire*.

import To bring media elements into your current working space. See also *capture, export*.

In point A placeholder used to mark a specific timecode as the starting point of a segment in a longer sequence. See *marker, Out point*.

interlaced video A technique used for television video formats, such as NTSC and PAL, in which each full frame of video actually consists of alternating lines taken from two separate fields captured at slightly different times. The two fields are then interlaced or interleaved into the alternating odd and even lines of the full video frame. When displayed on television equipment, the alternating fields are displayed in sequence, depending on the *field dominance* of the source material. See also *progressive video*.

inverse telecine The process used to reverse the effect of 3-2 pulldown, removing the extra fields inserted to stretch 24 frame per second film to 60 field per second interlaced video. See also *2-3/3-2 pulldown*.

ISO-9660   The file system used for CD-ROM. See also *UDF (Universal Disc Format)*.

JPEG   A still image file format developed by the Joint Photographic Experts Group that can compress photographic images into much smaller file sizes while sacrificing only a little image quality. Commonly used for photographs on web pages and in email. See also *GIF*.

layout   In DVD authoring, often used to describe the DVD creation step of combining the DVD content and navigational data into a DVD volume on hard disk. Layout multiplexes the video, audio, image, and subpicture streams, together with the navigational information, to create the DVD Volume format directories and files. Also, the result of the layout step—the DVD Volume on hard disk. See also *DVD Volume, format, multiplex, premaster*.

letterbox   A technique used to display a widescreen video image (with a 16:9 aspect ratio) on a standard television display (with a 4:3 aspect ratio). The widescreen image fills the width of the screen, with black bars above and below it. See also *aspect ratio, pan and scan*.

Line level   An analog audio connection intended for connecting interconnecting audio equipment, and without the amplification required to connect to speakers. See also *Mic*.

Linear PCM (LPCM)   See *PCM*.

link   A navigational connection between different elements of a DVD production, including menus and video clips. See also *navigation, path*.

lossless   Any compression scheme, especially for audio and video data, that uses a nondestructive method that retains all the original information, and therefore does not degrade sound or video quality.

lossy   Any compression scheme, especially for audio and video data, that removes some of the original information to significantly reduce the size of the compressed data. Lossy image and audio compression schemes, such as JPEG and MP3, try to eliminate information in subtle ways so that the change is barely perceptible, and sound or video quality is not seriously degraded.

Low-Frequency Effects (LFE)   A separate audio channel designed to carry low bass sounds, such as explosions and thunder. Used with multichannel surround-sound systems to separate these bass-only sounds that have no perceived directionality, and unburden the strongest bass main channels. Typically, this channel is routed to a subwoofer. This is the ".1" in Dolby Digital (AC-3) "5.1" channel audio.

luminance   The intensity or brightness of a video signal, usually represented by the letter Y. Video signals are split into separate luma and chroma (color) components for higher-quality and more efficient transmission and encoding. In YUV color format, for example, the color information stored in U and V (the color difference signals).

Macrovision APS (Analog Protection System)   The DVD Video copy-protection mechanism that prevents copying from a set-top DVD player to an analog videotape. This introduces distortions to the synchronization signals in the video output, so that video recorders cannot synchronize to the signal properly, although televisions will be able to display it correctly. See also *content protection*.

magnetic disk   Term used for storage media, such as hard disks and floppy discs, that record data using magnetic fields. See also *optical disc*.

marker   A placeholder used to mark a specific timecode in a sequence. Used to keep track of changes, events, or synchronization points in a longer sequence. See also *In point, Out point*.

master   To create the master mold used in manufacturing DVD (and CD) discs. See also *replication*.

MB   Megabytes—millions of bytes. In computer use, a megabyte actually represents the closest binary power of 2 to a million, or 1024 squared. See also *byte, GB*.

menu   The main mechanism for navigating DVD productions. Typically consists of a background (still image or motion video), title text, buttons to link to different elements of the DVD (menus or video tracks), and background audio. The viewer interacts with the menu by pressing the up, down, left, and right keys on the Remote Control to cycle through the buttons; and then presses Select to activate the currently highlighted button. See also *button, motion menu*.

Menu key   A dedicated key on DVD remote controls that typically returns playback to the main menu for the current section of the disc (that is, the current Video Title Set). The action of this key is defined by the DVD author. See also *Return key, Title key*.

Mic   Microphone audio input. See also *Line level*.

mini-DVD   A smaller-diameter DVD disc format, especially for use in portable camcorders. The disc diameter is 8cm (80mm), compared to 120mm (12cm) for full-size DVD discs.

mono   Monophonic audio—a single channel of audio. See also *stereo*.

motion menu   A DVD menu that incorporates motion video as the background image and in the thumbnail buttons to link to video tracks. The video is typically a short clip that repeats until a menu selection is made.

MOV   QuickTime Movie format. See also *QuickTime*.

MP3   An audio file format, especially popular for downloading songs from the web and for storing music in portable music players. Named for Moving Picture Experts Group (MPEG) 1, Layer 3. Uses lossy compression to significantly reduce file size, but often with little perceptible loss in sound quality. Used to store large song collections on hard disc, download audio to portable audio players, and save multiple hours of music to CD. Some consumer audio players and set-top DVD players can play MP3 audio files stored on CD-R/RW discs. See also *WAV*, *Windows Media Audio*.

MPEG   A family of popular multimedia file formats and associated compression schemes defined by the Moving Pictures Expert Group. MPEG-1 video was designed for use on CD-ROMs and provides picture quality somewhat comparable to VHS. MPEG-2 video was designed for consumer video and is used on DVD, and can provide high-quality full-screen full-rate video with smaller file sizes. MPEG-4 video is designed for a broad range of multimedia applications, and is used for web and wireless streaming video. MP3 is a commonly used audio compression format, especially for web downloads and portable music players.

MPEG-1   An older digital video compression format developed in the early 1990s by the Moving Picture Experts Group. MPEG-1 video was designed for lower-resolution video played from CD-ROM and provides picture quality some-what comparable to VHS (typically 352x240 resolution). Used for Video CD discs.

MPEG-2   A TV-quality digital video compression format developed in the mid-1990s by the Moving Picture Experts Group. MPEG-2 video provides high-quality full-screen full-rate video (720x480 resolutiosn for NTSC) with smaller file sizes than MPEG-1. Used for DVD discs, and also scales to high-definition resolution and bit rates.

MPEG-4   A digital multimedia compression format developed in the late 1990s by the Moving Picture Experts Group, that includes video, audio, and interactivity. MPEG-4 video is designed for interactive multimedia across networks, and works well for web and wireless streaming video.

MPEG audio   A multichannel, digital audio format created by Moving Picture Experts Group. One of the three required formats for PAL DVD-Video players. See also *Dolby Digital*, *PCM*.

multiangle video   DVD tracks can contain multiple video streams that can be switched between seamlessly. These tracks allow the user to choose from several different viewing angles when watching a concert. The DVD-Video format supports one main video track and up to eight alternate video streams. See also *video stream*.

multichannel audio   Audio stored in more than one component, typically representing different spatial positions, to be played on different speakers. Includes stereo (two-channel) and surround-sound audio.

multilanguage DVD   The DVD-Video format supports discs that can be played in multiple languages. Discs can contain different versions of material; each is tagged with an associated language code, including audio streams, subpicture streams for subtitles, and even menu paths for different languages. The user then can choose the desired material to view, or can select a language preference in the player setup menu.

multiplex   To combine multiple data streams into a single stream, typically by interleaving sequential elements from each stream. In DVD authoring, often used to describe combining the separate DVD content files and navigational data into finished DVD format. See also *format, layout*.

multi-story DVD   A DVD production with an alternate version of the same program material, accessed through user- and program-controlled conditional branching.

multistream audio   DVD presentations can contain multiple audio streams that can be switched between seamlessly. These are intended for uses such as multiple language support and commentaries. The DVD-Video format supports up to eight parallel audio streams. See also *audio stream, multilanguage DVD*.

navigation   The flow of playback through different elements of a DVD production—including menus, tracks, and chapters within video clips. Navigation can be explicitly controlled by the viewer by menu selections, can be defined when the production is authored (such as returning to a menu after playback reaches the end of a clip) or can be controlled dynamically by navigational commands. See also *link, path*.

navigation command   Programming instruction that can be authored into the DVD production and executed dynamically by the DVD player. These can be used to examine the current playback state; calculate, store, and retrieve values; and then alter the playback by selecting different streams and tracks based on user input, or even randomly. See also *script*.

non-seamless playback   A noticeable break or interruption during playback. DVD playback can have visible brief pauses in playback when moving between different tracks. For example, this can occur when the laser needs to move to a different portion of the disc or refocus on the second layer of the disc, or when the player needs to execute a navigation command. See also *seamless playback*.

NTSC   A television video format used in the United States and elsewhere. Displayed 525 lines of resolution at 60 fields per second, 30 frames per second (actually a fractional value near 29.97). Named for the National Television Standards Committee. See also *PAL*.

NTSC safe colors   Colors that are inside the safe region for NTSC television video. Title colors that are outside this range can display badly and bleed on NTSC televisions. See *safe area*.

NUON   An extension to DVD players with enhanced entertainment or game content.

optical disc   Removable storage medium, such as DVD and CD, that is read (and written) with laser light. See also *magnetic disk*.

Out point   A placeholder used to mark a specific timecode as the end point of a segment in a longer sequence. See *marker*, *In point*.

overscan   The outer edges of a video image that are typically cut off by consumer television sets to ensure that the image fills the entire display. See also *safe area*.

PAL   Acronym for Phase Alternation Line. A television video format used in Europe and elsewhere. Displayed with 625 lines of resolution at 50 fields per second, 25 frames per second. See also *NTSC*.

palette   In DVD-Video, a set of 16 colors available for use in subpictures. Can be defined for each program chain. Subpicture and subtitle images must be defined with only four colors, but these can be mapped to a palette color and contrast level (transparency) when the subpicture is displayed.

pan and scan   A technique used to crop a widescreen film (with a 16:9 aspect ratio) to store and display it at standard 4:3 aspect ratio. Instead of just cutting off the two sides of the widescreen image, an operator pans a 4:3 window within the full widescreen frame to show the most important speaker or action. See also *aspect ratio*, *letterbox*.

parental controls   The DVD-Video mechanism that permits a parent to prohibit a DVD player from playing DVD discs with more mature material. This feature depends on DVD discs being properly marked with an appropriate ratings level and then using the setup menu in the DVD player to restrict playback of movies above a specified level. See also *content protection*.

path   A flow of playback through different elements of a DVD production. Also, the order in which buttons on a menu highlight as the viewer presses the up, down, left, and right buttons on the DVD Remote Control. See also *link*, *navigation*.

PCM   Acronym for Pulse Code Modulation. An uncompressed (lossless) digital audio format. The format used for CD-Audio and one of the required audio formats for DVD-Video Players. See also *Dolby Digital*, *MPEG audio*.

perceptual compression   A compression technique that takes advantage of knowledge of how humans perceive; that is, by eliminating visual detail that the eye cannot easily see or audio frequencies that the ear cannot easily hear.

Phono connector   See *RCA connector*.

PICT   The standard Apple Macintosh still image picture file format.

pixel   The individual *picture elements*, or "dots" of color, that are arranged in a two-dimensional array to define a digital image or video frame. The dimensions or resolution of an image are described in terms of the horizontal and vertical pixel count.

playlist   Typically, a list of songs to be played in a specified order. Used to organize collections to download to a portable audio player or burn to a CD.

premaster   The process of preparing the disc image format ready to record to a DVD disc or to transfer to a replication facility for manufacturing. See also *format*, *layout*.

program (PG)   The DVD-Video data element within a program chain that typically contains a sequential piece of material, such as a video chapter. See also *cell*.

program chain (PGC)   The DVD-Video data element within a title that is the basic unit of playback used for both playback and navigation. A PGC can define a list of materials to be played in a specified order to present alternate versions of the same program material. The basic navigation of a DVD consists of playing each program chain (that is, a video clip), and then specifying pre- and post-commands to control the navigation between PGCs.

progressive scan   Video display in which the entire screen in refreshed (redrawn) at once. Typically used for computer monitors and high-end video systems. See also *interlaced video*.

progressive video   Video consisting of complete frames, not interlaced fields. Each individual frame is a coherent image captured by the camera at a single moment in time. See also *interlaced video*.

QuickTime   Popular multiplatform, multimedia movie file format from Apple Computers (.MOV).

RCA connector   A connector with a single central plug, commonly used for audio signals and composite and component video. Also called a phono connector. See also *BNC connector*, *F connector*, *FireWire connector*, *S-Video connector*.

record   For DVD or CD, to burn data to a recordable disc.

regional management   The DVD-Video anti-piracy mechanism that marks a disc as playable only on players in specific geographical regions of the world. See also *content protection*.

render   To generate a video production in its final form, including transitions, effects, and superimposed tracks.

replication   To manufacture DVD (and CD) discs in large quantities in a dedicated factory. Also includes mastering. See also *duplication*, *premaster*.

resolution   The dimensions of an image, in pixels, typically expressed as the number of horizontal pixels across and the number of vertical pixels down.

Return key   A dedicated key on DVD remote controls that is typically used to return back to the most recent menu from which the current menu was accessed. The action of this key is defined by the DVD author. See also *Menu key*, *Title key*.

RF video   Acronym for Radio Frequency. A composite video signal that has been modulated with audio onto a high-frequency radio wave that could be transmitted from an antenna. Typically connected to the antenna input of a TV receiver, and received on channel 3 or 4. The simplest and lowest-quality video signal connection. See also *component video*, *composite video*, *DV*, *S-Video*.

RGB   Acronym for Red, Green, Blue. Full-color video signal format, consisting of three elements. See also *YUV*.

rip   To extract data from a removable disc. Typically, to copy songs from a pre-recorded CD-Audio disc to hard disc to organize a collection, and play and burn personalized playlists.

SACD Acronym for Super Audio Compact Disc. A high-quality, audio format promoted by Sony and Philips in competition with DVD-Audio. Typically manufactured as a dual-layer disc, with a CD-Audio layer with a version of the album that can be played in standard CD players.

safe area Also known as the *safe zone*. Margins left around the edge of the image. Used when working with material intended for display on television. Safe margins keep titles from bleeding off the screen. See also *overscan*.

sample rate The rate at which samples of a continuous signal, such as music or a sound, are captured into a digital representation of the original signal. A higher audio sampling rate, with more samples per second, creates a more accurate representation of the original sound. See also *Hz*.

scale To reduce or enlarge an image or video sequence by squeezing or stretching the entire image to a smaller or larger image resolution.

scene A single video sequence, typically shot in one continuous take. For editing purposes, it is useful to capture or trim your video material so that each scene is marked or stored as an individual clip. See also *clip*.

Scene Index menu A DVD menu screen or linked set of screens that contains thumbnail buttons to link to each chapter or key scene within a video sequence. Commercial movies on DVD typically contain a Scene Index to jump directly to a specific scene; then play from that point to the end. Automated DVD authoring tools typically create Scene Index menus to access each clip included on a DVD. Also called Chapter Index menu.

script A list of programming instructions to be executed dynamically by the DVD player to change the playback behavior of the disc. See also *navigation command*.

SDDS Acronym for Sony Dynamic Digital Sound. A multichannel, surround-sound audio format used for cinemas. An optional format for DVD-Video. See also *Dolby Digital*, *DTS*.

seamless playback Continuous play without noticeable breaks or glitches. The DVD-Video format is designed to permit the user to switch seamlessly between alternate video, audio, and subtitle streams while playing a track. The streams must be authored in compatible formats. See also *non-seamless playback*.

set-top DVD player A consumer electronics hardware product that plays back DVD movies. The player box can connect to a television set, to an advanced digital or widescreen display, and to a surround-sound audio system. See also *DVD player application*, *DVD recorder*.

Setup menu   For set-top DVD players, a menu built in to the player hardware to access global system parameters, such as the preferred language and parental controls. For commercial movies on DVD, a menu that typically provides access to alternate audio formats, such as Dolby Digital 5.1 surround sound, alternate audio tracks with different languages, and subtitle text.

simulate   To preview the graphical look and interactive navigation of a DVD project. DVD authoring tools typically provide a built-in simulator to test the design before exporting to DVD format.

single-sided disc   A DVD disc with data on one side. The second side is typically used for a label, like a CD disc. The storage capacity of DVD formats is 4.7GB (actually billion bytes) per side. Also called DVD-5. See also *double-sided disc*, *dual-layer disc*.

slide show   A presentation of a sequence of still images that advance automatically after a specified duration, and can have an accompanying audio track. See also *still show*.

stereo   Two-channel audio, with left and right channels. See also *mono*, *surround sound*.

still frame   A single image, or single frame of a video clip.

still show   A presentation of a sequence of still images that must be advanced manually by the viewer by pressing a key on the Remote Control; does not have any audio track. See also *slide show*.

storyboard   In video production, a series of cartoon-like panels drawn to describe a movie, shot by shot. In video editing, an interface that allows you to organize the sequential flow of your production by arranging thumbnails of each video clip. See also *timeline*.

subpicture stream   Each DVD track can have accompanying subpicture streams that display along with the track. These are four-color graphics overlays used for button highlights on menus and for subtitles for video tracks. The DVD-Video format supports up to 32 subpicture streams per track. See also *subtitle stream*.

subtitle   A text overlay on video materials, typically used to display the audio dialog in various languages, or to transcribe hard-to-understand speech. These can be used much more generally in DVD productions to display other graphics. See also *subtitle stream*.

subtitle script   A timed list of subtitles to be displayed during the playback of track, synchronized to the video and audio streams. Typically contains the subtitle text (actually a graphics file), and the start and stop time within the track timecode.

subtitle stream   Each DVD track can have accompanying subtitle streams that display along with the track. Intended for uses such as allowing the user to choose from several different text translations of the audio dialog. Subtitles are actually implemented as subpicture streams of overlay graphics, so they can contain images as well as text. See also *subpicture stream*.

subwoofer   Dedicated speaker for low-frequency effects, such as rumbles and explosions. See also *surround sound*.

superimpose   To layer multiple tracks. To composite portions of multiple clips into the final production by overlaying clips with transparent regions to allow the underlying tracks to show through.

Super Video CD. See *SVCD*.

surround sound   Multichannel audio material designed to provide the effect of being in the middle of a collection of audio sources. Typically designed to be played through four or more speakers—placed to the left, center, and right—and in front and in back of the listener. See also *Dolby Digital*, *Dolby Headphone*, *virtual surround sound*.

SVCD   Acronym for Super Video CD. A higher-quality format for video on CD discs than Video CD. The SVCD format uses the same MPEG-2 video compression format as DVD, although at a lower resolution, to fit around 35 minutes of "near-DVD" quality material on a CD. Because many set-top DVD players do not support SVCD format, it is also not supported by some DVD authoring tools. See also *Video CD (VCD)*.

S-Video   A video signal that transmits the brightness (luminance or luma) and the color (chrominance or chroma) information separately. Actually uses a single cable, but with two wires in the cable. Because the luma and chroma are separate, S-Video provides higher quality than composite video. Requires a separate audio signal and connector. Also called Y/C, or sometimes (incorrectly) called S-VHS. See also *composite video*, *component video*, *DV*, *RF video*.

S-Video connector   A specialized connector used for S-Video signals. Contains multiple pins for the separate video components. See also *BNC connector*, *F connector*, *FireWire connector*, *RCA connector*, *S-Video*.

synchronize   To keep two sequences playing at the same rate (in sync). A slide show or a series of video clips can be synced to the beat on an audio track. A talking-head video needs to maintain lip-sync so that the audio matches the mouth movements of the speaker.

System Parameter (SPRM) Registers   Twenty-four built-in variables in DVD players that contain the current player settings. These can be used with scripts and navigational commands to program interactive behavior. See also *General Parameter (GPRM) Registers*.

TIFF   A lossless image file format designed for photographic images that compresses the image size while preserving all the image quality. The resulting files are therefore larger than those with JPEG compression, which sacrifices some detail to significantly reduce the image size.

timecode   An exact time used to identify a specific frame in a clip or production. Measured in hours, minutes, seconds, and frames. See also *duration*.

timeline   In video editing, an interface that allows you to assemble a collection of clips into a production with multiple overlapping tracks. A timeline provides a view of multiple sources being combined over time, with separate tracks for video, audio, and superimposed video, as well as transitions and effects. See also *storyboard*.

title   The DVD-Video data element within a title set (VTS) that contains a logical group of program material. Also used to describe the entire DVD production. See also *program chain (PGC)*.

Title key   A dedicated key on DVD remote controls that returns playback to the top or main menu for the disc. The action of this key is defined by the DVD author. See also *Menu key, Return key, Video Title Set*.

Title menu   The menu in a DVD production designated as the top or main menu for the disc. The Title menu is typically displayed when the disc first starts playing (sometimes after an introductory sequences), and contains navigational links to the contents of the entire disc. The viewer can access this menu at any time by pressing the Title key on the DVD remote control. See also *First Play*.

Top menu   See *Title menu*.

track   Typically used to describe a single sequential piece of material, such as a video clip or slide show, in a DVD project that is then connected by navigational links. A track contains a main video stream plus additional streams, including alternate multiangle video, audio, and subtitle streams. A track also can act as a menu, with subpicture button highlights.

transcode   To convert from one compression format to another (that is, from DV video from a camcorder to MPEG-2 for DVD). Preferably done intelligently to minimize loss of quality from repeated compression, and not requiring fully decompressing the input and then recompressing to the output.

transition   A visual effect to segue from the end of one clip or scene and the start of the next. The most basic transition is a cut, in which the last frame of one clip is immediately followed by the first frame of the next clip. More interesting transition effects include fades, dissolves, and wipes between adjacent clips.

trim   To cut out a segment of a clip by removing frames from the beginning and end. To adjust the In or Out points of a clip to identify the portion to be used in the final production.

UDF (Universal Disc Format)   The file system used for DVDs (technically, the condensed micro-UDF). Designed to be uniform across all DVDs and be flexible enough to support a wide variety of uses of DVD. See also *ISO-9660*, *UDF Bridge*.

UDF Bridge   A DVD file system combining the older ISO-9660 file system for CDs and micro-UDF for DVDs to provide backward compatibility for DVD players and computers.

USB (Universal Serial Bus)   A digital data interface standard providing a Plug-and-Play interface for personal computers. Typically used for lower-speed peripherals, such as mice, keyboards, printers, and scanners. Also used for interfacing to digital cameras. The existing USB 1 standard provides up to 12Mbps (million bits per second) data rate. The new USB 2 standard supports up to 480Mbps data rate. See also *FireWire*.

VBR   Acronym for Variable Bit Rate. A compression scheme in which each unit of input material can be compressed to different sizes. For MPEG-2 video, for example, this means that "easier" sequences (that is, with no motion) can compress to very small sizes, whereas "hard" sequences (with lots of motion and scene cuts) can compress to much larger sizes. VBR compression can take better advantage of the overall available bandwidth of a DVD player by allocating the available bits intelligently to the difficult parts of a sequence. See also *CBR*.

Video CD (VCD)   A consumer format for storing video presentations on CD discs. VCD can fit 74 minutes of "VHS-quality" video on a CD, but at lower video resolution than DVD using the older MPEG-1 compression format. The VCD format is especially popular in Asia as a format for distributing commercial movies and videos. Many DVD authoring tools provide the option to author to VCD format, and most DVD players can play the format. This provides an inexpensive option for sharing productions with most computers. Many set-top DVD players also can play VCDs. See also *DAT, DVD on CD, SVCD*.

Video for Windows   The media file format used with Microsoft Windows (.AVI). Supports many different video and audio compression formats (*codecs*). See also *Windows Media*.

Video Manager (VMG)   The DVD-Video data element that contains the global information and directory for the disc, including domains for multiple languages and regional and parental control settings. The VMG also typically contains the main title menu for navigating the entire disc, any introductory video clips, such as copyright notices. See also *Video Title Set (VTS)*.

Video Object (VOB)   An MPEG video program stream with multiplexed video, audio, subpictures, and control information. See also *DVD Volume*.

video stream   Each DVD-Video track is based on a main video stream, which can be motion video, a still image, or a series of stills. The track also can contain additional alternate video streams. The DVD-Video format supports one main video track and up to eight alternate video streams. See also *audio stream, multiangle video, track*.

Video Title Set (VTS)   The DVD-Video data element that contains a group of program material that shares the same menu hierarchy and basic data formats. Professional tools support multiple VTSs to organize the contents of a DVD into logical groups, and to include different kinds of material and formats on a single disc. See also *title, Video Manager (VMG)*.

VIDEO_TS   The root directory of a DVD-Video production as stored on a DVD disc. See also *AUDIO_TS, DVD Volume*.

virtual surround sound   Audio processing that creates a simulated surround-sound effect by converting a surround-sound signal into a stereo signal, either for playback on two speakers or especially for playback with stereo headphones. See also *Dolby Digital, Dolby Headphone, surround sound*.

VOB file   Video object file in the DVD-Video disc format. See also *DVD Volume*.

VTR   Acronym for Video Tape Recorder. Also called VCR (Video Cassette Recorder).

VTS file   Video Title Set files used to store the video contents (VOB files) and navigational information (IFO files) for each title in the DVD-Video disc format. See also *DVD Volume*.

watermark   A small, semitransparent graphic that identifies a scene or speaker. Many TV broadcasts use a watermark to let you know what channel you're watching.

WAV   The uncompressed Wave audio file format used with Microsoft Windows. See also *AIFF, MP3, WAV, Windows Media Audio*.

Web DVD   A general term for a DVD-Video disc with web-enhanced DVD content. May include web pages that combine local DVD video with current online content, or dynamic links from the DVD playback to online web content. See also *DVD@ACCESS, enhanced DVD*.

widescreen   A wide picture format for film at 16:9 aspect ratio. See also *aspect ratio*.

Windows Media   The multimedia platform built into Microsoft Windows, and a series of formats for storing and transmitting video and audio. Uses ASF, WMA, and WMF file types. See also *Video for Windows, Windows Media Audio*, and *Windows Media Video*.

Windows Media Audio (WMA)   The Microsoft Windows Media native audio file format. Used for compressing, storing, and organizing CDs and downloaded audio in albums on disk. Also used to download audio to portable audio players. Some consumer audio players and set-top DVD players can play WMA audio files stored on CD-R/RW discs. See also *MP3, WAV, Windows Media*.

Windows Media Video (WMV)   The Microsoft Windows Media format for compressed video and audio files. See also *Windows Media Audio*.

wipe   A video transition in which the new video physically moves into the frame while displacing the old video.

YUV   Full-color video signal format, consisting of three elements: Y (luminance), U, and V (chrominance). See also *RGB*.

DVD Authoring
Software Gallery

THIS APPENDIX PROVIDES A VISUAL GALLERY of software applications for desktop DVD authoring. Each application is shown with a representative screenshot and a brief description derived from the company's literature.

The applications are organized in the same grouping as used in the different parts of this book, from DVD players to consumer, to more professional authoring tools:

- DVD software players

- Integrated video editing with DVD authoring

- Automated DVD authoring

- Personal DVD authoring

- Professional DVD authoring

- Video-editing software

- Video compression and conversion software

These categories, as well as many of these tools, are described in more detail in the previous chapters. The products generally increase in capabilities and price range from one category to the next (the pricing is approximate as of mid-2002). The Macintosh products provided by Apple are included, along with a wide range of third-party tools for PC/Windows systems.

See the associated company web sites for more information on these applications. Many of these companies provide trial versions of these applications that can be downloaded from the Internet.

See Appendix B, "DVD References," for more references and web links for DVD technology and products.

Also see my Manifest Technology web site for updated links and references on DVD: www.manifest-tech.com

DVD Software Players

Software applications for playing DVDs on your computer, with enhanced viewing options and capabilities for exploring the DVD structure. Bundled free with operating systems, or third-party applications for $50 to $80.

Apple Computer—DVD Player 3 for Macintosh OS X

www.apple.com/dvd

www.apple.com/macosx

Macintosh DVD video player

Apple DVD Player version 3.1.1 released March 2002; Included with Macintosh OS X

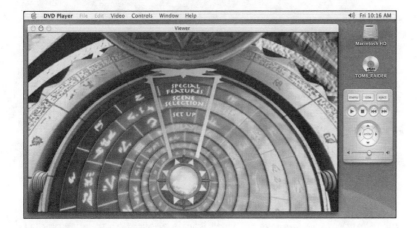

©Paramount Home Entertainment

Apple DVD Player is the Macintosh application for playing movies on DVD. It provides a clean-and-simple interface for controlling DVD playback on the Mac with a graphical controller, much like you are used to with a remote control for a set-top DVD player.

Rewritten for Mac OS X, the Apple DVD Player lets you control your viewing experience, just as if you were using a full-featured remote control with a standalone DVD player. You can access the movie chapter by chapter, freeze the action, zip forward and backward through the movie, play in slow motion, or step through the movie frame by frame.

DVD Player 3.1.1 adds features for DVD authoring, including the capability to select and play the contents of a VIDEO_TS folder from a local volume. It also adds AppleScript support for selection and playback of DVD content.

Microsoft Corp.—Windows Media Player for Windows XP

www.microsoft.com/windows/windowsmedia/players.asp

www.microsoft.com/windowsmedia

www.microsoft.com/windowsxp

All-in-one player and organizer for music and video, CDs and DVDs, Internet, and portable devices

Microsoft Windows Media Player version 8 is included with Microsoft Windows XP; Check Windows Update for latest version

©Paramount Home Entertainment

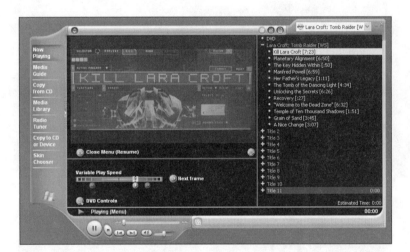

Microsoft Windows Media Player is an all-in-one application for playing digital media, accessing media over the Internet, and organizing and managing a media library. With audio CDs, Media Player can rip songs from CDs, download album information from online databases, and write playlists to CD and portable devices, from music players to Pocket PCs. With video, Media Player can download information from online databases, play local and streaming web video, and transfer video clips to Pocket PCs.

Windows Media Player for Windows XP extends the new interface design introduced with Windows Media Player 7. New features in the Windows XP Media Player include direct CD access from the My Music folder, MP3 encoding (using plug-ins), support for multiple CD and DVD drives, and DVD playback (using plug-ins).

CyberLink Corp.—PowerDVD XP 4

www.gocyberlink.com

Customizable DVD player with enhanced video and audio viewing features

CyberLink PowerDVD XP 4.0 released January 2002; Standard from $49 and Deluxe from $69

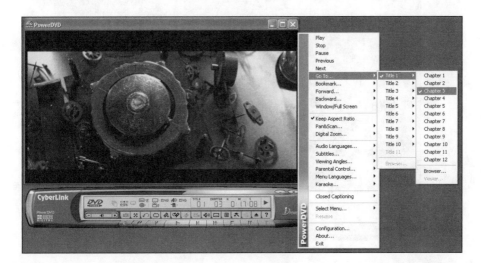

©Paramount Home Entertainment

CyberLink PowerDVD provides powerful tools for playing and exploring DVDs. It supports a wide range of video hardware acceleration, including dual-view monitors. It also supports surround-sound decoding, virtual surround sound, and audio enhancement. The Deluxe version supports DTS Digital Surround and SRS TruSurround XT audio enhancement.

For video playback, PowerDVD offers preset and adjustable contrast and color viewing controls, dual-view monitor support, digital zoom, and full-screen video playback. For audio playback, WinDVD offers dynamic range control, bass enhancement, and virtual surround sound through two speakers or using Dolby Headphone.

PowerDVD is compatible with a wide variety of DVD formats, including DVD-Video, Video CD (VCD 2.0), Super Video CD (SVCD), and the VR (Video Recording) format used on set-top DVD players. PowerDVD is also a general media player; and it plays a wide variety of video and audio files from hard disk, including AVI, QuickTime MOV, Windows Media, MPEG, and MP3.

InterVideo Corp.—WinDVD 4

www.intervideo.com

Customizable DVD player with enhanced video and audio viewing features

InterVideo WinDVD 4 released May 2002; Standard $49 and Plus $79

©Paramount Home
Entertainment

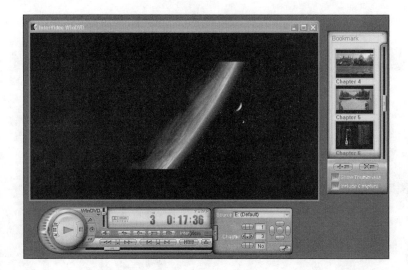

InterVideo WinDVD provides a flexible interface for playing and exploring DVD content. It includes extensive support for enhanced audio playback and a time stretching-feature to play back faster or slower while still preserving normal-sounding audio. The Plus version features include enhanced surround sound.

For video playback, WinDVD offers contrast and color controls, multiple monitor and TV out support, zoom and pan, and video playback as the desktop background. For audio playback, WinDVD offers dynamic range enhancement, dialog enhancement, audio equalization and effects, and virtual surround sound through two speakers or using Dolby Headphone.

WinDVD is compatible with a wide variety of DVD formats, including DVD-Video, Video CD (VCD 2.0), Super Video CD (SVCD), Audio CD, and the VR (Video Recording) format used on set-top DVD players. WinDVD also plays DVD, MPEG, MP3, and other video and audio files from hard disk.

InterActual Technologies—InterActual Player 2

www.interactual.com

Plays DVD-Video seamlessly integrated with web content stored on either the disc or the web

InterActual Player 2.0 released August 2000 (formerly PC Friendly); Included on retail movie DVDs

Many commercial movies on DVD include enhanced DVD-ROM features that are accessible only from a computer, including computer applications, web pages, links to additional online resources, and dynamic links between the DVD playback and online web content. InterActual is the leading provider of software and services for enhanced DVD content with commercial movies. The InterActual Player is included with the movie on each enhanced DVD.

InterActual Player is a software application that plays DVD-Video seamlessly integrated with a rich variety of HTML web content stored on either the disc or the web. Web links can be authored into the DVD-Video or embedded within the HTML content. These connections can be based on events that are user-initiated or triggered by the content itself. Fresh content can be provided online and blended with the DVD-Video content from the disc.

The InterActual Player 2.0 is fully backward-compatible with all PC friendly enabled titles, and offers support for the Macintosh, as well as Internet-connected set-top DVD players. It supports both DVD-Video and CD-Audio, and is DVD-Audio-ready. It also provides a customizable look through skins.

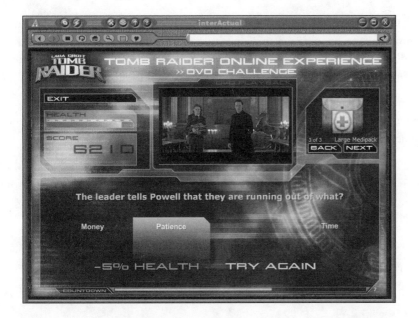

©Paramount Home Entertainment

One-K for Paramount Home Entertainment

Sonic CinePlayer 4

www.cineplayer.com

www.sonic.com

DVD player with high quality "High Definition" video decoder

Sonic CinePlayer 4.0 released June 2002 (formerly Ravisent); $49

©Paramount Home Entertainment

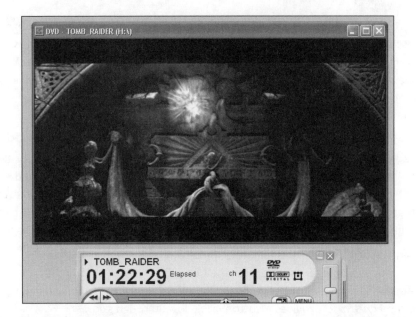

Sonic CinePlayer DVD brings the quality and excitement of high-end home theater systems to personal computers. CinePlayer extracts more picture detail from digital video, and displays it more accurately, resulting in full-frame rate DVD video with amazing clarity and detail.

CinePlayer 4.0 includes a new player application with "Retro" GUI, "High Definition" video decoder (displays resolutions as high as 1080i), and a modularized architecture tightly integrated into DirectX.

CinePlayer plays all DVD-ROM games and titles, supports Video CD 1.1 and 2.0, plays on any resolution or color depth video display, and supports Dolby Digital (AC-3), 5.1 channel Dolby Digital pass-through (S/PDIF), LPCM, MPEG-1 Layer 2, and MPEG-2 2-channel audio formats.

Consumer Video Editing with Automated DVD Authoring

Simplified video-editing tools with "consumerized" interfaces, and recently extended to include DVD authoring. Range from around $80 to $150.

CyberLink Corp.—PowerDirector 2

www.gocyberlink.com

Storyboard-based video-editor with a Disc Making Wizard

CyberLink PowerDirector 2.0 released February 2002; Standard $79 and Pro for DVD authoring $119

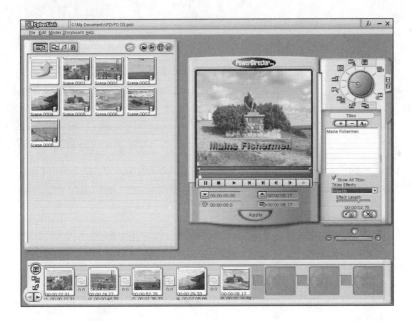

CyberLink PowerDirector 2.0 is a storyboard-based video editor. The Pro version includes an integrated Disc Wizard for creating productions on CD or DVD. PowerDirector has a visually simple interface, using the Modes Wheel in the top-right corner of the screen to select each kind of editing and to reveal the associated interface elements for that mode.

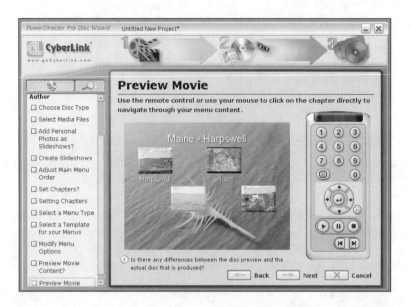

PowerDirector 2.0 Standard was designed as an advanced, yet easy-to-use video-editing software program. You can input video files from numerous sources, such as DV camcorders, camcorders, TV tuners, and more. PowerDirector offers an easy-to-use, drag-and-drop interface and an abundance of video-editing tools.

With the Disc Making Wizard in PowerDirector 2.0 Pro, you can take your movies, give them DVD menus and chapters, and then burn them onto CD or DVD.

InterVideo Corp.—WinProducer 3

www.intervideo.com

Timeline-based video editor with DVD authoring from the timeline

InterVideo WinProducer 3 released July 2002; CD $79 and DVD $149

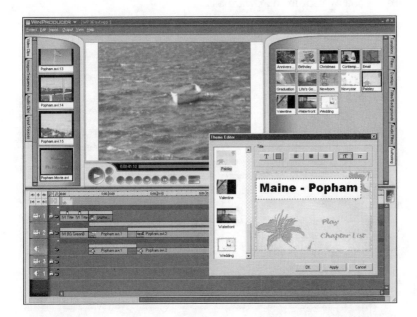

WinProducer provides a familiar timeline-based video-editing interface, in which you capture and import clips. You then assemble and edit your production by arranging clips on the timeline. For DVD authoring, instead of a separate DVD authoring component, WinProducer can create a CD or DVD directly from the production on the timeline by specifying a graphical theme for menus and defining chapter points in the production.

WinProducer 3 supports DivX, SVCD, VCD and DVD formats for importing, editing, and burning. WinProducer can import video from your camera or hard drive and instantly compress it into a high-quality MPEG file—saving space and ready to burn to DVD. It can combine video in MPEG-1, MPEG-2, MPEG-4, DV and AVI formats.

You can use drag-and-drop editing to add special effects, transitions, filters, fast/slow motion, titles, and picture in picture. Preview your work in the live editing window without waiting for long rendering times.

Pinnacle Systems—Studio 8

www.pinnaclesys.com

Consumer video editor with professional features and DVD-creation tools

Pinnacle Studio 8 released August 2002; Software $99 and bundled with FireWire, PC Card, or analog capture hardware $129

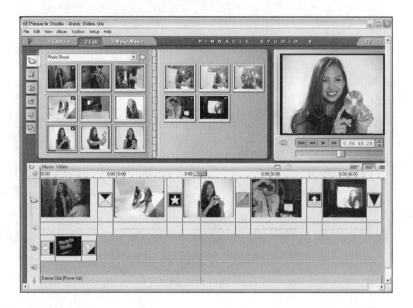

Pinnacle Studio combines a simple drag-and-drop interface with professional features such as fast/slow motion, custom audio, more than 100 transitions, advanced color correction, and contrast and brightness control. Studio includes SmartSound software that lets you select background music from a menu and automatically aligns musical soundtracks with the duration of the video.

Studio 8 adds real-time transcoding from DV to MPEG2, even more professional-quality effects and editing features, and DVD/VCD/SVCD-creation tools. Discs created with Studio version 8 can include menus with looping background music, moving video backgrounds, and moving video in the menu buttons. Users can easily create multiple linked and nested menus for complex interactivity.

Roxio—VideoWave 5 Power Edition

www.roxio.com

Consumer video editor with integrated DVD authoring

Roxio VideoWave 5 Power Edition released August 2002 (formerly MGI); $99

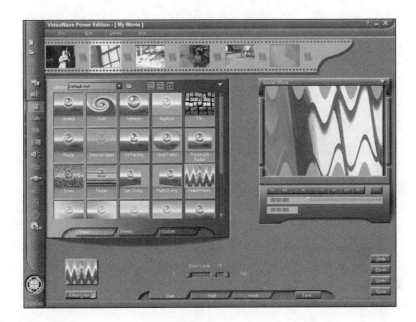

Roxio VideoWave 5 delivers a complete digital video experience in one easy-to-use program that is packed with professional-quality DVD authoring/recording and advanced web publishing capabilities. From business presentations to DVD home movies to streaming video, VideoWave guides you through the production process with ease.

VideoWave 5 Power Edition offers powerful professional tools for users who demand more control over their video projects. Users have complete access to a suite of high-end tools that can be applied to video with drag-and-drop ease. It also adds Media Library management and a simulation mode for DVD authoring.

Roxio—VideoWave Movie Creator

www.roxio.com

Automated movie creation and DVD authoring

Roxio VideoWave Movie Creator released August 2002; $79

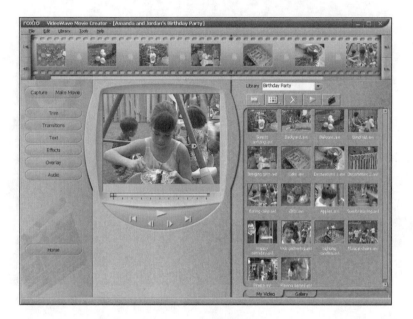

Roxio VideoWave Movie Creator allows consumers to create home movies in minutes, taking video from a camcorder to the PC, automatically set video to a music tune, and then burning them on Video CD or DVD.

VideoWave Movie Creator is ideal for creating short movies, which can be used as chapters for your DVD. Select from different styles that best fit your mood. Use Action style to create a music video, Personal to emphasize close-ups of people, or Nostalgia to give your movie a retro feel. With a few mouse clicks, one can transform raw video and a favorite song into a compelling movie with introductions, transitions, titles, and effects.

The program will guide you through the process while you choose introduction and ending templates, customize your titles, and drag and drop your video clips. And to edit and polish an existing movie further, easy-to-use editing tools will help you achieve impressive results. You can choose from dozens of templates for all occasions; add transitions; apply special effects and overlays; personalize text introductions, titles, and credits; edit music; and create DVD menus to easily navigate through the movie.

Ulead Systems—Ulead VideoStudio 6

www.ulead.com/vs

Consumer video editing with DVD/Video CD Authoring Wizard

Ulead VideoStudio 6 released January 2002; from $89

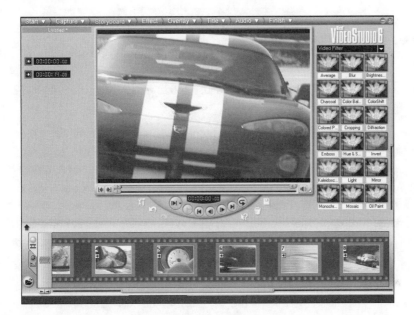

Ulead VideoStudio provides a wide range of video-editing tools to help you produce memorable movies. The DVD/Video CD Authoring Wizard provides ready-made templates to build interactive scene menus in just a few steps.

People with little or no experience in video editing will appreciate how easy it is to use VideoStudio. Trim video, add your own soundtrack, create compelling titles, and drop in stunning effects using an easy-to-learn interface that makes editing videos fun.

VideoWave 6 lets you grab DVD-ready MPEG video straight from your DV/D8 camcorder or other device. Enhanced Scene Detection automatically reads the timeline from your DV tape and cuts captured video into separate easy-to-manage files.

Automated DVD Authoring

Turn-key DVD authoring, direct from DV in to DVD out. Import and convert a wide variety of media formats. Template and wizard-based, automated menu layout, and some capability to edit and customize. Range from around $30 to $100.

MedioStream Inc.—NeoDVDstandard/Plus 4

www.mediostream.com

Home real-time "Direct-to-Disc" end-to-end DVD and VCD recording

MedioStream neoDVD 4.0 released August 2002; neoDVDstandard from $29 and neoDVDplus from $49

Designed specifically for the home user, MedioStream neoDVD Version 4.0 offers a complete, real-time, end-to-end software solution for consumers to easily capture, edit, compress, author, and burn DVDs or VCDs with their recordable CD and DVD drives. In addition, with features, such as "Direct-to-Disc" recording and "Smart Buffering", neoDVDstandard dramatically reduces the hard disk drive requirement for consumers to burn DVDs. The neoDVDplus version offers greater capability to customize and share personal videos with enhanced editing capabilities.

neoDVD 4.0 adds a new modular interface with the NEO Taskbar to provide direct access to key functions and options. It also adds support for DVD+RW Video Recording (VR) mode, permitting the same disk to be shared and edited across the PC and set-top video recorders. You then can edit a disc on either platform, adding and inserting new material and saving the changes back to the same disc.

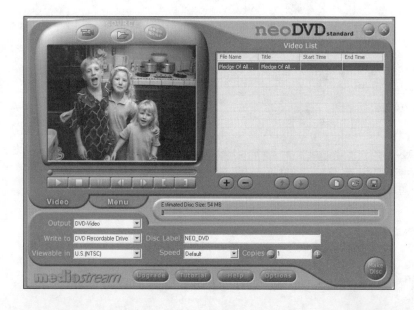

Pinnacle Systems—Express DV

www.pinnaclesys.com

Easy-to-use home CD- and DVD-creation software

Pinnacle Express 1.1 released April 2002; Express $49 and Express DV with FireWire card $79

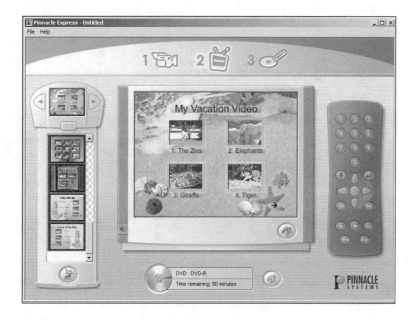

Pinnacle Express is the quickest and easiest way to watch your home movies or digital pictures on DVD. Simply connect your DV camcorder to your PC, and Pinnacle Express lets you capture video or digital still pictures, add menus and titles, and burn CDs or DVDs that play in your set-top DVD Player. Pinnacle Express will also import AVI files.

With its built-in scene detection, Express automatically generates a scene index so that you can instantly go to any spot in your video. After your video has been captured, you can burn a disc right away and watch it in your DVD player, or you can personalize your project by adding Hollywood-style menus and effects. Express allows you to add fades, titles, music, and professional-looking scene menus. Pinnacle Express enables you to import still photos and build interactive slide shows.

Sonic Solutions—MyDVD 4

www.mydvd.com

www.sonic.com

DVD recording and editing application for personal computers

Sonic MyDVD 4.0 released July 2002; Plus $79 and Video Suite $99

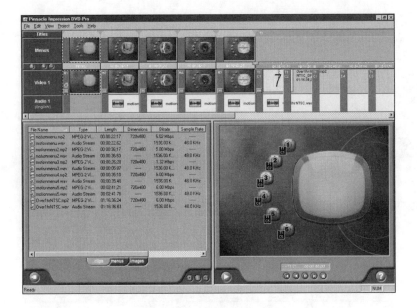

Sonic MyDVD is a personal DVD-authoring tool for recording, editing, and sharing video content on recordable DVD and CD discs. MyDVD allows you to easily author full DVD productions from your video, including graphical menus with thumbnail buttons to play your clips.

You can import clips from media files on your hard disk, or you can capture clips directly within MyDVD. MyDVD then automatically lays out the menu structure and navigation for your clips. You can add chapter points and create a hierarchy of nested menus.

MyDVD can burn your productions to DVD or Video-CD (VCD) format. MyDVD also can record "Direct-to-DVD" from DV to DVD.

MyDVD 4.0 adds a new user interface, motion menus, and slide shows. MyDVD creates OpenDVD-compliant discs, DVD titles that can be opened and re-edited as a new project.

Ulead Systems—DVD MovieFactory

`www.ulead.com/dmf`

Consumer wizard-style DVD-authoring program for burning movies onto DVDs or CDs

Ulead DVD MovieFactory released October 2001; $44

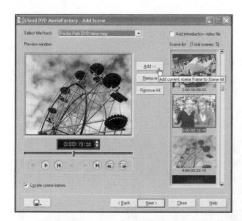
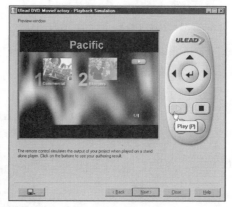

Ulead DVD MovieFactory gives home and office users an affordable and simple solution for sharing high-quality videos on DVDs and CDs. DVD MovieFactory employs an intuitive wizard-style authoring workflow that makes placing home movies onto DVD and CD media a simple, enjoyable camcorder-to-DVD experience.

With DVD MovieFactory, video novices and enthusiasts can create interactive, professionally designed scene selection menus with two layers of navigation. Ulead provides a wide variety of template themes, and users can even design their own backgrounds for maximum personalization and impact. Adding background music to enhance menus is simple using MP3, WAV, or MPEG Audio files. DVD MovieFactory supports multiple movie projects, so users can present multiple movies on a single disc. The software also makes DVD menu organization flexible—with a main menu of all available movies on a disc plus a scene menu to navigate within each video clip. Users may also add an introductory video to their projects so that a video will play before the chapter menu appears.

Personal DVD Authoring

Simplified DVD authoring—working at an "abstraction layer" to hide the details and some capabilities of the full DVD-Video specification. Provides automated layout and built-in templates with more capability to customize the design. Range from around $300 to $600.

Apple Computer—iDVD 2

www.apple.com/idvd

Creates professional-looking DVDs in a few simple steps

Apple iDVD 2 for Mac OS X released October 2001, 2.1 upgrade released July 2002; $19 upgrade

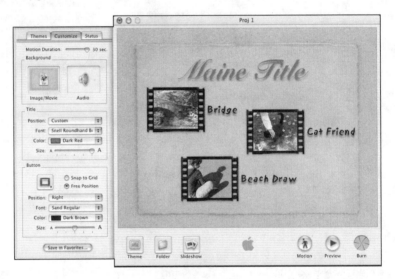

With its fast MPEG encoder and QuickTime support, Apple iDVD 2 for Mac OS X gives you the tools to create top-notch, professional-looking DVDs in a few simple steps.

Assemble your content by simply dragging and dropping your QuickTime files into the streamlined iDVD interface. Drag and drop your digital images into iDVD to make a slide show. Use one of the built-in still menu themes, or create your own using your digital images.

iDVD 2 lets you create motion menus and motion buttons using video clips as menu backgrounds and button images. The iDVD 2.1 updater adds hybrid DVD-ROM data support, AppleScript support, enhancements to the burning process, and general performance improvements.

Sonic Solutions—DVDit! 2.5

www.dvdit.com

www.sonic.com

Powerful yet accessible application for publishing video productions on DVD

Sonic DVDit! 2.5 released November 2001; Standard Edition $299 and Professional Edition $599

DVDit! is a powerful yet accessible application for publishing video productions on DVD. Combining a simple and straightforward user interface with Sonic's award-winning DVD-formatting technology, DVDit! gives video professionals, graphic designers, artists, and video enthusiasts the power to create interactive DVD content on their PC.

DVDit! offers drag-and-drop ease for creating simple productions—with nested menus with links to video and still image clips, and automatic conversion from AVI and QuickTime movie formats. DVDit! also provides access to more sophisticated DVD designs, with custom buttons and titles, a video timeline for setting chapter points, explicit control of navigational links, and the capability to play unattended by automatically linking between menus and clips. It supports advanced DVD features, including control over compression bit rates, widescreen video format, Dolby Digital stereo audio, and writing the final production to DLT tape for professional mastering.

DVDit! PE, the professional edition, adds support for widescreen video, Dolby Digital audio, and mastering to DLT tape.

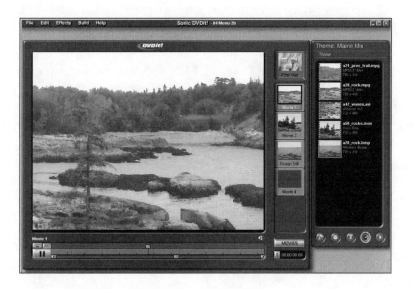

Ulead Systems—Ulead DVD Workshop

www.ulead.com/dws

Powerful DVD authoring software for creative video professionals and enthusiasts

Ulead DVD Workshop released June 2002; from $279

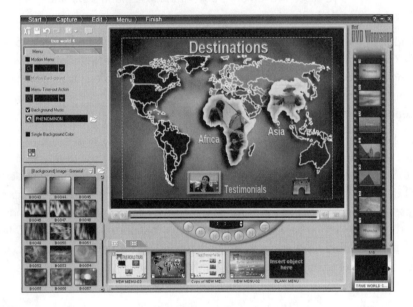

Ulead DVD Workshop is a powerful yet flexible DVD-authoring software designed for creative video professionals and enthusiasts. You can capture DVD-ready MPEG video; build dynamic still and motion menus; and create interactive DVD, VCD, and SVCD movies.

Output sophisticated DVDs, VCDs, and SVCDs with features such as motion menus, special text effects, and highlight color customization. Create instant photo slide shows with still images and audio. Set auto-play navigation controls so that videos/slide shows jump to other target videos/menus when finished playing.

Professional DVD Authoring

Hands-on DVD authoring with support for almost all DVD-Video features: menu and button graphics, multiple video and audio streams, subtitles, navigational links, scripts, and Dolby audio. Requires materials to be prepared and converted to DVD formats. From around $1000.

Apple Computer—DVD Studio Pro 1.5

www.apple.com/dvdstudiopro

DVD authoring for creative professionals, not DVD technicians

Apple DVD Studio Pro 1.5 for Mac OS X released April 2002; $999

With Apple DVD Studio Pro, you can create DVDs that take advantage of every feature outlined in the DVD-Video standard. Taking over where video-editing applications, such as Final Cut Pro leave off, DVD Studio Pro handles the MPEG encoding, menu creation, asset organization, linking, and output formatting that are required to produce DVD-Video discs.

DVD Studio Pro provides advanced features for menu and button design, video chapters and linked story clips, multiple alternate streams, slide shows, scripts, and web links. You can visualize the structure of your project in a variety of ways, and DVD Studio Pro has real-time previewing to see how your project looks and operates.

DVD Studio Pro 1.5 adds the capability to import marker points from Final Cut Pro 3.0.2 to use as chapter points in your DVD.

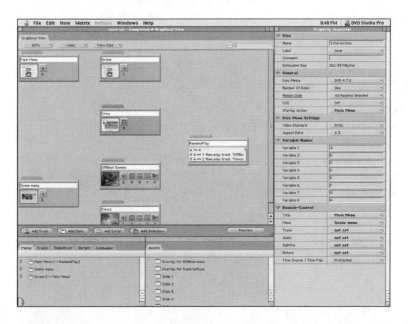

Pinnacle Systems—Impression DVD-Pro 2.2

www.pinnaclesys.com

Professional software to create compelling, interactive DVD titles

Pinnacle Impression DVD-Pro 2.2 released June 2002; $599

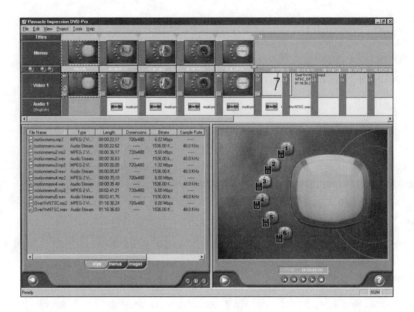

Pinnacle Impression DVD-Pro is designed for video editors. It combines an intuitive timeline-editing interface for drag-and-drop editing with complete professional DVD authoring features.

Impression DVD-Pro provides unlimited menus or submenus for navigation, and supports full motion, animated menus.

Impression DVD-Pro supports multiple streams, including multiple video angles, up to 32 subtitle tracks, and up to eight audio streams for multiple language or soundtrack support.

Pinnacle Impression DVD-Pro 2.2 adds DV AVI file import, and output to DVD-R/RW and DVD+RW discs.

Sonic Solutions—ReelDVD 3

www.sonic.com/products/reeldvd

www.sonic.com

Professional-level DVD authoring tool designed for corporate video projects

Sonic ReelDVD 3.0 released summer 2002; $1500

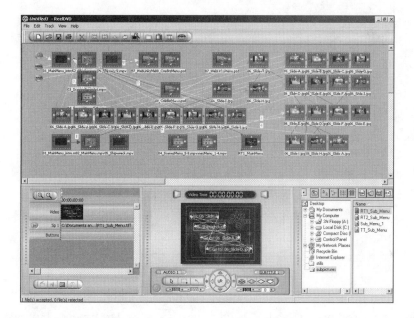

Sonic ReelDVD is a professional-level authoring tool designed specifically for independent and corporate video projects. ReelDVD uses a convenient drag-and-drop interface and simple workflow to provide access to a focused set of advanced features designed for its target audience, without attempting to support the full-feature set of the DVD-Video standard.

The key DVD features that ReelDVD offers include multiple audio and subtitle tracks; and explicit control over layered video, images, menu buttons, and subtitles.

Built upon the same DVD formatting technology from Sonic Scenarist for feature film authoring, ReelDVD combines the strength of professional-level software with a friendly user interface and simple workflow.

ReelDVD 3.0 adds support for up to eight audio streams and 32 subtitle streams.

Sonic Solutions—Scenarist 2.6

www.sonic.com

The standard for feature film DVD production on Windows

Scenarist 2.6 released February 2002; from $10,000–$30,000

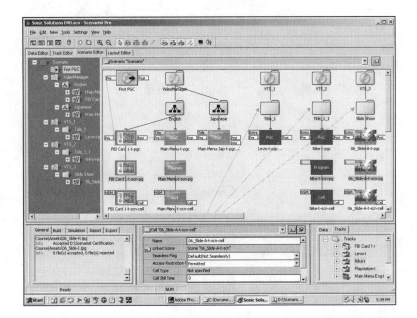

Scenarist is a comprehensive DVD authoring system used to produce Hollywood DVD titles for commercial release. Scenarist provides complete control over DVD authoring by working directly with the low-level components of the DVD-Video specification.

DVD features provided by Scenarist include nonseamless and seamless multiangle switching, karaoke support, and active subpictures.

The Sonic product line of professional authoring tools includes the following:

- Sonic DVD Fusion—for multimedia professionals on Macintosh

- Sonic DVD Producer—for multimedia professionals on Windows

- Sonic DVD Creator—for feature film DVD production on Macintosh

- Sonic Scenarist—for feature film DVD production on Windows

Video-Editing Software

Stand-alone video-editing tools from bundled consumer tools to higher-end professional tools from up to $1000.

Apple Corp.—iMovie 2

www.apple.com/imovie

Consumer digital video-editing software

Apple iMovie 2 released July 2000; Bundled with Macintosh systems

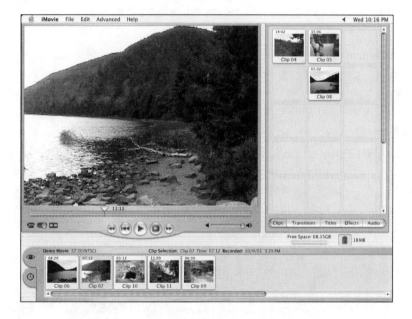

Apple iMovie 2 is the next version of the world's most popular, easy-to-use consumer digital video-editing software. iMovie 2 features a refined user interface with Mac OS X-like design elements, dramatically improved audio-editing capabilities, enhanced controls for titling and transitions, and powerful new special effects.

iMovie 2's new features include a richer, more intuitive user interface, an effects panel, and more control over audio. Users can import video from a digital video camcorder directly into their FireWire-enabled Mac system and then rearrange clips and add special effects, such as cross dissolves and scrolling titles. Finished iMovies can be stored on the computer, transferred back to a camcorder for viewing on a standard TV, or shared with friends and family via a personal web site.

Apple Corp.—Final Cut Pro 3

www.apple.com/finalcutpro

Professional nonlinear editor with real-time preview

Apple Final Cut Pro 3 released December 2001, 3.0.2 update released
May 2002; $999

Final Cut Pro 3 is the only professional nonlinear editor available that lets you
work in the entire range of professional editing formats—from DV to SD and
HD—within the same affordable application. Final Cut Pro 3 allows you to seamlessly work in different modes (editing, effects, and trimming modes, for example).
And with Final Cut Pro's G4 real-time effects, you don't need PCI hardware to
preview transitions and effects in real-time.

Apple Final Cut Pro 3 is the industry's first video-editing solution to deliver
professional-quality, real-time effects without the addition of specialized hardware.
Tapping the powerful video-processing capabilities of the PowerPC G4 processor's
Velocity Engine, the new G4 real-time effects in Final Cut Pro 3 deliver the produc-
tivity and creativity of real-time to a much broader audience of video editors.

Final Cut Pro 3 also debuts OfflineRT, an offline format that holds up to five times
as much footage as the DV format, and has new professional color-correction
tools previously available only in solutions costing tens of thousands of dollars
more. Final Cut Pro 3.0.2 addresses performance and reliability issues and adds
chapter and compression marker export support for DVD Studio Pro 1.5.

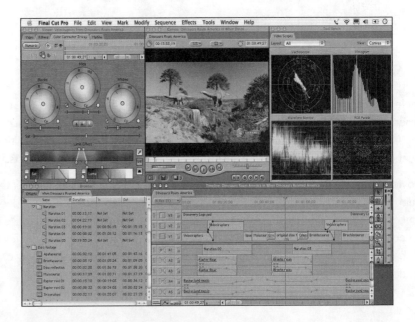

Microsoft Corp.—Windows Movie Maker for Windows XP

www.microsoft.com/windowsxp/moviemaker www.microsoft.com/windowsmedia
www.microsoft.com/windowsxp

Basic Windows XP video editor, with DV capture and Windows Media output

Included with Windows XP

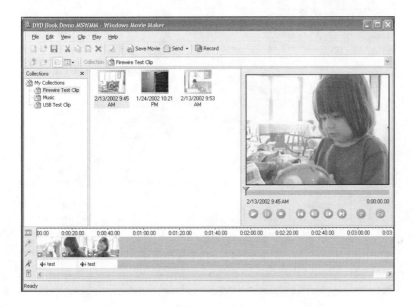

Microsoft Windows Movie Maker is the basic video-editing tool built into recent versions of Windows. With Movie Maker for Windows XP, you can import media files, capture video from DV camcorders or record from other devices, and import and edit clips into projects. You can then export your movie to a video file, copy it to a portable device, or post it to a web site.

You can import video, audio, and still images in a variety of formats. You also can capture video, audio, and stills from any available input devices, including digital and analog sources. Movie Maker can record to files from digital camcorders with FireWire or USB connections.

Adobe Systems—Adobe Premiere 6.5

www.adobe.com/products/premiere

Professional, digital video-editing software for video and business professionals

Premiere 6.5 released August 2002; $549

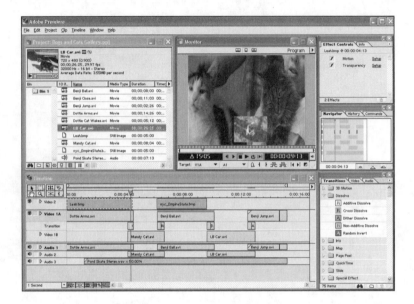

Adobe Premiere allows video and business professionals to quickly and easily edit digital video on a desktop, and publish it to the web in multiple formats—including RealNetworks RealMedia, Microsoft WindowsMedia, and Apple QuickTime. Premiere addresses the needs of the professional by providing major enhancements to the digital video-editing process—from capturing video to editing to final project export. It offers built-in cross-platform support for a large selection of DV devices; professional-editing tools including an audio mixer; and seamless integration with other Adobe applications, including Adobe After Effects, Adobe Photoshop, Adobe Illustrator, and Adobe GoLive.

Premiere 6.5 adds support for Mac OS X and Windows XP, with real-time software preview of edits, effects, titles, and transitions. You can import and edit files in Windows Media format, and export in MPEG-2 format directly for DVD authoring. Premiere 6.5 also adds a sophisticated new Adobe Title Designer with professional typographical controls.

Pinnacle Systems—Edition

www.pinnaclesys.com

Professional video editing and DVD authoring for corporate and video professionals

Pinnacle Edition released July 2002; $699

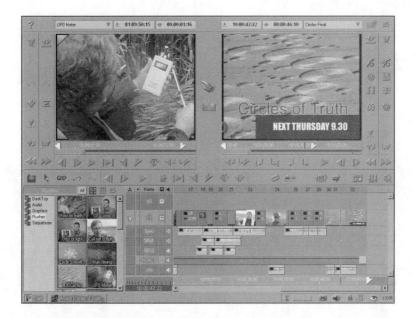

Pinnacle Edition is a powerful professional video-editing and DVD-authoring software product that provides a complete solution for corporate and event video professionals, educators, and dedicated hobbyists who want high-quality and comprehensive content-creation capabilities.

Edition includes Pinnacle's new nonlinear editing software application, along with Hollywood FX software for special effects and TitleDeko RT software for graphics. Edition can burn play-at-once DVDs and SVCDs directly from the timeline, or export the timeline as MPEG-2 for DVD authoring with the included Impression DVD Pro.

Background processing allows work to continue on the project while the application renders even the most complex effects. Edition is built on broadcast technology, with an advanced subpixel processing engine that goes beyond any other desktop video-editing products to offer options that guarantee broadcast quality for 2D/3D digital video effects, color correction tools, and slow-motion capabilities.

Ulead Systems—Ulead MediaStudio Pro 6.5

www.ulead.com/msp

Professional digital video-editing package with full DV and MPEG-2 support

MediaStudio Pro 6.5 released August 2001; Director's Cut from $199 and full version from $495

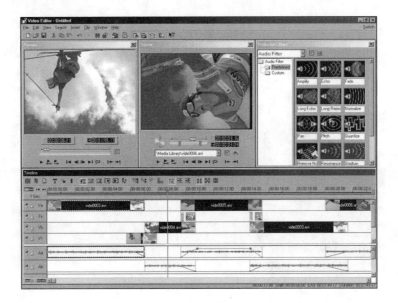

Ulead MediaStudio Pro 6.5 is a complete digital video-editing package with full DV and MPEG-2 support. Six well-integrated modules bring you sophisticated, multi-track video editing, video capture, audio editing, powerful video painting, vector graphics creation, and even built-in DVD/VCD authoring.

MediaStudio Pro 6.5 consists of five components: Video Capture, Video Editor, Video Paint (rotoscoping), CG Infinity (vector-based graphics for animated titles and graphics), and Audio Editor.

MediaStudio 6.5 Director's Cut does not include the rotoscoping program Video Paint or the vector graphics program CG Infinity.

Index

G

H-I

VOICES THAT MATTER

HOW TO CONTACT US

VISIT OUR WEB SITE

WWW.NEWRIDERS.COM

On our web site, you'll find information about our other books, authors, tables of contents, and book errata. You will also find information about book registration and how to purchase our books, both domestically and internationally.

EMAIL US

Contact us at: **nrfeedback@newriders.com**

- If you have comments or questions about this book
- To report errors that you have found in this book
- If you have a book proposal to submit or are interested in writing for New Riders
- If you are an expert in a computer topic or technology and are interested in being a technical editor who reviews manuscripts for technical accuracy

Contact us at: **nreducation@newriders.com**

- If you are an instructor from an educational institution who wants to preview New Riders books for classroom use. Email should include your name, title, school, department, address, phone number, office days/hours, text in use, and enrollment, along with your request for desk/examination copies and/or additional information.

Contact us at: **nrmedia@newriders.com**

- If you are a member of the media who is interested in reviewing copies of New Riders books. Send your name, mailing address, and email address, along with the name of the publication or web site you work for.

BULK PURCHASES/CORPORATE SALES

The publisher offers discounts on this book when ordered in quantity for bulk purchases and special sales. For sales within the U.S., please contact: Corporate and Government Sales (800) 382-3419 or **corpsales@pearsontechgroup.com**. Outside of the U.S., please contact: International Sales (317) 581-3793 or **international@pearsontechgroup.com**.

WRITE TO US

New Riders Publishing
201 W. 103rd St.
Indianapolis, IN 46290-1097

CALL/FAX US

Toll-free (800) 571-5840
If outside U.S. (317) 581-3500
Ask for New Riders
FAX: (317) 581-4663

New Riders

WWW.NEWRIDERS.COM

Solutions from experts you know and trust.

www.informit.com

- OPERATING SYSTEMS
- WEB DEVELOPMENT
- PROGRAMMING
- NETWORKING
- CERTIFICATION
- AND MORE...

Expert Access.
Free Content.

New Riders has partnered with **InformIT.com** to bring technical information to your desktop. Drawing on New Riders authors and reviewers to provide additional information on topics you're interested in, **InformIT.com** has free, in-depth information you won't find anywhere else.

- **Master the skills you need, when you need them**

- **Call on resources from some of the best minds in the industry**

- **Get answers when you need them, using InformIT's comprehensive library or live experts online**

- **Go above and beyond what you find in New Riders books, extending your knowledge**

As an **InformIT** partner, **New Riders** has shared the wisdom and knowledge of our authors with you online. Visit **InformIT.com** to see what you're missing.

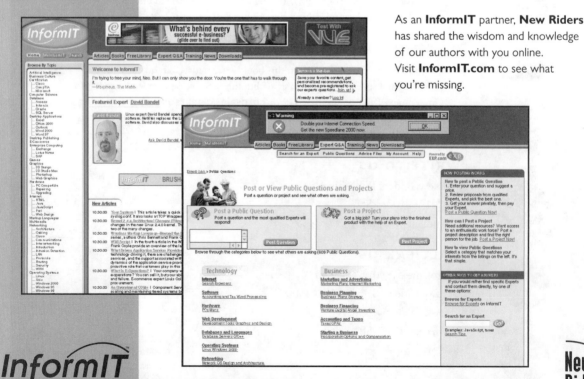

Publishing the Voices that Matter

OUR AUTHORS

PRESS ROOM

| web development | design | photoshop | new media | 3-D | server technologies |

EDUCATORS

ABOUT US

CONTACT US

You already know that New Riders brings you the **Voices That Matter**. But what does that mean? It means that New Riders brings you the Voices that challenge your assumptions, take your talents to the next level, or simply help you better understand the complex technical world we're all navigating.

Visit **www.newriders.com** to find:

- ▸ **10% discount** and **free shipping** on all book purchases
- ▸ Never before published chapters
- ▸ Sample chapters and excerpts
- ▸ Author bios and interviews
- ▸ Contests and enter-to-wins
- ▸ Up-to-date industry event information
- ▸ Book reviews
- ▸ Special offers from our friends and partners
- ▸ Info on how to join our User Group program
- ▸ Ways to have your Voice heard

New Riders

WWW.NEWRIDERS.COM

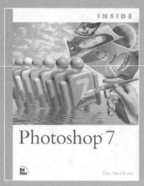
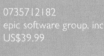
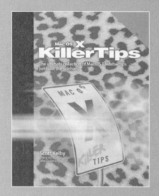
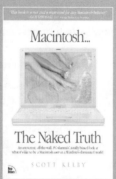
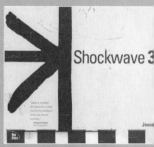
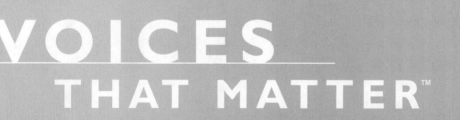